Pregnancy and Heart Disease

Editors

MELINDA B. DAVIS

KATHRYN J. LINDLEY

CARDIOLOGY CLINICS

www.cardiology.theclinics.com

February 2021 • Volume 39 • Number 1

ELSEVIER

1600 John F. Kennedy Boulevard • Suite 1800 • Philadelphia, Pennsylvania, 19103-2899

http://www.theclinics.com

CARDIOLOGY CLINICS Volume 39, Number 1
February 2021 ISSN 0733-8651, ISBN-13: 978-0-323-80926-9

Editor: Joanna Collett
Developmental Editor: Julia McKenzie

Cardiology Clinics (ISSN 0733-8651) is published quarterly by Elsevier Inc., 360 Park Avenue South, New York, NY 10010-1710. Months of issue are February, May, August, and November. Business and Editorial Offices: 1600 John F. Kennedy Blvd., Ste. 1800, Philadelphia, PA 19103-2899. Customer Service Office: 3251 Riverport Lane, Maryland Heights, MO 63043. Periodicals post-age paid at New York, NY and additional mailing offices. Subscription prices are $359.00 per year for US individuals, $929.00 per year for US institutions, $100.00 per year for US students and residents, $445.00 per year for Canadian individuals, $962.00 per year for Canadian institutions, $466.00 per year for international individuals, $962.00 per year for international institutions, $100.00 per year for Canadian students/residents and $220.00 per year for international students/residents. To receive student/resident rate, orders must be accompanied by name of affiliated institution, data of term, and the *signature* of program/residency coordinator on institution letterhead. Orders will be billed at individual rate until proof of status is received. Foreign air speed delivery is included in all *Clinics* subscription prices. All prices are subject to change without notice. **POSTMASTER:** Send address changes to *Cardiology Clinics*, Elsevier Health Sciences Division, Subscription Customer Service, 3251 Riverport Lane, Maryland Heights, MO 63043. **Customer Service: 1-800-654-2452 (U.S. and Canada); 314-447-8871 (outside U.S. and Canada). Fax: 314-447-8029. E-mail: journalscus-tomerservice-usa@elsevier.com (for print support); journalsonlinesupport-usa@elsevier.com (for online support).**

Reprints. For copies of 100 or more, of articles in this publication, please contact the Commercial Reprints Department, Elsevier Inc., 360 Park Avenue South, New York, NY 10010-1710. Tel.: 212-633-3874; Fax: 212-633-3820; E-mail: reprints@elsevier.com.

Cardiology Clinics is also published in Spanish by McGraw-Hill Interamericana Editores S. A., P.O. Box 5-237, 06500, Mexico D. F., Mexico; in Portuguese by Reichmann and Alfonso Editores Rio de Janeiro, Brazil; and in Greek by Dimitrios P. Lagos, 8 Pondon Street, GR115-28 Ilissia, Greece.

Cardiology Clinics is covered in *MEDLINE/PubMed (Index Medicus), Excerpta Medica, The Cumulative Index to Nursing and Allied Health Literature* (CINAHL).

Contributors

ALINA BRENER, MD
Division of Cardiology, University of Illinois at Chicago, Chicago, Illinois, USA

JOAN BRILLER, MD, FACC, FASE, FAHA
Division of Cardiology, University of Illinois at Chicago, Chicago, Illinois, USA

TIMOTHY B. COTTS, MD
Clinical Associate Professor, Director, Adult Congenital Heart Disease, Departments of Internal Medicine and Pediatrics, University of Michigan, University of Michigan Congenital Heart Center, C.S. Mott Children's Hospital, Ann Arbor, Michigan, USA

CHRISTOPHER DeZORZI, MD
University of Missouri-Kansas City School of Medicine, Saint Luke's Mid America Heart Institute, Kansas City, Missouri, USA

BRITTANY DIXON, MD
Division of Cardiovascular Medicine, Department of Medicine, Washington University School of Medicine, St Louis, Missouri, USA

ERIKA J. DOUGLASS, MPH
Cardiovascular Research Liaison, Department of Cardiovascular Medicine, Mayo Clinic, Jacksonville, Florida, USA; DrPH Candidate, Department of Environmental Health and Engineering, Johns Hopkins Bloomberg School of Public Health, Baltimore, Maryland, USA

KAREN L. FLORIO, DO, FACOG
Saint Luke's Hospital of Kansas City, Heart Disease in Pregnancy Program, University of Missouri-Kansas City School of Medicine, Kansas City, Missouri, USA

ANNA GRODZINSKY, MD, MS
Saint Luke's Mid America Heart Institute and Muriel Kauffman Women's Heart Center, Kansas City, Missouri, USA

APURVA M. KHEDAGI, MS
Columbia University Vagelos College of Physicians and Surgeons, New York, New York, USA

LISA D. LEVINE, MD, MSCE
Assistant Professor of Obstetrics and Gynecology, Director of the Pregnancy and Heart Disease Program, Department of Obstetrics and Gynecology, Maternal and Child Health Research Center, University of Pennsylvania Perelman School of Medicine, Philadelphia, Pennsylvania, USA

JENNIFER LEWEY, MD, MPH
Assistant Professor of Medicine, Director of Women's Cardiovascular Health, Co-director of the Pregnancy and Heart Disease Program, Division of Cardiology, Department of Medicine, University of Pennsylvania Perelman School of Medicine, Philadelphia, Pennsylvania, USA

ANTHONY MAGALSKI, MD, FACC, FAHA, FASE, FHFSA
University of Missouri-Kansas City School of Medicine, Saint Luke's Mid America Heart Institute, Kansas City, Missouri, USA

COLLEEN A. McEVOY, MD
Division of Pulmonary and Critical Care Medicine, Department of Medicine, Washington University School of Medicine, St Louis, Missouri, USA

KRASIMIRA MIKHOVA, MD
Department of Medicine, Cardiovascular Division, John T. Milliken Department of Medicine, Washington University School of Medicine, St Louis, Missouri, USA

CHARISHMA NALLAPATI, MD
Department of Medicine, University of Florida College of Medicine, Gainesville, Florida, USA

ANNA C. O'KELLY, MD, MPhil
Department of Medicine, Massachusetts General Hospital and Harvard Medical School, Boston, Massachusetts, USA

KI PARK, MD
Division of Cardiovascular Medicine, University of Florida College of Medicine, Gainesville, Florida, USA

SARA SABERI, MD, MS
Clinical Assistant Professor, Department of Internal Medicine, Division of Cardiovascular Medicine, University of Michigan School of Medicine, Ann Arbor, Michigan, USA

KATHERINE B. SALCICCIOLI, MD
Fellow, Adult Congenital Heart Disease,
Department of Internal Medicine, University of
Michigan, University of Michigan Congenital
Heart Center, C.S. Mott Children's Hospital,
Ann Arbor, Michigan, USA

LAURA SCHMIDT, MD
Saint Luke's Mid America Heart Institute and
Muriel Kauffman Women's Heart Center,
Kansas City, Missouri, USA

NANDITA SCOTT, MD
Division of Cardiology, Cardiovascular Disease
and Pregnancy Program, Massachusetts
General Hospital and Harvard Medical School,
Boston, Massachusetts, USA

GARIMA SHARMA, MD, FACC
Division of Cardiology, Johns Hopkins
Ciccarone Center for Prevention of
Cardiovascular Disease, Johns Hopkins
School of Medicine and Hospital, Baltimore,
Maryland, USA

CANDICE K. SILVERSIDES, MD
Division of Cardiology, University of Toronto
Pregnancy and Heart Disease Research
Program, Mount Sinai and Toronto General
Hospitals, Toronto, Ontario, Canada

SANDEEP SODHI, MD
Assistant Professor, Cardiovascular Division,
Electrophysiology, John T. Milliken
Department of Internal Medicine, Washington
University School of Medicine, St Louis,
Missouri, USA

**KATHLEEN SWEARINGEN, MSN, APRN,
FNP-C**
Saint Luke's Hospital of Kansas City, Heart
Disease in Pregnancy Program, Kansas City,
Missouri, USA

AMANDA K. VERMA, MD
Division of Cardiovascular Medicine,
Department of Medicine, Washington
University School of Medicine, St Louis,
Missouri, USA

DOMINIQUE S. WILLIAMS, MD
Assistant Professor, Cardiovascular Division,
John T. Milliken Department of Internal
Medicine, Washington University School of
Medicine, St Louis, Missouri, USA

EMILY WILLIAMS, MD
University of Missouri-Kansas City School of
Medicine, Kansas City, Missouri, USA

DOREEN DEFARIA YEH, MD
Division of Cardiology, Cardiovascular Disease
and Pregnancy Program, Massachusetts
General Hospital and Harvard Medical School,
Boston, Massachusetts, USA

WENDY YING, MD
Division of Cardiology, Johns Hopkins
Ciccarone Center for Prevention of
Cardiovascular Disease, Johns Hopkins
School of Medicine and Hospital, Baltimore,
Maryland, USA

Contents

Preface: Cardio-Obstetrics: An Emerging Field to Improve Maternal Mortality   xiii

Melinda B. Davis and Kathryn J. Lindley

Cardiovascular Contribution to Maternal Mortality   1

Anna Grodzinsky and Laura Schmidt

The United States is the only industrialized nation with an increasing maternal mortality. Many factors contribute to this worrisome US trend; among them, social and demographic factors, and congenital and acquired cardiac conditions. Cardiovascular disease is the leading cause of maternal mortality, and adverse outcomes related to cardiovascular disease disproportionately affect black and Hispanic mothers. This article addresses knowledge gaps related to the treatment of heart disease in pregnancy, initiatives to address these gaps, and guidelines and best practices surrounding the care of women affected by cardiovascular disease and their babies affected by cardiovascular disease.

The Importance of Cardiovascular Risk Assessment and Pregnancy Heart Team in the Management of Cardiovascular Disease in Pregnancy   7

Garima Sharma, Wendy Ying, and Candice K. Silversides

Pregnancy-related maternal morbidity and mortality is increasing because of complications from cardiovascular disease. Pregnancy results in physiologic changes that can adversely impact the cardiovascular system and lead to adverse pregnancy outcomes. A multidisciplinary pregnancy heart team is essential to safely navigate women with heart disease through pregnancy. This role of the pregnancy heart team is to offer preconception counseling, determine pregnancy risks and educate women about those risks, develop a comprehensive antenatal and delivery plan, and ensure appropriate postpartum follow-up. These steps are important to improve cardiovascular outcomes in pregnancy.

Cardiovascular Testing and Imaging in Pregnant Women   21

Alina Brener and Joan Briller

Cardiovascular disease is a major contributor to maternal morbidity and mortality and frequently preventable. Women with known cardiovascular disease should undergo cardiac evaluation before pregnancy. Many women with pregnancy-associated cardiac complications are not previously known to have cardiac disease. Women at high risk or who have signs or symptoms suggestive of heart failure, angina, or arrhythmias should undergo prompt evaluation. This article describes various diagnostic imaging modalities that can be used in pregnancy, including indications, strengths, and limitations.

Cardiovascular Medications in Pregnancy: A Primer   33

Karen L. Florio, Christopher DeZorzi, Emily Williams, Kathleen Swearingen, and Anthony Magalski

Cardiovascular disease and cardiovascular disease–related disorders remain among the most common causes of maternal morbidity and mortality in the United

States. Due to increased rates of obesity, delayed childbearing, and improvements in medical technology, greater numbers of women are entering pregnancy with pre-existing medical comorbidities. Use of cardiovascular medications in pregnancy continues to increase, and medical management of cardiovascular conditions in pregnancy will become increasingly common. Obstetricians and cardiologists must familiarize themselves with the pharmacokinetics of the most commonly used cardiovascular medications in pregnancy and how these medications respond to the physiologic changes related to pregnancy, embryogenesis, and lactation.

Pregnancy in Women with Adult Congenital Heart Disease   55

Katherine B. Salciccioli and Timothy B. Cotts

Women with congenital heart disease are pursuing pregnancy in increasing numbers. Counseling about genetic transmission, medication management, maternal and fetal risks, and maternal longevity should be initiated well before pregnancy is considered. Although preconception medical and surgical optimization as well as coordinated multidisciplinary care throughout pregnancy decrease maternal and fetal risks, the rate of complications remains increased compared with the general population. Lesion-specific risk stratification and care throughout pregnancy further improve outcomes and decrease unnecessary interventions.

Arrhythmias and Pregnancy: Management of Preexisting and New-Onset Maternal Arrhythmias   67

Dominique S. Williams, Krasimira Mikhova, and Sandeep Sodhi

Arrhythmias are the most common cardiovascular complication of pregnancy in women with and without structural heart disease. Appropriate maternal diagnosis and management is of utmost importance to optimize maternal and fetal outcomes. A multidisciplinary care approach with cardiology, maternal fetal medicine, anesthesia, and pediatrics is important for preconceptional, pregnancy, and delivery planning.

Hypertensive Disorders of Pregnancy   77

Apurva M. Khedagi and Natalie A. Bello

Hypertension is the most common medical disorder occurring during pregnancy and a leading cause of maternal and perinatal morbidity and mortality. Accurate blood pressure measurement and the diagnosis and treatment of hypertensive disorders during pregnancy and in the postpartum period are pivotal to improve outcomes. This article details hemodynamic adaptations to pregnancy and provides an approach to the prevention, diagnosis, and management of hypertensive disorders of pregnancy (HDP) and hypertensive emergencies. In addition, it reviews optimal strategies for the care of women with hypertension during the fourth trimester and beyond to minimize future cardiovascular risk.

Ischemic Heart Disease in Pregnancy   91

Charishma Nallapati and Ki Park

The reported incidence of ischemic heart disease in pregnancy is 2.8 to 6.2 per 100,000 pregnancies. Although additional factors, such as maternal diabetes, obesity, and hypertension, are risk factors for ischemic heart disease, pregnancy itself more than doubles the risk for acute myocardial infarction. Given the increasing clinical importance of ischemic heart disease during pregnancy, this article addresses underlying pathophysiology, risk stratification, screening, and diagnosis of ischemic heart disease, as well as recommendations for management of acute myocardial infarction during pregnancy and the early postpartum period.

Pulmonary Arterial Hypertension in Pregnancy   109

Wenners Ballard III, Brittany Dixon, Colleen A. McEvoy, and Amanda K. Verma

Pulmonary arterial hypertension is a rare disease that predominantly affects women. The pathophysiology of the disease is complex, with both genetic and hormonal influences. Pregnancy causes significant physiologic changes that may not be well tolerated with underlying pulmonary arterial hypertension, in particular leading to volume overload and increased pulmonary pressures. A multidisciplinary approach and careful monitoring are essential for appropriate management of pulmonary arterial hypertension during pregnancy. Nonetheless, outcomes are still poor, and pregnancy is considered a contraindication in patients with pulmonary arterial hypertension.

Peripartum Cardiomyopathy   119

Erika J. Douglass and Lori A. Blauwet

Peripartum cardiomyopathy (PPCM) is a form of heart failure that occurs toward the end of pregnancy or in the months following pregnancy and is marked by left ventricular systolic dysfunction. The cause of PPCM remains unknown and there is no diagnostic test specific to PPCM. Outcomes vary and include complete left ventricular recovery, persistent cardiac dysfunction, transplant, and death. Numerous advances have been made in understanding this disease, but many knowledge gaps remain. This article reviews recent data and recommendations for clinical practice in addition to highlighting the multiple knowledge gaps related to PPCM that warrant further investigation.

Hypertrophic Cardiomyopathy in Pregnancy   143

Sara Saberi

Hypertrophic cardiomyopathy (HCM) is the most common genetic cardiac condition and highly heterogeneous. Echocardiography and genetic and clinical screening have led to detection in women of childbearing age. Maternal and fetal outcomes among women with HCM are favorable. Genetic counseling is recommended. Prepregnancy clinical evaluation and risk assessment are paramount in ensuring optimal outcomes. Most women carry moderate risk of morbidity, have clinical evaluations and echocardiography each trimester, and deliver vaginally. Those who are symptomatic or have significant left ventricular outflow obstruction or recurrent arrhythmias prior to pregnancy are at higher risk and should be monitored at least monthly.

Valvular Heart Disease in Pregnancy   151

Jennifer Lewey, Lauren Andrade, and Lisa D. Levine

Valvular heart disease (VHD) is generally well tolerated during pregnancy; however, the dramatic changes in hemodynamics that occur during pregnancy can lead to clinical decompensation in high-risk women. Women with VHD considering pregnancy should undergo preconception counseling with a high-risk obstetrician and cardiologist to review the maternal, fetal, and obstetric risks of pregnancy and delivery. Vaginal delivery is recommended for most women with VHD. Given the complexity of managing VHD during pregnancy, women should be managed by a multidisciplinary Pregnancy Heart Team during pregnancy, consisting of a high-risk obstetrician, cardiologist, and cardiac anesthesiologist.

Delivering Coordinated Cardio-Obstetric Care from Preconception through Postpartum   **163**

Anna C. O'Kelly, Nandita Scott, and Doreen DeFaria Yeh

Coordinated preconception through postpartum cardio-obstetrics care is necessary to optimize both maternal and fetal health. Maternal mortality in the United States is increasing, largely driven by increasing cardiovascular (CV) disease burden during pregnancy and needs to be addressed emergently. Both for women with congenital and acquired heart disease, CV complications during pregnancy are associated with increased future risk of CV disease. Comprehensive cardio-obstetrics care is a powerful way of ensuring that women's CV risks before and during pregnancy are appropriately identified and treated and that they remain engaged in CV care long term to prevent future CV complications.

CARDIOLOGY CLINICS

FORTHCOMING ISSUES

May 2021
Mitral Valve Disease
Takeshi Kitai, *Editor*

August 2021
Nephrocardiology
Parta Hatamizadeh, *Editor*

RECENT ISSUES

November 2020
Coronary Artery Disease
Alberto Polimeni, *Editor*

August 2020
Adult Congenital Heart Disease
Curt J. Daniels, *Editor*

SERIES OF RELATED INTEREST

Cardiac Electrophysiology Clinics
Heart Failure Clinics
Interventional Cardiology Clinics

THE CLINICS ARE AVAILABLE ONLINE!
Access your subscription at:
www.theclinics.com

Preface

Cardio-Obstetrics: An Emerging Field to Improve Maternal Mortality

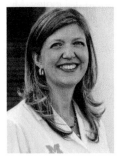 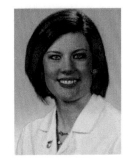

Melinda B. Davis, MD   Kathryn J. Lindley, MD
Editors

With steadily rising maternal morbidity and mortality in the United States, there is an urgent need to address the root causes. Cardiovascular disease is the leading cause of maternal deaths, many of which are preventable. Hemodynamic changes of pregnancy include significant increases in cardiac output, blood volume, and heart rate, as well as changes in systemic vascular resistance and increased oxygen consumption. This hemodynamic stress can unmask previously subclinical cardiovascular disease and contribute to complications, including arrhythmias, hypertensive disorders, heart failure, and ischemic events. Women who suffer adverse pregnancy outcomes are also at increased risk for future cardiovascular disease.

The subspecialty field of Cardio-Obstetrics has grown rapidly to address an emerging population of women needing advanced care. More women with complex congenital heart disease have now survived into reproductive years and require advanced subspecialty care. In addition, increasing numbers of women are presenting with acquired heart disease and cardiovascular risk factors during pregnancy, contributing to higher morbidity and mortality than congenital heart disease. The complexities of managing cardiovascular conditions throughout the pregnancy continuum require multidisciplinary communication among the Pregnancy Heart Team, including obstetricians, maternal-fetal medicine specialists, cardiologists, anesthesiologists, and many other subspecialists and team members.

The following issue of *Cardiology Clinics* highlights several of the most important clinical and systematic aspects of the subspecialty of Cardio-Obstetrics with a series of articles authored by expert leaders in this field. Understanding the cardiovascular contribution to maternal mortality, particularly in the context of social and demographic inequalities, sets the background for further study and multicenter collaboration. Several risk assessment tools can be used to counsel women with known preexisting cardiovascular disease, which should be implemented by the Pregnancy Heart Team, consisting of a dedicated and experienced multidisciplinary group of specialists, as outlined in this special issue. Additional knowledge about appropriate and safe cardiovascular testing and imaging during pregnancy as well as the use of

Cardiol Clin 39 (2021) xiii–xiv
https://doi.org/10.1016/j.ccl.2020.10.001
0733-8651/21/© 2020 Published by Elsevier Inc.

medications during pregnancy and lactation is essential.

Specific diseases that require dedicated attention during pregnancy are also described in detail in this issue, including congenital heart disease, arrhythmias, hypertensive disorders, ischemic heart disease, pulmonary arterial hypertension, peripartum cardiomyopathy, hypertrophic cardiomyopathy, and valvular heart disease. Finally, delivering coordinated care by the Pregnancy Heart Team and establishing and developing programs of excellence will be explored. These topics are important to cardiologists, obstetricians, maternal-fetal medicine specialists, anesthesiologists, pharmacists, nurses, advanced practice providers, and trainees interested in the complex multidisciplinary field of Cardio-Obstetrics.

Melinda B. Davis, MD
1500 East Medical Center Drive
SPC 5853
Ann Arbor, MI 48109-5853, USA

Kathryn J. Lindley, MD
660 South Euclid Avenue
CB 8086
St Louis, MO 63110, USA

E-mail addresses:
davismb@med.umich.edu (M.B. Davis)
kathryn.lindley@wustl.edu (K.J. Lindley)

Cardiovascular Contribution to Maternal Mortality

Anna Grodzinsky, MD, MS*, Laura Schmidt, MD

KEYWORDS

• Cardiovascular • Cardio-obstetrics • Maternal mortality

KEY POINTS

- The United States is the only industrialized nation with an increasing maternal mortality.
- Many factors contribute to this worrisome US trend; among them, social and demographic factors, and congenital and acquired cardiac conditions.
- Cardiovascular disease is the leading cause of maternal mortality, and adverse outcomes related to cardiovascular disease disproportionately affect black and Hispanic mothers.

INTRODUCTION

The United States is the only industrialized nation with an increasing maternal mortality.[1] According to a January 2020 report from the Centers for Disease Control and Prevention (CDC) National Vital Statistics System, the 2018 maternal mortality was 17.4 maternal deaths per 100,000 live births (**Fig. 1**). This figure included deaths during pregnancy, at birth, and within 42 days of birth. The statistic placed the United States last among similarly wealthy countries; if this CDC figure is compared with other countries in the World Health Organization's latest maternal mortality ranking, the United States would rank 55th, just behind Russia (17 per 100,000) and just ahead of Ukraine (19 per 100,000). If the comparison is limited to those similarly wealthy countries, the United States would rank 10th out of 10 countries. Maternal and fetal outcomes remain key metrics of population health, and there is a growing recognition of this problem and renewed urgency to address it.

There has been heightened media coverage surrounding the many drivers (among them, sociodemographic factors, congenital and acquired cardiac conditions) that contribute to this worrisome US trend. These stories included the ProPublica/National Public Radio's Lost Mothers investigation, *Time* magazine's "Why are U.S. Mothers Still Dying in Childbirth," and USA Today's "Deadly Deliveries," highlighting the key factors contributing to maternal mortality in the United States.[2,3] It is important to extend on several of the key contributors to high maternal morbidity and mortalities in the United States. First, clinicians have been limited in their ability to recognize and report pregnancy-associated mortality. Before 2003, there was no mandate to include pregnancy-associated deaths on death certificates. Once this mandate was in place, the addition of this field was not standardized for several years, contributing to barriers in accurate reporting.[4] Clinicians have also been limited in their access to large-scale, representative, granular data surrounding the care patterns and outcomes of pregnant women with heart disease. Second, underinsurance and lack of access to care (importantly, in the postpartum period) remain key and difficult-to-address systemic contributors.[5,6] This situation is particularly distressing because early and consistent prenatal (and subsequent postnatal) care favorably affect the lives of mothers and babies.[7]

Saint Luke's Mid America Heart Institute and Muriel Kauffman Women's Heart Center, 4401 Wornall Road, Kansas City, MO 64111, USA
* Corresponding author.
E-mail address: agrodzinsky@saint-lukes.org

Cardiol Clin 39 (2021) 1–5
https://doi.org/10.1016/j.ccl.2020.09.001

U.S Maternal Mortality Ratio Compared to Industrialized Countries with 300,000+ Births, 2017–2018

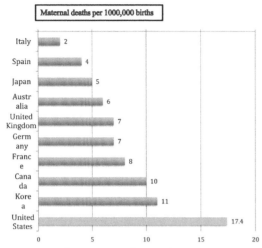

Maternal deaths per 1000,000 births

Italy	2
Spain	4
Japan	5
Australia	6
United Kingdom	7
Germany	7
France	8
Canada	10
Korea	11
United States	17.4

Fig. 1. Trends in maternal mortality, 2000 to 2017. (*Data from* Trends in maternal mortality 2000 to 2017: estimates by WHO, UNICEF, UNFPA, World Bank Group and the United Nations Population Division. Geneva: World Health Organization; 2019. Licence: CC BY-NC-SA 3.0 IGO; and Hoyert DL, Miniño AM. Maternal Mortality in the United States: Changes in Coding, Publication, and Data Release, 2018. National Vital Statistics Report 2020;69(2):1–16.)

The key cause of maternal mortality in the United States is cardiovascular disease,[8] which is driven not only by the growing population of adults with congenital heart conditions desiring pregnancy but also by higher incidence of traditional cardiovascular risk factors (hypertension, diabetes, obesity) in young women. The epidemic of obesity also contributes to cardiovascular risk factors in pregnancy. Women with obesity face a higher risk of hypertensive disorders of pregnancy as well as gestational diabetes.[9] Fetal complications may include congenital birth defects and increased risk of stillbirth.[9] Both obese women and their children are at risk of diabetes later in life, with its associated risk of vascular disease.

Further, there are significant racial disparities in maternal mortality. In California, African American women represent only 6% of all deliveries, but 22% of all pregnancy-related deaths.[10] Across the United States, African American women have a 3.4-fold higher risk of dying in the intrapartum and postpartum periods compared with their white counterparts.[11] This disparity is even more pronounced in the older maternal population, with black women more than 40 years of age having the highest rate of dying, at 192 per 100,000. The most recent morbidity and mortality report published by the CDC found that more black women are dying in the postpartum period compared with other racial groups, which could be attributable to loss of affordable health insurance or access to care after the 6-week postpartum visit. These concerning trends highlight the need to better understand the social determinants of health and barriers to appropriate care. These social determinants include clinical factors (workforce shortages, low patient volume, and the opioid epidemic) and social determinants of health (transportation, housing, poverty, food security, racism, violence, and trauma).[12]

The American College of Obstetrics and Gynecology has attempted to address some of these issues by implementing new guidelines for postpartum care.[13] Traditionally, bundled coverage for postpartum care included only a 1-time visit at 6 weeks. However, most maternal deaths occur in the 42 to 365 days after delivery; this high-risk time frame occurs after health insurance coverage for many patients has been discontinued. As of May 2019, it is recommended that women with any pregnancy-associated complication, including hypertension, diabetes, or underlying cardiovascular risk factors, now be seen within the first week postpartum.[14] California remains an outlier in the maternal mortality statistics, having enjoyed a marked decline in the maternal mortality since 2006. Since 2006, California has reduced the maternal mortality by 57% and, for African Americans, by 50%. The driver of this improvement has been the state's concerted effort to reduce the maternal death rate by initiating a statewide, pregnancy-associated maternal mortality review committee and contracting with the California Maternal Quality Care Collaborative to investigate the primary causes of maternal death.[15] This collaborative, including nearly 200 hospitals representing ~95% of births in the state, developed evidence-based tool kits to address the most common causes of maternal mortality, and they continue to build on these data. From the California collaborative data, and according to the American College of Obstetricians and Gynecologists (ACOG) Committee on Safety and Quality Improvement statement, outcomes improve when obstetric care is standardized.[16]

The California data and the pregnancy mortality surveillance system data have provided important insights into the causes of maternal mortality. Although cardiovascular disease accounts for only 4% of all pregnancies in the United States, it causes or is associated with 26% of all deaths, surpassing traditional causes, including hypertensive disorders, hemorrhage, and embolic events.[17,18] Most of these deaths occur during the intrapartum and postpartum time frame. Briller and Geller[8] reported that there were 636 deaths in Illinois from 2002 to 2011 of pregnant women or within 1 year postpartum. One-hundred and forty women (22.2%) died of cardiovascular causes. Women with cardiovascular mortality were likely to be older and die postpartum. The most common causes were related to acquired cardiovascular disease (97.1%) compared with congenital heart disease (2.9%). Strikingly, studies evaluating the preventability of maternal deaths have deemed that up to 68% of these deaths were potentially preventable.[17] From the 2018 CDC Foundation Nine Maternal Mortality Review Committees report, assessing preventability is a priority because it is critical to informing and prioritizing potential actions. Using data from the nine committees, these analyses found that 63% of pregnancy-related deaths were preventable. The years of deaths included within this analysis were variable: Colorado 2008 to 2012; Delaware 2009 to 2015; Georgia 2012 to 2014; Hawaii 2015; Illinois 2015; North Carolina 2014 to 2015; Ohio 2008 to 2015; South Carolina 2014 to 2017; Utah 2014. Now that maternal mortality review committees are established within at least 42 states (CDC), clinicians may continue to evaluate preventability and better understand additional leading causes of pregnancy-related deaths in an effort to address the root causes of severe maternal morbidity and mortality. In the United States, the challenge in caring for this high-risk group of women is the lack of large-scale, representative, real-world data guiding management. Previously established risk models (such as the CARPREG or ZAHARA risk models) may be used to identify patients who will require further surveillance or who should be counseled regarding avoidance of pregnancy altogether, but these risk stratification models were developed largely from European and Canadian patient cohorts and may not be generalizable to American women, where the rates of traditional cardiovascular risk factors and acquired cardiovascular disease are more common than those of their Canadian European counterparts.

The explanation of these adverse outcomes is complex, and, within this issue, this article discusses knowledge gaps related to the treatment of heart disease in pregnancy and initiatives to address these gaps, and highlights guidelines and best practices surrounding the care of women and their babies affected by cardiovascular disease.

CARDIOVASCULAR COMPLICATIONS AND ADVERSE MATERNAL OUTCOMES

Although social and demographic determinants of health remain paramount drivers of outcomes, cardiovascular conditions complicating pregnancy are the leading cause of maternal mortality in the United States.[17,18] Most of these deaths occur during the intrapartum and postpartum period; in an analysis of Illinois, greater than 90% of maternal deaths caused by cardiovascular disease could be attributed to acquired heart disease.[8]

Acquired and congenital heart conditions, as well as preeclampsia, are the leading causes of maternal morbidity and mortality.[17,18] In the United States, older age at pregnancy, along with a higher burden of traditional risk factors for coronary heart disease and heart failure, further increases the risk of adverse pregnancy outcomes. Given the advances of cardiac surgeries and pediatric care, there are more adults living with congenital heart conditions in the United States than there are children.[19] Many of these adults desire pregnancy, and providers are working to navigate and optimize the care of these patients. Given the hemodynamic changes of pregnancy, it is clear that patients with certain underlying cardiovascular conditions are at higher risk of decompensating during pregnancy.

- Hemodynamic changes during pregnancy in patients with structurally normal hearts include[20] (**Fig. 2**):
  - Cardiac output increases by ∼50%
  - Blood volume increases by 30% to 50%
  - Heart rate increases by at least 15 to 20 beats/min
  - Blood pressure decreases by 5 to 10 mm Hg in midpregnancy
  - System vascular resistance decreases
  - Oxygen consumption increases by 20%
  - Red blood cell mass increases by 15% to 20%

Because of these hemodynamic changes during pregnancy, labor, and delivery, planning surrounding preconception counseling and management during pregnancy and the postpartum period must be prioritized. Ideally, this occurs within a combined cardio-obstetrics clinic or via a cardio-obstetric team approach.[21]

It is also now understood that adverse pregnancy outcomes (eg, small-for-gestational-age infants, preterm birth, hypertensive disorder of pregnancy) confer a higher risk of subsequent maternal cardiovascular risk factors as well as overt conditions such as coronary heart disease,

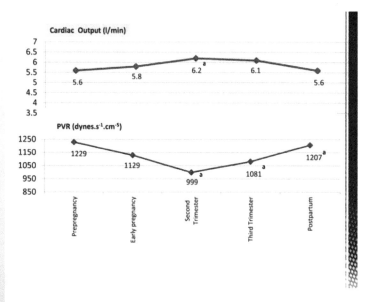

Fig. 2. Detailed hemodynamics were longitudinally studied in 54 women with normal pregnancies preconception and then at 6, 23, and 33 weeks during pregnancy and 16 weeks postpartum. [a]$P<.05$ versus previous value. (*From* Sanghavi M, Rutherford JD. Cardiovascular physiology of pregnancy. Circulation 2014;130(12):1004; with permission.)

heart failure, and valvular disease.[22] These later cardiovascular diagnoses are made on average 10 years after delivery, much earlier than would typically be suspected.[22]

Cardiovascular guidelines identify preeclampsia, eclampsia, and gestational hypertension as independent risk factors for vascular disease later in life. The presence of these hypertensive disorders of pregnancy increases the risk of vascular events in the 10 years after delivery, a risk factor as strong as the presence of diabetes. With this in mind, clinicians need to be alert to identifying hypertensive disorders of pregnancy in their patients, and encourage lifestyle changes to help mitigate these risk factors.

There have been more recent calls for prospective research addressing care patterns and outcomes of pregnant women with cardiovascular disease and their babies. There is a multidisciplinary network that has been working to develop the foundation for the first multisite, prospective US registry focused on better understanding these patients' care patterns, quality of life, and outcomes over time.

The scope of the topic of cardiovascular conditions complicating pregnancy is broad and this issue features topics covering each major component of management of cardiovascular conditions in pregnancy and underscores the role and importance of the emerging cardio-obstetrics subspecialty.

FUTURE DIRECTIONS

This article recognizes the importance of acquired and congenital cardiovascular conditions'

contribution to maternal morbidity and mortality. There is a new and growing network of providers within maternal fetal medicine, cardiology, anesthesia, and perinatology working collaboratively to build a research infrastructure in order to answer key questions related to the care patterns, quality-of-life metrics, and long-term outcomes of mothers with cardiovascular conditions in the preconception period, during pregnancy, in the postpartum period, and for several years beyond. It is hoped that this foundational research will extend to include more sites across the country to provide representative data that will be generalizable to patients across the country, and will also allow the ability to validate current risk models that exist outside of the United States and to better understand patient perceptions of care. It is hoped that, empowered with more information, clinicians will be able to counsel patients more confidently not only about how their cardiac conditions may affect their pregnancies but also how pregnancy may affect their cardiac conditions. With time, it is hoped to deliver data to support the standardization and enhancement of the care of women with cardiovascular conditions in pregnancy and their babies.

CLINICS CARE POINTS

- Among industrialized nations, the United States has the highest maternal mortality, estimated at 17.4 maternal deaths per 100,000 live births. Profound racial disparities persist: African American patients' risk of dying surrounding pregnancy is 3.4 times that of white women.

- Acquired and congenital heart disease are leading causes of severe maternal morbidity and mortality in the United States, accounting for ∼one-quarter of pregnancy-related deaths.
- A growing research alliance is collaborating to address key gaps in knowledge surrounding the preconception period, antenatal care, delivery planning and outcomes, postpartum care, and long-term outcomes of women with heart disease in pregnancy and their babies.

DISCLOSURE

The authors have no disclosures, nor any commercial or financial conflicts of interest.

REFERENCES

1. Centers for Disease Control and Prevention. Pregnancy mortality surveillance system. 2019. Available at: http://www.cdc.gov/reproductivehealth/maternal infanthealth/pmss.html. Accessed July 1, 2020.
2. Young A. Deadly deliveries. USA Today 2019.
3. Nina Martin EC, Freitas A. Lost mothers. New York: ProPublica; 2017.
4. Horon IL. Underreporting of maternal deaths on death certificates and the magnitude of the problem of maternal mortality. Am J Public Health 2005;95(3): 478–82.
5. Stevenson AJF-VI, Allgeyer RL, Schenkkan P, et al. Effect of removal of Planned Parenthood from the Texas women's health program. N Engl J Med 2016;374(9):853–60.
6. Liptak A. Supreme court appears sharply divided as it hears Texas Abortion Case. New York: Times; Aahwnc; 2016.
7. Moaddab ADG, Brown H, Bateni ZH, et al. Health care disparity and pregnancy-related mortality in the United States, 2005-2014. Obstet Gynecol 2018;131(4):707–12.
8. Briller JKA, Geller SE. Maternal cardiovascular mortality in Illinois, 2002-2011. Obstet Gynecol 2017; 129:819–26.
9. Leddy MA, Power ML, Schulkin J. The impact of maternal obesity on maternal and fetal health. Rev Obstet Gynecol 2008;1(4):170–8.
10. Main EKMC, Morton CH, Holtby S, et al. Pregnancy-related mortality in California. Obstet Gynecol 2015; 125(4):938–47.
11. Leise KL, Mogos M, Abboud S, et al. Racial and ethnic disparities in severe maternal morbidity in the United States. J Racial Ethn Health Disparities 2019;6(4):790–8.
12. Kozhimannil KB, Interrante JD, Henning-Smith C, et al. Rural-urban differences in severe maternal morbidity and mortality in the US, 2007-15. Health Aff (Millwood) 2019;38(12):2077–85.
13. ACOG Committee Opinion No. 736. Optimizing postpartum care. Obstet Gynecol 2018;131(5): e140–50.
14. Hollier LM, Martin JN Jr, Connolly H. ACOG practice bulletin No. 212: pregnancy and heart disease. Obstet Gynecol 2019;133(5):e320–56. APBNPahdOG.
15. Available at: https://www.cmqcc.org. Accessed July 1, 2020.
16. Committee Opinion No. 629. Clinical guidelines and standardization of practice to improve outcomes. Obstet Gynecol 2015;125(4):1027–9.
17. Review to action. Report from nine maternal mortality review committees. Available at: https://reviewtoaction.org/Report_from_Nine_MMRCs. Accessed July 1, 2020.
18. Creanga ASC, Seed K, Callaghan W. Pregnancy-related mortality in the United States, 2011-2013. Obstet Gynecol 2017;130(2):366–73.
19. Gilboa SM, Devine OJ, Kucik JE, et al. Congenital heart defects in the United States: estimating the magnitude of the affected population in 2010. Circulation 2016;134(2):101–9.
20. Sanghavi M, Rutherford JD. Cardiovascular physiology of pregnancy. Circulation 2014;130(12): 1003–8.
21. Silversides CGJ, Mason J, Sermer M, et al. Pregnancy outcomes in women with heart disease. The CARPREG II study. J Am Coll Cardiol 2018;71: 2419–30.
22. Lane-Cordova AD, Khan SS, Grobman WA, et al. Long-term cardiovascular risks associated with adverse pregnancy outcomes: JACC review topic of the week. J Am Coll Cardiol 2019;73(16): 2106–16.

The Importance of Cardiovascular Risk Assessment and Pregnancy Heart Team in the Management of Cardiovascular Disease in Pregnancy

Garima Sharma, MD[a],*, Wendy Ying, MD[a], Candice K. Silversides, MD[b]

KEYWORDS

- Cardiovascular disease • Pregnancy heart team • Cardiovascular risk
- Adverse pregnancy outcomes

KEY POINTS

- Multidisciplinary team-based care is the cornerstone of management of cardiovascular disease in pregnancy.
- Understanding and anticipating how the physiologic changes of pregnancy may impact underlying cardiovascular status is important when addressing pregnancy risks in women with cardiac disease. Women with preexisting cardiac disease, prior adverse pregnancy outcomes, and traditional cardiovascular risk factors should undergo careful prepregnancy counseling and have antenatal surveillance once pregnant.
- Incorporating validated risk scores, lesion-specific information, imaging parameters, biomarkers, and patient-specific details can help identify women at highest risk, plan appropriate pregnancy care, and improve outcomes.
- Close postpartum follow-up for women with maternal placental syndromes, gestational diabetes, and other adverse pregnancy outcomes provides a unique opportunity to continue monitoring and implement guideline-directed strategies to reverse long-term cardiovascular complications.

INTRODUCTION

Cardiovascular disease (CVD) is the most common cause of pregnancy-related maternal mortality in the United States.[1] According to data from the Healthcare Cost and Utilization Project's National Inpatient Sample, hospital admissions in pregnant women with CVD increased by 25% from 2003 to 2012.[2] Additionally, the incidence of major adverse cardiac events and arrhythmias also increased. especially in women with pulmonary hypertension or cardiomyopathy.[2] Large cohort studies of pregnancies in women with heart disease report cardiac complication rates of 10% to 15%, of which 4% are serious or life threatening.[3,4] These numbers are likely to increase, because in the past two decades, deliveries among women with

[a] Division of Cardiology, Johns Hopkins Ciccarone Center for Prevention of Cardiovascular Disease, Johns Hopkins University School of Medicine and Hospital, 1800 Orleans Street, Zayed 7125s, Baltimore, MD 21287, USA;
[b] Division of Cardiology, University of Toronto Pregnancy and Heart Disease Research Program, Mount Sinai and Toronto General Hospitals, 700 University Avenue, Room 3-913, Toronto, Ontario M5G 1Z5, Canada
* Corresponding author.
E-mail address: gsharma8@jhmi.edu
Twitter: @GarimaVSharmaMD (G.S.); @WendyYingMD (W.Y.); @CandiceSilvers1 (C.K.S.)

Cardiol Clin 39 (2021) 7–19
https://doi.org/10.1016/j.ccl.2020.09.002

congenital heart disease (CHD) increased by 34.9%, a greater rise than the 21.3% increase observed in the general population, likely from advances in pediatric cardiac surgery and cardiac care.[5] This group of women are also more likely to have comorbidities, including pulmonary hypertension, congestive heart failure, coronary artery disease, arrhythmias, thromboembolic events, preeclampsia and placenta previa.[6] Importantly, among pregnancies complicated by serious cardiac events, almost 50% are preventable, highlighting the need for early recognition, risk stratification, and management of CVD in pregnancy.[7]

Adverse pregnancy outcomes (APO), such as maternal placental syndromes (preeclampsia, hypertensive disorders of pregnancy [HDP], preterm birth, and small for gestational age baby) and gestational diabetes (GDM), are increasingly recognized to be associated with future maternal cardiometabolic risk and CVD.[8–10] Although the pathogenetic mechanisms of how these conditions result in long-term cardiovascular damage are unclear, at least one explanation is that pregnancy may unmask preexisting elevated CVD risk.[8]

Although pregnancy in women with heart disease is associated with significant morbidity, most women have a safe pregnancy if they have appropriate prepregnancy evaluation and pregnancy care by an experienced pregnancy heart team (PHT). The understanding of pregnancy risk and how to care for women with CVD during pregnancy has evolved over the past two decades.[11,12] Prediction of maternal cardiac complications in women with heart disease is enhanced by integration of general, lesion-specific, and delivery of care variables.[4] A multidisciplinary approach to the care of patients improves outcomes and facilitates a consistent and clear message for the patient (and those caring for each patient). The PHT needs to address risk stratification and management of complications during pregnancy, and risks in the postpartum period.[13,14] In this review, we discuss (1) the multiorgan physiologic changes in pregnancy that can result in decompensation in women with preexisting CVD, (2) an approach to risk stratification in women with heart disease, and (3) the role of multidisciplinary team–based care (**Fig. 1**).

PHYSIOLOGIC CHANGES IN PREGNANCY

The pregnant mother undergoes significant anatomic and physiologic changes to nurture and accommodate the developing fetus. These changes begin after conception and affect every organ system in the body.[15] For most women

experiencing an uncomplicated pregnancy, these changes resolve after pregnancy with minimal residual effects (**Table 1**). However, these changes can exacerbate underlying CVD in pregnancy and result in significant maternal morbidity and mortality.[16,17] One of the most important aspects of antenatal care is to assess the impact that these changes could have on existing CVD. This in turn can help guide antenatal follow-up, timing of interventions or medications when needed, and mitigate decompensation.

Changes in the Cardiovascular System

Hemodynamic changes in pregnancy are largely caused by an increase in the cardiac output (CO) by 30% to 50%, secondary to increased stroke volume (SV) and, to a lesser extent, heart rate (HR).[17,18] CO rises early in pregnancy and plateaus between the second and third trimester. The systemic vascular resistance (SVR) decreases until the second trimester and then starts to increase until term.[17] HR increases progressively throughout the pregnancy by 10 to 20 bpm, reaching a maximum in the third trimester. The overall change in HR represents a 20% to 25% increase over baseline.[19–21] Although plasma volume and SVR increase, pulmonary capillary wedge pressure and central venous pressure do not increase significantly.[22] Pulmonary vascular resistance, like SVR, decreases during pregnancy. Maternal hemodynamics during labor are influenced by active stage labor, pain, analgesia, and anesthesia and this can have a profound effect on the existing CVD, especially because of large volume shifts. CO increases by 30% during the active stage of labor. Uterine contractions lead to an autotransfusion of 300 to 500 mL of blood back into the circulation and the sympathetic response to pain and anxiety further elevate the HR and blood pressure. All of these changes can result in acute decompensation or heart failure in women with left-sided valvular obstructive lesions (aortic and mitral stenosis) or right ventricular dysfunction in setting of severe pulmonary hypertension. Following delivery, there is an immediate rise in CO caused by relief of the inferior vena cava obstruction and contraction of the uterus, which empties blood into the systemic circulation. CO starts to decline within about 1 hour of delivery.[18] During this early postpartum period, the transfer of fluid from the extravascular space increases venous return and SVR further especially consequential in those with CVD and therefore these patients are most at risk of pulmonary edema during the second stage of labor and the immediate postpartum period. Cardiac changes can take

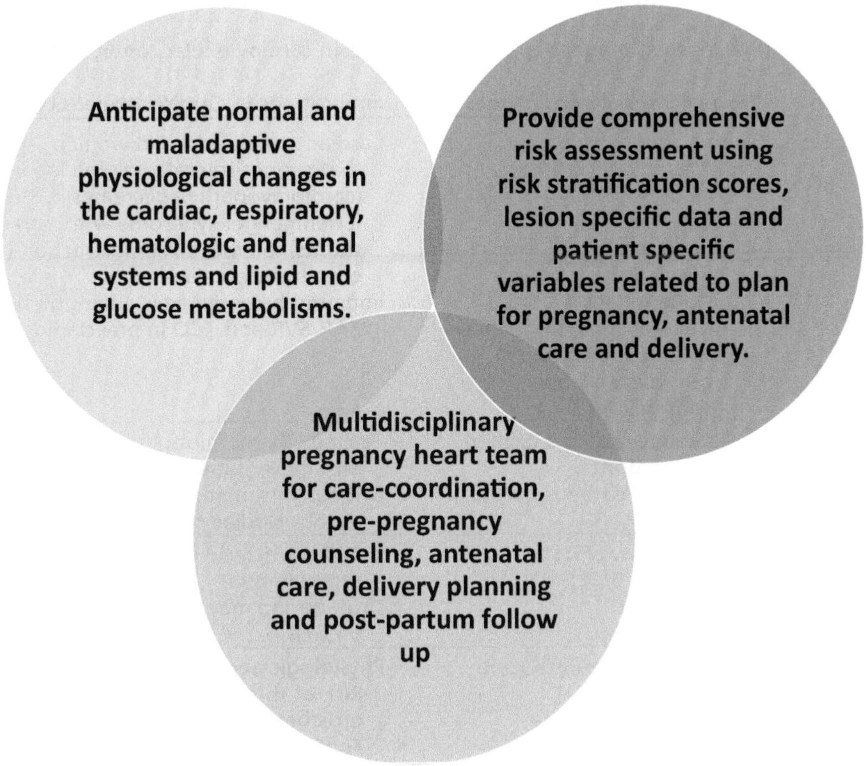

Anticipate normal and maladaptive physiological changes in the cardiac, respiratory, hematologic and renal systems and lipid and glucose metabolisms.

Provide comprehensive risk assessment using risk stratification scores, lesion specific data and patient specific variables related to plan for pregnancy, antenatal care and delivery.

Multidisciplinary pregnancy heart team for care-coordination, pre-pregnancy counseling, antenatal care, delivery planning and post-partum follow up

Fig. 1. Comprehensive approach to cardiovascular risk stratification in pregnancy.

6 months to return to normal (prepregnancy values). Some pathologic changes (eg, hypertension in preeclampsia) may take much longer.[23]

Changes in the Respiratory System

During a normal pregnancy, there is an increase in oxygen demand caused by a 15% increase in the metabolic rate and 20% increase in the oxygen consumption.[22,24] There is maternal hyperventilation caused by a 40% to 50% increase in minute ventilation, mostly because of an increase in tidal volume, rather than in the respiratory rate. This causes arterial Po_2 to increase and arterial Pco_2 to fall, with a compensatory fall in serum bicarbonate to 18 to 22 mmol/L resulting a mild fully compensated respiratory alkalosis (arterial pH, 7.44).[22] Diaphragmatic elevation in late pregnancy results in decreased functional residual capacity, but peak expiratory flow rate and forced expiratory volume in 1 second are unaffected by pregnancy. There is also a subjective feeling of breathlessness without hypoxia in pregnancy. This is most common in the third trimester but may start at any time during gestation, and may be worse at rest and improve with mild activity.[22] In patients with severe restricted lung disease, the ability to increase their ventilation is limited and their lung

function and oxygen saturation needs to be monitored.[25] In patients with preeclampsia, there is an increase in minute ventilation because of increase in concentration of blood leptin (a ventilation-stimulating hormone) and decrease in vital capacity caused by pharyngeal edema, weight gain with higher adiposity around the neck, and overall decrease exercise tolerance, which can worsen the respiratory status.[26]

Changes in the Hematologic System

Plasma volume increases proportionally more than the red blood cell mass, resulting in a "physiologic anemia" from hemodilution, with hemoglobin levels as low as 11 g/dL considered physiologic.[18] There are significant increases in total blood volume, plasma volume, and red blood cell mass during pregnancy.[17,18,27] Normal pregnancy is accompanied by changes in the coagulation and fibrinolytic systems. These include increases in several clotting factors (I, II, VII, VIII, IX, and XII), a decrease in protein S levels, and inhibition of fibrinolysis.[28] As gestation progresses, there is also a significant fall in the activity of activated protein C, an important anticoagulant. Thus, pregnancy alters the balance within the coagulation system in favor of clotting, predisposing the

Table 1
Normal physiologic changes in pregnancy and implications in cardiovascular conditions

Organ System	Normal Physiologic Changes	Implications in Cardiovascular Conditions
Cardiovascular system	During pregnancy: ↑ Plasma flow (75%) ↑CO (30%–50%) ↓ SVR and PVR During labor: ↑ CO by 30% in active stage of labor Increased circulating blood volume (300–500 mL) caused by uterine contractions	Cardiac complications in women with lesions that cannot tolerate volume loading (cardiomyopathy), decreases in SVR (Eisenmenger syndrome with intracardiac shunts), or with fixed obstruction (aortic or mitral stenosis) Impaired hemodynamic adaptation ↑MAP, SVR and ↓CO in preeclampsia
Respiratory system	↑Metabolic rate and oxygen consumption Mild compensated respiratory alkalosis	Feeling of breathlessness during pregnancy ↑ Minute ventilation in preeclampsia Difficulty intubating in those who develop serious cardiac complications
Renal system	↑ Plasma flow (75%) ↑ GFR (40%–50%) ↑ Proteinuria	↓ GFR ↓ Uric acid clearance ↑ Proteinuria in preeclampsia Drug dosing may need to be adjusted based on GFR
Hematologic system	↑Plasma volume (50%) and red cell mass ↑ Coagulation factors ↓ Protein C Compression of the inferior vena cava	Physiologic anemia ↑ Risk of thromboembolism in women with prosthetic heart valves, atrial fibrillation, Fontan circulation ↓Lifespan of platelets in and hemolysis in severe preeclampsia (HELLP syndrome)
Lipid metabolism	↑Triglycerides, total cholesterol (50%) and in LDL (50%) and ↓HDL	↑Dyslipidemia with ↓ HDL ↑Free fatty acids in preeclampsia Existing maternal dyslipidemia is associated with adverse pregnancy outcomes
Glucose metabolism	↑Insulin resistance, mild diabetogenic state	Gestational diabetes

Abbreviations: ↓, decrease; ↑, increase; CO, cardiac output; GFR, glomerular filtration rate; HDL, high-density lipoprotein cholesterol; HELLP, hemolysis elevated liver enzymes and low platelets; LDL, low-density lipoprotein cholesterol; MAP, mean arterial pressures; PVR, pulmonary vascular resistance; SVR systemic vascular resistance.

pregnant and postpartum woman to venous thrombosis and other thromboembolic complications.[22] There is an increased risk for thromboembolism during pregnancy because of lower extremity venous stasis resulting from inferior vena caval compression by the gravid uterus and because of a hypercoagulable state caused by an increase in vitamin K–dependent clotting factors and a reduction in free protein S.[29] The issue of hypercoagulability is of particular relevance for women with mechanical heart valves, atrial fibrillation, Fontan circulation, or previous thromboembolic events.

Changes in the Renal System

In a normal pregnancy, there is substantial activation of the renin-angiotensin-aldosterone system, which occurs early in pregnancy, with increases in plasma volume starting at 6 to 8 weeks and rising progressively until 28 to 30 weeks.[30] The decrease in SVR and vasodilation that is seen in early pregnancy results in a 50% increase in renal plasma flow and glomerular filtration rates (GFR) by the end of the first trimester, resulting in decreases in serum creatinine, urea, and uric acid values.[31] Changes in GFR, and changes in the volume of distribution, are important to consider when dosing cardiac medications during pregnancy. In preeclampsia, there is maladaptation of the renin-angiotensin-aldosterone system caused by an increase in SVR and decrease in CO, resulting in decrease in GFR and decreased secretion of uric acid leading to hyperuricemia and exaggerated urinary excretion of proteins.[32]

Changes in the Lipid Metabolism

There is an increase in total serum cholesterol and triglyceride levels mainly as a result of increased synthesis by the liver and decreased lipoprotein lipase activity, resulting in decreased catabolism of adipose tissue. Maternal hypertriglyceridemia is a characteristic feature during pregnancy and corresponds to an accumulation of triglycerides not only in very-low-density lipoprotein but also in low- and high-density lipoprotein.[33] Low-density lipoprotein cholesterol levels also increase and reach 50% at term. High-density lipoprotein increase in the first half of pregnancy and fall in the third trimester but concentrations are 15% higher than nonpregnant levels. Increased triglyceride levels provide for the mother's energy needs and increase in low-density lipoprotein cholesterol is important for placental steroidogenesis. Dyslipidemia in pregnancy is associated with APOs with direct implications on perinatal outcomes.[34] It is prudent to screen women with existing lipid disorders, ideally before conception or at the initial obstetric visit. Abnormal lipids should be treated with diet, exercise, and weight management and bile acid sequestrants in severe cases. In general, statins and other cholesterol medications, such as ezetimibe, are not used during pregnancy and lactation.[35]

Changes in the Glucose Metabolism

During pregnancy, there is a mild diabetogenic state, characterized by increased insulin secretion and increased insulin sensitivity in early pregnancy, followed by progressive insulin resistance.[36] Physiologic pancreatic β-cell hyperplastic adaptation allows for shunting of glucose to the fetus while maintaining maternal nutrition. Maternal insulin resistance begins in the second trimester and peaks in the third trimester. Maladaptive changes in the maternal system that occur in GDM, such as lipotoxicity, inflammation and oxidative stress, and impairments in adipokine and placental signaling, are associated with impaired β-cell adaptation.[37] In the presence of preexisting maternal obesity or excessive gestational weight gain, insulin secretion becomes insufficient to overcome insulin resistance, resulting in hyperglycemia and glucose intolerance that is characteristic of GDM.[38] Preconception counseling, early antenatal risk assessment, and comprehensive health education strategies are helpful strategies to mitigate GDM.

COMPONENTS OF ANTENATAL RISK ASSESSMENT

Ideally, the maternal cardiovascular risk assessment should occur in the preconception phase, because this allows for informed and shared decision making about pregnancy. The prepregnancy encounter should include education about maternal and perinatal risks, optimization of maternal cardiac status, careful review of potentially teratogenic medications with switches to alternatives when necessary, and a discussion about what to expect during pregnancy. Potential risks for women with heart disease and their babies include: maternal and perinatal mortality; maternal cardiac complications, such as heart failure and arrhythmias; obstetric complications, such as postpartum bleeding, preterm birth, and growth restriction; transmission of CHD to offspring; and the potential negative impact of pregnancy on long-term maternal cardiac health.[16,39] Recognition of underlying comorbidities that can result in complications is also important so that early guideline-directed preventative strategies are implemented. For example, women with high-risk features for developing preeclampsia, such as advanced maternal age, prior history of preeclampsia, or diabetes, should be started on low-dose aspirin by 12 to 14 weeks.[40]

Maternal Cardiovascular Risk Assessment

For women with existing CVD including CHD, several risk prediction models have been developed to identify poor maternal cardiac outcomes. The three most commonly known are the CARPREG (Cardiac Disease in Pregnancy), the ZAHARA (Zwangerschap bij vrouwen met een Aangeboren HARtAfwijking-II), and the modified World Health Organization (WHO) risk models (**Table 2**).[3] The three risk models are described next. These risk scores are used as a starting point for risk estimation. Additional variables that are incorporated into risk assessment includes lesion-specific risks; cardiac imaging data (MRI, computed tomography); exercise test results; biomarkers levels, such as brain natriuretic peptide; and other patient-specific information including patient compliance and access to care.

Modified World Health Organization classification

Based on expert consensus, a British Working Group classified pregnancy risk in women with heart disease using modified WHO classification categories[41]: class I (conditions associated with no detectable increased risk of maternal mortality and no/mild increase in morbidity), class II (conditions with small increased risk of maternal mortality or moderate increase in morbidity), class III (conditions with significantly increased risk of maternal mortality or severe morbidity), and class IV (conditions with extremely high risk of maternal

Table 2
Comparison of cardiovascular risk assessment scores and classifications

Modified WHO Classification	ZAHARA Risk Score (Weighted Risk Score Based on Factors of Poor Predictive Outcomes)	CARPEG II Risk Predictors (Weighted Risk Score Based on Lesion, Imaging Parameters and Patient Factors)
Class I: No detectable increase in maternal mortality and no/mild increase in morbidity (uncomplicated and repaired ASD, VSD, PDA, and MVP, atrial and ventricular ectopic beats) Class II: Small increase in maternal mortality and moderate increase in morbidity (Unoperated ASD, VSD, TOF, and ventricular arrhythmias. Depending on the individual mild LV dysfunction, HCM, Marfan without aortic dilatation, repaired coarctation of aorta)	Mechanical valve prosthesis (4.25) Evidence of left-side obstruction (aortic valve peak gradient >50 mm Hg or AVA <1.0 cm^2 (2.50) History of arrhythmia (1.50) Use of cardiac medication prepregnancy (1.50) Repaired and unrepaired cyanotic heart disease (1.0) Moderate to severe atrioventricular valve dysfunction (possibly related to underlying LV dysfunction) (0.75) Baseline NYHA functional classification > II (0.75)	Prior cardiac events or arrhythmias (3) NYHA functional class III-IV or cyanosis (3) Mechanical valve (3) Systemic LV dysfunction (EF <55%) (2) High-risk valve disease (2) Pulmonary hypertension (RVSP >49 mm Hg (2) High-risk aortopathy (2) Coronary artery disease (2) No prior cardiac intervention (1) Late pregnancy assessment (1)
Class III: Significantly increased maternal mortality and morbidity. (Mechanical valve, systemic right ventricle, Fontan circulation, unrepaired cyanotic heart disease, aortic root dilatation in Marfan and bicuspid valve) Class IV: Extremely high-risk maternal mortality and morbidity (Cardiomyopathy with LVEF <30%, pulmonary hypertension, native severe coarctation, severe mitral and aortic stenosis)	Weighted risk score: Maternal cardiovascular complications risk: <0.5 points = 2.9%, 0.5–1.5 points = 7.5% 1.51–2.50 points = 17.5% 2.51–3.5 points = 43.1% >3.5 points = 70%	Weighted risk score: Maternal cardiac complications risk: 0–1 = 5% 2 = 10% 3 = 15% 4 = 22% >4 = 41%
Maternal cardiovascular complication risks: class I, 2.5%–5%; class II, 5.7%–10.5%; class II-III, 10%–19%; class III, 19%–27%; class IV, 40%–100%		

Abbreviations: ASD, atrial septal defect; AVA, aortic valve area; CARPREG, cardiac disease in pregnancy; HCM, hypertrophic cardiomyopathy; LVEF, left ventricular ejection fraction; PDA, patent ductus arteriosus; RVSP, right ventricular systolic pressure; TOF, teratology of Fallot; VSD, ventricular septal defect; ZAHARA, Zwangerschap bij vrouwen met een Aangeboren HARtAfwijking-II.

Adapted from Balci A, Sollie-Szarynska KM, Van Der Bijl AGL, et al. Prospective validation and assessment of cardiovascular and offspring risk models for pregnant women with congenital heart disease. Heart 2014;100(17):1375; with permission.

mortality or severe morbidity; pregnancy is contra-indicated) (see **Table 2**). The 2018 American College of Cardiology/American Heart Association Guideline for the Management of Adults with Congenital Heart Disease[42] and the 2018 European Society of Cardiology Guidelines for the Management of Cardiovascular Diseases during Pregnancy[43] recommend the modified WHO classification to predict cardiovascular risk. One criticism of the WHO classification is that it provides a large risk margin for class IV lesions and does not take the patient's clinical characteristics into consideration; nevertheless, the designation of specific cardiac conditions that are considered contraindications for pregnancy is helpful for the clinician.

ZAHARA score

The ZAHARA risk score is a weighted scoring system to predict adverse maternal cardiac events in pregnant women with CHD.[44] The investigators identified eight predictors of poor outcomes: the presence of mechanical heart valve (4.25 points), severe left heart obstruction (mean aortic pressure gradient >50 mm Hg or aortic valve area <1.0 cm^2) (2.50 points), history of arrhythmias and cardiac medication use before pregnancy (1.50 points each), history of cyanotic heart disease (uncorrected or corrected) (1.00 points), moderate-to-severe pulmonary or systemic atrioventricular valve regurgitation, and symptomatic heart failure before pregnancy (New York Heart Association [NYHA] functional class ≥II) (0.75 points each). The score was divided into five categories of risk based on accrued points (see **Table 2**).[44]

CARPREG I and CARPREG II score

The original CARPREG risk score was a four-point risk score developed to predict maternal cardiac complications in women with heart disease. The four variables were equally weighted and included: (1) prior cardiac events, (2) poor NYHA functional class (NYHA class III or IV) or cyanosis, (3) impaired systemic ventricular function (ejection fraction <40%), and (4) left-sided obstruction (mitral valve area of <2 cm^2, aortic valve area of <1.5 cm^2, or peak left ventricular outflow gradient >30 mm Hg).[11] Higher risk scores were associated with higher risk of maternal cardiac complications.

The CARPREG II risk score, based on outcomes data from 1938 pregnancies in women with heart disease at two large Canadian hospitals, identified 10 risk predictors of maternal cardiac complications.[4] In contrast to the ZAHARA population, the CARPREG II study included a more diverse cardiac population that included women with CHD

(63.7%), acquired heart disease (22.9%), cardiac arrhythmias (13.4%), mild left ventricular dysfunction (13.6%), and coronary artery disease (2%).[4] The CARPREG II risk score is a weighted risk score, which includes the original four CARPREG risk predictors, and six additional risk predictors. These include five general cardiac predictors (prior cardiac events or arrhythmias, poor functional class or cyanosis, high-risk valve disease/left ventricular outflow tract obstruction, systemic ventricular dysfunction, no prior cardiac interventions); four lesion-specific predictors (mechanical valves, high-risk aortopathies, pulmonary hypertension, coronary artery disease); and one predictor related to delivery of care (late pregnancy assessment) (see **Table 2**).[4] Women with a score greater than 4 had a risk of maternal cardiac complications of more than 40%, and even women in the lowest risk group (score of 0 or 1) had a 5% risk of cardiac complications.

Genetic Counseling

Genetic counseling is an important component of prenatal counseling in women with inherited CVD. For women with inherited genetic disease, a three-generation family history, including details on consanguinity, should be obtained.[45] Genetic evaluation should be made available to all women with CHD, particularly those who are syndromic or who have a family history of CHD; women with inherited arrhythmias, aortopathies, or cardiomyopathies; and women with known autosomal-dominant or recessive conditions.[45,46] The risk of inheriting CHD for the fetus from an affected mother is between 2% and 3% in simple valvular disease; 3% and 6% in complex CHD; and up to 50% in autosomal-dominant syndromes, such as Noonan or Marfan.[47,48]

Antenatal Surveillance

Based on the results of individualized risk assessment, the frequency of antenatal surveillance can be planned. Pregnancy surveillance should include a history and physical examinations, electrocardiograms and transthoracic echocardiograms, basic metabolic profile, complete blood count, and further testing as needed (ie, potential stress testing, cardiac MRI). However, close attention is essential, because some testing modalities involve radiation and therefore may be contraindicated during pregnancy. The goal is to optimize the patient's cardiovascular status. Careful considerations should be given to medications associated with embryopathy and they should be discontinued before pregnancy. For women on anticoagulation for prosthetic valves and other conditions requiring anticoagulation, guideline-directed recommendations of changing to lower-molecular-weight heparin or continuing with warfarin if the recommended dose is less than 5 mg should be followed.[43]

Delivery Planning

Vaginal delivery remains the optimal method of delivery in most women with heart disease.[49] A Registry of Pregnancy and Cardiac disease (ROPAC) study of in 1262 women with cardiac disease showed that a planned caesarean delivery did not confer any maternal health advantages over planned vaginal delivery, but was associated with an adverse fetal outcome.[50] There is consensus that a planned vaginal birth for most women with CVD, including those with high-risk disease, is safe,[51] Cesarean delivery is generally reserved for obstetric indications, such as breech presentation, failure to progress, placenta previa, or some abnormal fetal HR patterns.[42] Cesarean delivery is necessary in women who have not stopped oral anticoagulation before delivery or in those with acute or chronic aortic dissection. Many experts recommend cesarean delivery in women with Marfan syndrome who have a dilated aorta (>45 mm) or those with intractable heart failure.[16,39,52] The risks of cesarean delivery include: general anesthesia and the risk of hemodynamic instability associated with intubation and the anesthetic agent; blood loss of at least twice that associated with vaginal delivery in some cases, especially in those patients on anticoagulation; and risk of postoperative wound infections. Other labor and delivery considerations include the location of delivery (intensive care unit vs labor and delivery), need for monitoring (oxygen saturation monitors, telemetry monitoring), mode of delivery (vaginal vs cesarean, Valsalva or second-assisted stage), timing of delivery, anesthetic approach (regional vs general), and postdelivery follow-up plans.

COMPONENTS OF POSTPARTUM RISK ASSESSMENT AND FOLLOW-UP

There is increasing focus on extending comprehensive care and close follow-up in the postpartum period. The weeks following birth are a critical period for a woman and her infant, setting the stage for long-term health and well-being. The American College of Obstetrics and Gynecology has released guidelines to optimize the health of women and infants in the postpartum phase and recommended that it should become an ongoing process, rather than a single encounter, with

services and support tailored to each woman's individual needs.[53] Women are encouraged to have contact with their obstetrician-gynecologists or other obstetric care providers within the first 3 weeks postpartum.[53] On-going care for complications and postoperative issues should continue until these issues are resolved (**Fig. 2**).[53] Detailed screening for postpartum depression, hypertension, and chronic disease management should include a full assessment of physical, social, and psychological well-being, including the following domains: mood and emotional well-being; breast-feeding, contraception, and birth-control; sleep and fatigue; physical recovery from birth; exercise recommendations; chronic disease management; and health maintenance.[53] Women with chronic medical conditions, such as hypertensive disorders, obesity, diabetes, dyslipidemia, and ischemic or structural heart disease, should be counseled regarding the importance of timely follow-up with their cardiologists or primary care providers for ongoing coordination of care. For women with peripartum cardiomyopathy, aortopathies, and other complex cardiovascular conditions, immediate close follow-up with echocardiograms may be required.[43,52] The postpartum period offers an excellent time to discuss the possibility of future pregnancy and the likelihood of late cardiovascular risk in women with APOs.[13] This is especially important, because APOs are thought to unmask a woman's preexisting cardiovascular risk and act as a harbinger for long-term CVD.[32] Additionally, APOs may be the manifestation of the first diagnosis of a woman's CVD made in pregnancy, particularly chronic hypertension diagnosed as HDP or type 2 diabetes diagnosed as GDM. Unique considerations exist relating to the specific type of underlying CVD and APO. For example, in patients with pre-eclampsia who develop chronic hypertension, a detailed cardiovascular risk assessment in the postpartum time frame with atherosclerotic cardiovascular risk score and focused interventions on improving diet, lifestyle, exercise, and glucose control in those that have these risk factors can lead to improved health literacy and reduction of cardiovascular risk burden.[54] Several centers throughout the United States and Canada have reported on multidisciplinary maternal health clinics for women with APOs, such as HDP.[55,56] There are several care models incorporating in-person and telehealth visits for implementation of preventative measures, such as home blood pressure and weight monitoring, nutritional referral, exercise recommendations, and other cardiometabolic risk-reduction methods.[57,58] Women should also be counseled about safe contraceptive options.

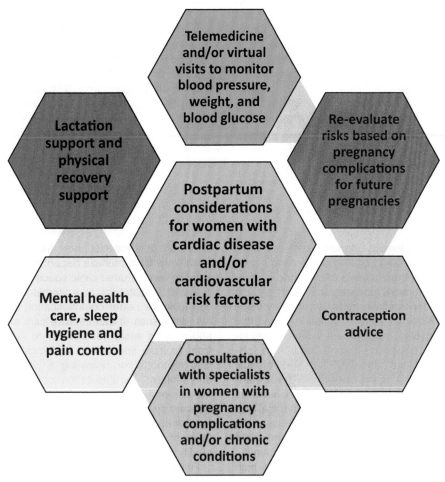

Fig. 2. Postpartum considerations in cardiovascular patients.

ROLE OF MULTIDISCIPLINARY PREGNANCY HEART TEAM

The rising prevalence of cardiovascular conditions complicating pregnancy and the contribution of advancing maternal age, chronic cardiovascular risk factors (eg, maternal obesity, chronic hypertension, sleep apnea, dyslipidemia, and diabetes), and known CVD has led to need for multidisciplinary care models to improve preconception counseling and screening for women.[13,59] More recently, this high-risk care coordination has been endorsed by the national scientific societies and there have been joint presidential statements urging comanagement.[60] The need for multidisciplinary care between cardiologists and obstetricians is supported by best practice statements from the American Heart Association and the American College of Obstetrics and Gynecology.[14] Drawing on this expert opinion and with growing evidence of heart centers for women, we advocate for the assembly of a similar multidisciplinary team

for the management of women with CVD in pregnancy.[61]

Members of the Pregnancy Heart Team

Multidisciplinary teams include, at a minimum, a core group of providers from cardiology, obstetrics or maternal fetal medicine, anesthesia, and nursing. Providers should all have expertise in the management of CVD in pregnancy. Other medical specialists (ie, hematologists), geneticists, neonatologists, cardiac interventionalists or surgeons, pharmacists, and social workers can also serve as additional key members.[62] Optimal team-based care involves regular multidisciplinary meetings, during which time these key stakeholders discuss patient management, treatment of complications, and delivery plans (**Fig. 3**).[62]

Specific Goals of the Pregnancy Heart Team

There are several specific goals that a PHT can aim to achieve (see **Fig. 3**). First, the PHT can

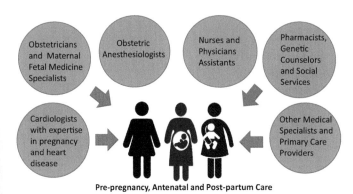

Pre-pregnancy, Antenatal and Post-partum Care

Fig. 3. Composition of the pregnancy heart team and specific goals. Specific goals of the pregnancy heart team: (1) improve the quality of care and establish safety protocols; (2) provide prepregnancy counseling, cardiovascular risk assessment, and pregnancy management with shared decision making; (3) develop detailed delivery plans; (4) organize multidisciplinary conferences for cross-specialty training and education; and (5) ensure postpartum cardiovascular risk assessment and close monitoring of those with chronic conditions.

create and implement standardized protocols aimed at improving quality and safety and reducing preventable causes of obstetric complications and maternal morbidity.[60,63] A list of such causes has been defined by the Alliance for Innovation on Maternal Health, a national maternal safety and quality improvement initiative, and includes maternal venous thromboembolism, obstetric hemorrhage, and HDP.[64] One potential benefit of the PHT is the opportunity for a standardized approach to pregnancy care. Checklists and protocols are known to reduce medical and surgical errors and offer similar benefits over the longitudinal care of a woman's pregnancy.[65–69] Protocols may include workflows to identify, educate, and manage women who are at high risk for APO and maternal morbidity and mortality.

Second, the PHT can risk stratify patients to identify women at high risk of developing cardiac complications, direct antenatal surveillance, and coordinate plans for a safe labor and delivery. Care may include referrals to other specialists and staff. Treatment plans should be clearly recorded into medical records with clear delineation as to the provider responsible for each action item. This provides patients with a uniform approach to counseling and ensures comfort among delivering obstetricians at a given institution when managing these high-risk women in labor. Additionally, the multidisciplinary PHT can help to formulate a birth plan. Given the unpredictable nature of labor, each patient needs a documented delivery plan that outlines mode of delivery, location of delivery, labor analgesia plan, and intrapartum monitoring needs that is accessible to all members of the clinical team. Postpartum follow-up for certain high-risk conditions could also be protocolized to ensure optimal postpartum care.

The logistics of developing a PHT may be a barrier in some institutions. Initiating such an effort requires substantial support from an organizational level from multiple departments. If feasible, establishing a shared clinic space between cardiology and obstetrics or maternal-fetal medicine can facilitate better communication between the two disciplines. It can improve care coordination and make it easier for patients to see providers from multiple specialties. Additionally, standardized methods for reviewing a patient's history and uniform documentation can help coalesce the different practice patterns of providers from different specialties and improve efficiency. Identification of quality metrics a priori to the implementation of a PHT is crucial and lays a foundation for quality improvement assessments.

Finally, the PHT can improve the training and education of residents and fellows. Trainees will be exposed to multidisciplinary clinics and patient conferences, which can provide a forum for discussions of diagnostic and treatment plans in this complex population. Although the primary purpose of these meetings is to optimize care for patients, these meetings also contribute to the continuing education and help to develop rapport among members of the team. Exposure to multidisciplinary care of the pregnant patient with heart is recommended by the Core Cardiovascular Training Statement 4 as part of the fundamental training for cardiology fellows.[70]

SUMMARY

For women with heart disease, pregnancy poses a hemodynamic stress. The increasing burden of CVD in young women of childbearing age has contributed to an increase in maternal morbidity and mortality in the United States. An understanding of the physiologic changes of pregnancy and how they impact women with heart disease is crucial when caring for this group of women. Optimizing the care of pregnant women with CVD necessitates a multidisciplinary PHT. The PHT consists of specialists from cardiology, obstetrics and maternal fetal medicine, obstetric anesthesia, and nursing supports and provides standard approaches to antenatal, intrapartum, and postpartum care. The PHT also facilitates opportunities for cross-disciplinary education and to bridge the disciplines of cardiology and obstetrics and gynecology.

CLINICS CARE POINTS

- For women with existing CVD, risk prediction models, including the modified WHO, CAR-PREG II, and ZAHARA scores, should be used to estimate risk of maternal cardiac outcomes and formulate individualized plans for pregnancy, antenatal care, and delivery.
- Multidisciplinary care teams comprised of cardiology and obstetric team members should be utilized for management of patients with CVD in pregnancy.
- Standardized protocols aimed at specific preventable causes of obstetric complications and maternal morbidity can be important in improving quality and safety during pregnancy.
- Women who experience adverse pregnancy outcomes should undergo comprehensive postpartum follow up, with cardiovascular risk assessment focused on prevention of future atherosclerotic cardiovascular disease.

DISCLOSURE

Drs G. Sharma, W. Ying, and C.K. Silversides have no relevant disclosures.

REFERENCES

1. Creanga AA, Syverson C, Seed K, et al. Pregnancy-related mortality in the United States, 2011-2013 HHS public access author manuscript. Obstet Gynecol 2017. https://doi.org/10.1097/AOG.0000000000002114.
2. Lima FV, Yang J, Xu J, et al. National trends and in-hospital outcomes in pregnant women with heart disease in the United States. Am J Cardiol 2017. https://doi.org/10.1016/j.amjcard.2017.02.003.
3. Balci A, Sollie-Szarynska KM, Van Der Bijl AGL, et al. Prospective validation and assessment of cardiovascular and offspring risk models for pregnant women with congenital heart disease. Heart 2014. https://doi.org/10.1136/heartjnl-2014-305597.
4. Silversides CK, Grewal J, Mason J, et al. Pregnancy outcomes in women with heart disease: the CAR-PREG II study. J Am Coll Cardiol 2018. https://doi.org/10.1016/j.jacc.2018.02.076.
5. Opotowsky AR, Siddiqi OK, D'Souza B, et al. Maternal cardiovascular events during childbirth among women with congenital heart disease. Heart 2012. https://doi.org/10.1136/heartjnl-2011-300828.
6. Schlichting LE, Insaf TZ, Zaidi AN, et al. Maternal comorbidities and complications of delivery in pregnant women with congenital heart disease. J Am Coll Cardiol 2019. https://doi.org/10.1016/j.jacc.2019.01.069.
7. Pfaller B, Sathananthan G, Grewal J, et al. Preventing complications in pregnant women with cardiac disease. J Am Coll Cardiol 2020. https://doi.org/10.1016/j.jacc.2020.01.039.
8. Grandi SM, Filion KB, Yoon S, et al. Cardiovascular disease-related morbidity and mortality in women with a history of pregnancy complications: systematic review and meta-analysis. Circulation 2019. https://doi.org/10.1161/CIRCULATIONAHA.118.036748.
9. Wu P, Gulati M, Kwok CS, et al. Preterm delivery and future risk of maternal cardiovascular disease: a systematic review and meta-analysis. J Am Heart Assoc 2018. https://doi.org/10.1161/JAHA.117.007809.
10. Wu P, Haththotuwa R, Kwok CS, et al. Preeclampsia and future cardiovascular health: a systematic review and meta-analysis. Circ Cardiovasc Qual Outcomes 2017. https://doi.org/10.1161/CIRCOUTCOMES.116.003497.
11. Siu SC, Sermer M, Colman JM, et al. Prospective multicenter study of pregnancy outcomes in women with heart disease. Circulation 2001. https://doi.org/10.1161/hc3001.093437.
12. Ruys TPE, Cornette J, Roos-Hesselink JW. Pregnancy and delivery in cardiac disease. J Cardiol 2013. https://doi.org/10.1016/j.jjcc.2012.11.001.
13. Sharma G, Lindley K, Grodzinsky A. Cardio-obstetrics: developing a niche in maternal cardiovascular health. J Am Coll Cardiol 2020. https://doi.org/10.1016/j.jacc.2020.02.019.
14. Grodzinsky A, Florio K, Spertus JA, et al. Importance of the cardio-obstetrics team. Curr Treat Options Cardiovasc Med 2019. https://doi.org/10.1007/s11936-019-0789-1.
15. Lockitch G. Clinical biochemistry of pregnancy. Crit Rev Clin Lab Sci 1997. https://doi.org/10.3109/10408369709038216.
16. Elkayam U, Goland S, Pieper PG, et al. High-risk cardiac disease in pregnancy: Part I. J Am Coll Cardiol 2016. https://doi.org/10.1016/j.jacc.2016.05.048.
17. Ouzounian JG, Elkayam U. Physiologic changes during normal pregnancy and delivery. Cardiol Clin 2012. https://doi.org/10.1016/j.ccl.2012.05.004.
18. Sanghavi M, Rutherford JD. Cardiovascular physiology of pregnancy. Circulation 2014. https://doi.org/10.1161/CIRCULATIONAHA.114.009029.
19. Mahendru AA, Everett TR, Wilkinson IB, et al. A longitudinal study of maternal cardiovascular

function from preconception to the postpartum period. J Hypertens 2014. https://doi.org/10.1097/HJH.0000000000000090.

20. Clapp JF, Capeless E. Cardiovascular function before, during, and after the first and subsequent pregnancies. Am J Cardiol 1997. https://doi.org/10.1016/S0002-9149(97)00738-8.

21. Grindheim G, Estensen ME, Langesaeter E, et al. Changes in blood pressure during healthy pregnancy: a longitudinal cohort study. J Hypertens 2012. https://doi.org/10.1097/HJH.0b013e32834f0b1c.

22. Soma-Pillay P, Nelson-Piercy C, Tolppanen H, et al. Physiological changes in pregnancy. Cardiovasc J Afr 2016. https://doi.org/10.5830/CVJA-2016-021.

23. Buddeberg BS, Sharma R, O'Driscoll JM, et al. Cardiac maladaptation in term pregnancies with preeclampsia. Pregnancy Hypertens 2018. https://doi.org/10.1016/j.preghy.2018.06.015.

24. Silversides CK, Colman JM. Physiological changes in pregnancy. In: Oakley C, Warnes CA, editors. Heart disease in pregnancy: 2nd edition. Malden, Mass; Oxford, UK: Blackwell Pub./BMJ Books; 2007. p. 6-17. https://doi.org/10.1002/9780470994955.ch2.

25. Lapinsky SE, Tram C, Mehta S, et al. Restrictive lung disease in pregnancy. Chest 2014. https://doi.org/10.1378/chest.13-0587.

26. Da Silva EG, De Godoy I, De Oliveira Antunes LC, et al. Respiratory parameters and exercise functional capacity in preeclampsia. Hypertens Pregnancy 2010. https://doi.org/10.3109/10641950902779271.

27. Chesley LC. Plasma and red cell volumes during pregnancy. Am J Obstet Gynecol 1972. https://doi.org/10.1016/0002-9378(72)90493-0.

28. Bremme KA. Haemostatic changes in pregnancy. Best Pract Res Clin Haematol 2003. https://doi.org/10.1016/S1521-6926(03)00021-5.

29. Dresang LT, Fontaine P, Leeman L, et al. Venous thromboembolism during pregnancy. Am Fam Physician 2008. https://doi.org/10.1097/00006254-199701000-00024.

30. Lumbers ER, Pringle KG. Roles of the circulating renin-angiotensin-aldosterone system in human pregnancy. Am J Physiol Regul Integr Comp Physiol 2014. https://doi.org/10.1152/ajpregu.00034.2013.

31. Cheung KL, Lafayette RA. Renal physiology of pregnancy. Adv Chronic Kidney Dis 2013. https://doi.org/10.1053/j.ackd.2013.01.012.

32. Hauspurg A, Ying W, Hubel CA, et al. Adverse pregnancy outcomes and future maternal cardiovascular disease. Clin Cardiol 2018. https://doi.org/10.1002/clc.22887.

33. Herrera E. Lipid metabolism in pregnancy and its consequences in the fetus and newborn. Endocrine 2002. https://doi.org/10.1385/ENDO:19:1:43.

34. Shen H, Liu X, Chen Y, et al. Associations of lipid levels during gestation with hypertensive disorders of pregnancy and gestational diabetes mellitus: a prospective longitudinal cohort study. BMJ Open 2016. https://doi.org/10.1136/bmjopen-2016-013509.

35. Goldberg AC, Hopkins PN, Toth PP, et al. Familial hypercholesterolemia: screening, diagnosis and management of pediatric and adult patients: clinical guidance from the National Lipid Association Expert Panel on Familial Hypercholesterolemia. J Clin Lipidol 2011. https://doi.org/10.1016/j.jacl.2011.03.001.

36. Angueira AR, Ludvik AE, Reddy TE, et al. New insights into gestational glucose metabolism: lessons learned from 21st century approaches. Diabetes 2015. https://doi.org/10.2337/db14-0877.

37. Moyce BL, Dolinsky VW. Maternal β-cell adaptations in pregnancy and placental signalling: implications for gestational diabetes. Int J Mol Sci 2018. https://doi.org/10.3390/ijms19113467.

38. Boyle KE, Hwang H, Janssen RC, et al. Gestational diabetes is characterized by reduced mitochondrial protein expression and altered calcium signaling proteins in skeletal muscle. PLoS One 2014. https://doi.org/10.1371/journal.pone.0106872.

39. Elkayam U, Goland S, Pieper PG, et al. High-risk cardiac disease in pregnancy: Part II. J Am Coll Cardiol 2016. https://doi.org/10.1016/j.jacc.2016.05.050.

40. ACOG practice bulletin No. 202: gestational hypertension and preeclampsia. Obstet Gynecol 2019. https://doi.org/10.1097/AOG.0000000000003018.

41. Thorne S, MacGregor A, Nelson-Piercy C. Risk of contraception and pregnancy in heart disease. Heart 2006. https://doi.org/10.1136/hrt.2006.095240.

42. Stout KK, Daniels CJ, Aboulhosn JA, et al. 2018 AHA/ACC guideline for the management of adults with congenital heart disease: a report of the American College of Cardiology/American Heart Association Task Force on Clinical Practice Guidelines. Circulation 2019. https://doi.org/10.1161/CIR.0000000000000603.

43. Regitz-Zagrosek V, Roos-Hesselink JW, Bauersachs J, et al. 2018 ESC Guidelines for the management of cardiovascular diseases during pregnancy. Eur Heart J 2018. https://doi.org/10.1093/eurheartj/ehy340.

44. Drenthen W, Boersma E, Balci A, et al. Predictors of pregnancy complications in women with congenital heart disease. Eur Heart J 2010. https://doi.org/10.1093/eurheartj/ehq200.

45. Canobbio MM, Warnes CA, Aboulhosn J, et al. Management of pregnancy in patients with complex congenital heart disease: a scientific statement for Healthcare Professionals from the American Heart Association. Circulation 2017. https://doi.org/10.1161/CIR.0000000000000458.

46. Shum KK, Gupta T, Canobbio MM, et al. Family planning and pregnancy management in adults with

congenital heart disease. Prog Cardiovasc Dis 2018. https://doi.org/10.1016/j.pcad.2018.08.001.

47. Burn J, Brennan P, Little J, et al. Recurrence risks in offspring of adults with major heart defects: results from first cohort of British collaborative study. Lancet 1998. https://doi.org/10.1016/S0140-6736(97) 06486-6.

48. Whittemore R, Wells JA, Castellsague X. A second-generation study of 427 probands with congenital heart defects and their 837 children. J Am Coll Cardiol 1994. https://doi.org/10.1016/0735-1097(94) 90392-1.

49. Scott NS. Management of cardiovascular disease during pregnancy. US Cardiol Rev 2018. https://doi.org/10.15420/usc.2018.8.1.

50. Ruys TPE, Roos-Hesselink JW, Pijuan-Domènech A, et al. Is a planned caesarean section in women with cardiac disease beneficial? Heart 2015. https://doi.org/10.1136/heartjnl-2014-306497.

51. Easter SR, Rouse CE, Duarte V, et al. Planned vaginal delivery and cardiovascular morbidity in pregnant women with heart disease. Am J Obstet Gynecol 2020. https://doi.org/10.1016/j.ajog.2019.07.019.

52. ACOG practice bulletin No. 212: pregnancy and heart disease. Obstet Gynecol 2019. https://doi.org/10.1097/AOG.0000000000003243.

53. ACOG committee opinion no. 736: optimizing postpartum care. Obstet Gynecol 2018;131(5): e140–50. https://doi.org/10.1097/AOG.0000000000002633.

54. Arnett DK, Blumenthal RS, Albert MA, et al. 2019 ACC/AHA guideline on the primary prevention of cardiovascular disease: a report of the American College of Cardiology/American Heart Association Task Force on clinical practice guidelines. J Am Coll Cardiol 2019. https://doi.org/10.1016/j.jacc.2019.03.010.

55. Smith GN. The maternal health clinic: improving women's cardiovascular health. Semin Perinatol 2015. https://doi.org/10.1053/j.semperi.2015.05.012.

56. Celi AC, Seely EW, Wang P, et al. Caring for women after hypertensive pregnancies and beyond: implementation and integration of a postpartum transition clinic. Matern Child Health J 2019. https://doi.org/10.1007/s10995-019-02768-7.

57. Hauspurg A, Lemon LS, Quinn BA, et al. A postpartum remote hypertension monitoring protocol implemented at the hospital level. Obstet Gynecol 2019. https://doi.org/10.1097/AOG.0000000000003479.

58. DeNicola N, Grossman D, Marko K, et al. Telehealth interventions to improve obstetric and gynecologic health outcomes: a systematic review. Obstet Gynecol 2020. https://doi.org/10.1097/AOG.0000000000003646.

59. Easter SR, Valente AM, Economy KE. Creating a multidisciplinary pregnancy heart team. Curr Treat Options Cardiovasc Med 2020. https://doi.org/10.1007/s11936-020-0800-x.

60. Brown HL, Warner JJ, Gianos E, et al. Promoting risk identification and reduction of cardiovascular disease in women through collaboration with obstetricians and gynecologists: a presidential advisory from the American Heart Association and the American College of Obstetricians and Gynecologists. Circulation 2018. https://doi.org/10.1161/CIR.0000000000000582.

61. Lundberg GP, Mehta LS, Sanghani RM, et al. Heart centers for women historical perspective on formation and future strategies to reduce cardiovascular disease. Circulation 2018. https://doi.org/10.1161/CIRCULATIONAHA.118.035351.

62. Davis MB, Walsh MN. Cardio-obstetrics. Circ Cardiovasc Qual Outcomes 2019. https://doi.org/10.1161/circoutcomes.118.005417.

63. Mann S, Hollier LM, McKay K, et al. What we can do about maternal mortality, and how to do it quickly. N Engl J Med 2018. https://doi.org/10.1056/NEJMp1810649.

64. Mahoney J. The alliance for innovation in maternal health care: a way forward. Clin Obstet Gynecol 2018. https://doi.org/10.1097/GRF.0000000000000363.

65. Bernstein PS, Martin JN, Barton JR, et al. National partnership for maternal safety. Obstet Gynecol 2017. https://doi.org/10.1097/AOG.0000000000002115.

66. Semrau KEA, Hirschhorn LR, Kodkany B, et al. Effectiveness of the WHO Safe Childbirth Checklist program in reducing severe maternal, fetal, and newborn harm in Uttar Pradesh, India: study protocol for a matched-pair, cluster-randomized controlled trial. Trials 2016. https://doi.org/10.1186/s13063-016-1673-x.

67. Markow C, Main EK. Creating change at scale: quality improvement strategies used by the California maternal quality care collaborative. Obstet Gynecol Clin North Am 2019. https://doi.org/10.1016/j.ogc.2019.01.014.

68. Bernstein PS, Martin JN, Barton JR, et al. Consensus bundle on severe hypertension during pregnancy and the postpartum period. J Midwifery Womens Health 2017. https://doi.org/10.1111/jmwh.12647.

69. D'Alton ME, Friedman AM, Smiley RM, et al. National partnership for maternal safety: consensus bundle on venous thromboembolism. Obstet Gynecol 2016. https://doi.org/10.1097/AOG.0000000000001579.

70. Halperin JL, Williams ES, Fuster V, et al. ACC 2015 core cardiovascular training statement (COCATS 4) (revision of COCATS 3). J Am Coll Cardiol 2015. https://doi.org/10.1016/j.jacc.2015.03.017.

Cardiovascular Testing and Imaging in Pregnant Women

Alina Brener, MD, Joan Briller, MD*

KEYWORDS

- Cardiovascular imaging • Pregnancy • Echocardiography • ECG • MRI • Ionizing radiation
- Cardiac catheterization • Coronary angiography

KEY POINTS

- All women with known cardiac disease, women are at increased risk for underlying cardiac complications, and pregnant women with symptoms that may reflect cardiac decompensation should undergo evaluation of cardiovascular status.
- Physiologic changes that accompany pregnancy affect normal findings during evaluation.
- Echocardiography is the most commonly used modality for evaluation.
- Additional testing with cardiac MRI, computed tomography scan, nuclear testing, and coronary angiography may be required in selected patients.

INTRODUCTION

Cardiovascular diseases (CVD) are leading contributors to increasing maternal morbidity and mortality.[1,2] Older maternal age, social disparities, obesity, and chronic conditions such as diabetes and hypertension are potential driving mechanisms, especially for acquired ischemic disease and cardiomyopathy.[1,2] Increasing numbers of women with congenital heart disease survive to reproductive age and are at risk of pregnancy complications. Emerging countries have different profiles with higher frequencies of rheumatic heart disease, undetected congenital heart defects (HDs), human immunodeficiency virus (HIV)/acquired immunodeficiency syndrome (AIDS), Chagas disease, and sarcoid.[3–5] Maternal morbidity and mortality reviews suggest that many serious pregnancy-associated cardiac complications are preventable and could be reduced with improved health care provider management and earlier recognition.[6–8]

All women with known CVD ideally undergo evaluation before pregnancy, which allows for informed maternal decision making, optimization of maternal and fetal risk, and generation of a multidisciplinary pregnancy heart team.[9] However, many women do not carry a known cardiovascular diagnosis and symptoms of heart failure, chest discomfort, palpitations, or syncope should prompt urgent and thorough evaluation. The California Maternal Quality Care Cooperative has developed a screening algorithm that could prevent most maternal deaths.[10] The American College of Obstetrics and Gynecology now recommends that this tool be used to assess all women during pregnancy and postpartum to assess for cardiac risk.[11] Red flags that should trigger emergent evaluation include shortness of breath at rest, severe orthopnea, resting heart rate greater than 120 beats/min, systolic blood pressure (BP) greater than 160 mm Hg, increased respiratory rate greater than or equal to

Division of Cardiology, University of Illinois at Chicago, 840 South Wood Street (MC 715), Chicago, IL 60612, USA
* Corresponding author.
E-mail address: briller@uic.edu
Twitter: @UICDom (J.B.)

Cardiol Clin 39 (2021) 21–32
https://doi.org/10.1016/j.ccl.2020.09.003

30 breaths/min, and O_2 saturation less than or equal to 94%.[10,11] Other factors should prompt urgent screening even in the absence of known disease or red flags. These factors are shown in **Fig. 1**.

Signs and symptoms of normal pregnancy may overlap with pathologic changes, making differentiation problematic. Moreover, some imaging modalities pose maternal or fetal risk. Interpretation of results may be limited by the structural and anatomic changes that develop across the pregnancy continuum. This article reviews indications, advantages and disadvantages, and risks of various cardiac diagnostic modalities, and the effect of pregnancy on normal findings. These data are summarized in **Table 1**.

BIOMARKERS
Natriuretic Peptides

Indications
Natriuretic peptides (brain natriuretic peptide [BNP] and N-terminal proBNP [NT-ProBNP]) should be measured in the setting of new clinical symptoms compatible with heart failure, at baseline assessment in patients who are high risk of cardiac decompensation based on screening algorithms, and serially to follow women with known disease or at risk of decompensation.

Advantages and disadvantages
Natriuretic peptide levels typically increase during pregnancy and early after delivery but remain within the normal range.[12] Increased levels are reported during pregnancy in both systolic and diastolic heart failure and in hypertensive disorders of pregnancy, including preeclampsia.[13-15] Increasing levels can predict adverse events and normal levels help exclude cardiac decompensation.[15] A limitation is the inverse relationship with body mass index, which may reduce sensitivity in obese gravidas.[16]

Cardiac troponins

Indications
Evaluation of symptoms of chest discomfort suggestive of acute coronary syndrome or other cause of myocardial injury.

Advantages and disadvantages
Troponins are sensitive and specific biomarkers for myocardial injury. However, troponin levels may be increased in some women with preeclampsia and other conditions associated with increased troponin level outside of pregnancy, such as pulmonary embolism and chronic kidney disease.[17,18] Abnormal values should prompt additional investigation.

CARDIAC DIAGNOSTIC TESTING
Electrocardiogram

Indications
Performance of a 12 lead electrocardiogram (ECG) is indicated for women with known or suspected cardiovascular disease.[19]

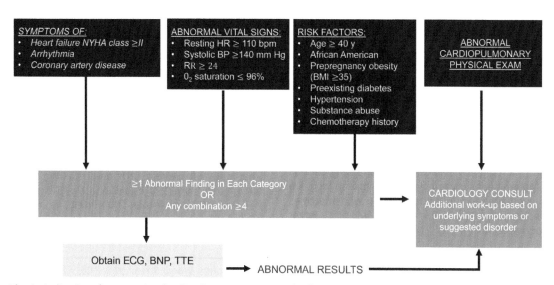

Fig. 1. Indications for screening for CVD in pregnancy. BMI, body mass index; BNP, brain natriuretic peptide; ECG, electrocardiogram; HR, heart rate; NYHA, New York Heart Association; RR, respiration rate; TTE, transthoracic echocardiogram (*Adapted from* ©California Department of Public Health, 2017; supported by Title V funds. Developed in partnership with California Maternal Quality Care Collaborative Cardiovascular Disease in Pregnancy and Postpartum Taskforce. Visit www.CMQCC.org for detail.)

Table 1
Common diagnostic modalities in pregnancy

Diagnostic Test	Information Provided	Advantages	Limitations
ECG	Assessment: • Arrhythmias • Heart blocks • Acute coronary syndrome	• Radiation free • Easily accessible	• Not always sensitive for specific cause • May not be abnormal if performed when asymptomatic
TTE	Assessment: • Ventricular function • Valvular abnormalities • Congenital heart disease • Estimation of cardiac pressures and hemodynamics • Measurement of aorta	• Radiation free • Safe • Easily accessible	• Moderate intraobserver and interobserver variability • Hemodynamic changes during pregnancy affect measurements • Image quality depends on body habitus and acoustic windows
Transesophageal echocardiography	• Used to aid in percutaneous interventions • Evaluation of aortic dissection • Evaluation of prosthetic valve thrombosis	• Radiation free	• Increased risk of aspiration • Requires sedation
Cardiac magnetic resonance	Assessment • Complex structural heart disease • Aortopathies • Aortic dissection • Right ventricular structure and function	• Radiation free • High-resolution images • Less intraobserver and interobserver variability than TTE	• After 20 wk of gestation, patients need to lie in left lateral position because of uterine compression of the IVC, resulting in alterations to cardiac output • Gadolinium avoided during pregnancy
Computer tomography	Assessment: • Anomalous coronary • Spontaneous coronary artery dissection (for follow-up) • Pulmonary embolism	• High-resolution images	• Ionizing radiation exposure

(continued on next page)

Table 1
(continued)

Diagnostic Test	Information Provided	Advantages	Limitations

Stress testing	Indications
	• Chest pain
	• Coronary artery disease
	• Functional capacity
		• Usually performed with echo imaging	• Contraindications:
			  ○ Hemodynamically significant heart disease
			  ○ Incompetent cervix/cerclage
			  ○ Multiple gestation at risk for premature labor
			  ○ Persistent second-trimester or third-trimester bleeding
			  ○ Placenta previa after 26 wk of gestation
			  ○ Premature labor during the current pregnancy
			  ○ Ruptured membranes
			  ○ Preeclampsia-induced /pregnancy-induced hypertension

Coronary angiography	Assessment of acute coronary syndromes Adjunct to percutaneous intervention	• Allows for diagnostic and therapeutic intervention	• Ionizing radiation exposure • Vascular access complications
Ventilation-perfusion scintigraphy	Second line for pulmonary embolism evaluation	• If CT is contraindicated for evaluation of pulmonary embolism	• Usually higher fetal ionization exposure than CTPA

Abbreviations: CTPA, computed tomographic pulmonary angiography; ECG, electrocardiogram; IVC, inferior vena cava; TTE, transthoracic echocardiogram.

Advantages and disadvantages

Electrocardiography is affordable, noninvasive, and readily available. It is an independent marker of myocardial disease reflecting electrophysiologic, anatomic, metabolic, and hemodynamic alterations. However, diagnosis of structural changes, such as myocardial infarction, hypertrophy, valvular heart disease, and congenital heart disease is by inference. The same ECG may be recorded in patients with different underlying disorders and the procedure is not always sensitive for specific disorders.[19,20]

Pregnancy-related findings

Normal pregnancy-associated changes include an increase in heart rate, nonspecific ST and T changes, and prolongation of the QT interval. Heart rate typically increases approximately 10 to 15 beats/min, especially in late pregnancy.[21,22] The absolute value of the QT interval is increased throughout pregnancy compared with nonpregnant controls, but, when corrected for heart rate, typically remains within the normal range ($\leq$460 milliseconds). The QRS axis typically is shifted, most commonly leftward, because of uterine enlargement. Isolated premature ectopic beats are common.[21,23] Significant increases in corrected QT and otherwise unexplained increased heart rates greater than those anticipated should prompt further investigation.[24]

Transthoracic Echocardiography

Indications

Transthoracic echocardiography plays a pivotal role in the evaluation of ventricular function, valvular abnormalities, congenital heart disease, and hemodynamics during pregnancy, with similar indications to those outside of pregnancy.[25] Echocardiography is appropriate for patients with known cardiac disease and commonly plays a role in prepregnancy counseling.[9,11] Serial echocardiography during the pregnancy continuum provides additional information in women at risk of decompensation, especially in cardiomyopathy, aortopathies, and valvular heart disease.[9,26–28] Suggested frequency is shown in **Table 2**. It is frequently used for symptomatic gravidas as an initial screening tool and for women with multiple risk factors for underlying cardiac disease.[11]

Advantages and disadvantages

Transthoracic echocardiography is an affordable, safe, and a convenient tool for evaluation of cardiac hemodynamics, structure, and function.[29] However, technically adequate imaging is more difficult during pregnancy because the heart is more horizontal, the gravida may be more tachypneic, and some imaging planes (such as subcostal views) may be more difficult to obtain. Hemodynamic parameters change throughout pregnancy, resulting in a moving target. Small numbers of patients studied, different patient positioning (lateral vs supine), and use of postpartum values as surrogates for prepartum hemodynamics have resulted in heterogeneity in published findings. Patient results need to be interpreted in the context of each individual case. Use of agitated saline contrast has not been systematically studied but is generally considered safe.[30] Similarly, safety of echo contrast agents such as perflutren lipid microspheres or perflutren protein type A have not been studied during pregnancy but these agents may be used if there is clear maternal benefit.[31]

Pregnancy-related findings

There are substantial changes in preload and afterload with pregnancy. Blood volume increases early in pregnancy and systemic vascular resistance decreases because of the increased capacitance of the uteroplacental bed resulting increased cardiac output.[32,33] Increased cardiac output is attributed to the combination of increased stroke volume and heart rate.[34,35] Reports of changes in ejection fraction are variable, with some studies showing no change and others a small increase or decrease.[36] Interestingly, there might be racial differences in response.[37] Studies addressing myocardial contractility also show conflicting results.[38–40] Most hemodynamic alterations return to baseline by several weeks postpartum.[34]

All cardiac chambers enlarge during both systole and diastole.[37] Increased cardiac chamber dimensions are thought to be caused by cardiac remodeling as a consequence of volume-overload state.[39] Enlargement is accompanied by eccentric hypertrophy.[34,36,41]

Diastolic function also changes in normal pregnancy. The ratio of early diastolic mitral inflow velocity to late diastolic mitral inflow velocity (E/A ratio) is decreased with normal early diastolic mitral inflow velocity (E wave) and reflects increased volume load and heart rate. Early mitral annular velocity ratio (E/e') is typically preserved, suggesting that left ventricular end-diastolic pressure remains normal.[42–45] Melchiorre and colleagues[39] performed echocardiographic analysis in healthy women during pregnancy, finding diastolic abnormalities and impaired myocardial relaxation in 17.9% and 28.4% respectively.

Transvalvular flow velocities increase because of increased heart rate, cardiac output, and volume during pregnancy. Velocity-derived

Table 2
Suggested frequency of transthoracic echocardiography in select diseases during pregnancy

Disease Process	TTE Frequency
Aortic disease associated with: • Marfan syndrome • Ehlers-Danlos syndrome • Loeys-Dietz syndrome • Turner syndrome • Bicuspid aortic valve	• Every trimester in aortic diameter ≤ 40 mm • Every 4–6 wk and 6 mo postpartum if aortic diameter ≥40 mm, progressive dilatation, or a history of aortic surgery for aortic dilatation or dissection
Mitral stenosis	• Mild/moderate: every trimester and before delivery • Severe: 4–8 wk
Aortic stenosis	• Severe: 4–8 wk
Mechanical prosthetic valves	• Up to monthly or with symptom development
Hypertrophic cardiomyopathy	• Every trimester
Recurrent pregnancy with history of peripartum cardiomyopathy	• End of the first and second trimesters, 1 mo before delivery, after delivery before hospital discharge, 1 mo postpartum, and at any time if symptoms develop

Data from Refs.[9,27,28]

measurements (eg, peak and mean gradients) do not correlate as well with degree of valvular stenosis as in the nonpregnant state.[46] However, calculated valve areas can still be used to assess valve severity.[36,46] Mild degrees of valvular regurgitation are common.[47]

Similarly, measurement of pulmonary pressure using the Bernoulli equation is more problematic during pregnancy because this is a flow-derived measure. Estimated pulmonary artery systolic pressure may be overestimated because of increased cardiac output and may require confirmation by right heart catheterization.[48]

Echocardiography may be helpful to risk stratify women with hypertensive disorders of pregnancy. Increased left ventricle (LV) mass and vascular resistance are the most consistent findings, present in both gestational hypertension and preeclampsia.[49] Diastolic abnormalities are exaggerated in preeclampsia and may reflect higher LV filling pressure.[49] Women with early-onset preeclampsia (<34 weeks) have significantly higher E/e' compared with late-onset subgroups.[49]

Myocardial mechanics is an area of interest for future research but currently is not commonly used clinically. Global longitudinal strain and global area strain decrease in later trimesters, which may reflect changes in ventricular sphericity from volume loading returning to baseline postpartum.[34,50] Strain abnormalities have been associated with adverse prognosis in peripartum cardiomyopathy and congenital aortic stenosis.[51,52]

Focused clinician-performed transthoracic echocardiography has proved to be useful in differentiating life-threatening causes of hypotension at the time of delivery.[53]

Transesophageal Echocardiography

Indications
Transesophageal echocardiography (TEE) is indicated as an adjunctive procedure when additional imaging of cardiac structures is required that cannot be obtained with surface transthoracic imaging when it will aid in patient management. Examples include evaluation for endocarditis, prosthetic function, cardiac embolic source, aortic dissection, or before cardiac interventions such as balloon mitral valvuloplasty or percutaneous valve insertion.

Advantages and disadvantages
TEE is considered relatively safe in pregnancy, but sedation increases maternal risk of aspiration and respiratory complications.[54] Agents used for moderate sedation may also enter the fetal circulation.[54] Help from anesthesia colleagues should be considered for airway management, especially later in pregnancy. Fetal monitoring should also be considered once viability is achieved.

Exercise Stress Testing

Indications
Exercise testing is indicated for evaluation of functional status, ischemia, arrhythmias, and prognosis in the setting of heart failure and congenital

heart disease. Estimation of functional capacity is a critical component in assessing pregnancy risk, especially in patients with known disease. It should be considered prepregnancy for risk stratification, may be used during pregnancy in asymptomatic women who present with known disease to assess risk of continuation, and may be helpful for diagnosis of symptoms.[9,31,55]

Advantages and disadvantages

Exercise testing is considered safe in pregnancy.[56–58] Exercise does not seem to be associated with increased risk of miscarriage.[9] Moderate exercise does not affect fetal umbilical artery flow and fetal responses to strenuous exercise seem to be minimal and transient, and seem not to affect fetal outcomes.[56,58,59] However, certain obstetric conditions are contraindications to performing stress testing. These conditions include incompetent cervix or presence of a cerclage, multiple gestation pregnancy at risk for premature labor, second-trimester or third-trimester bleeding, placenta previa, premature labor during the current pregnancy, ruptured membranes, preeclampsia, or uncontrolled pregnancy-induced hypertension.[60] If there is doubt about obstetric safety, discussion with the patient's obstetric provider is warranted.

Imaging modalities improve the sensitivity and specificity of the standard ECG and allow for the visualization of ventricular function.[61] Given the high frequency of ECG changes during pregnancy, the authors typically perform stress testing in conjunction with imaging using the echocardiographic approach to avoid the radiation exposure that would accompany nuclear imaging. Guidelines recommend submaximal exercise testing to 80% of maximum predicted heart rate in asymptomatic patients with known CVD.[9,31] In our stress laboratory, we perform symptom-limited testing using a modified Bruce protocol with a low threshold for discontinuation in women with exertional symptoms. Safety of dobutamine stress echocardiographic testing during pregnancy has not been documented; this is typically avoided.[9,31]

Cardiac Magnetic Resonance

Indications

Cardiac magnetic resonance (CMR) results in high-resolution, ionizing radiation–free images allowing detailed three-dimensional measurements and hemodynamic assessment. CMR-derived data are frequently the gold standard for evaluation of congenital HD, aortopathies, right ventricular function, and tissue characterization with late gadolinium enhancement (LGE) for patients with ischemia, myocarditis, and some cardiomyopathies, such as cardiac sarcoidosis, amyloidosis, and endomyocardial fibrosis. Accordingly, CMR with or without gadolinium, depending on indication, is frequently appropriate for prepregnancy counseling. During pregnancy, CMR without gadolinium (discussed later) is advised when other noninvasive testing does not provide definitive diagnosis and it is preferable to avoid ionizing radiation. Although transthoracic echocardiography is more frequently used for serial assessment during pregnancy, CMR plays an occasional role and may be a substitute for TEE in the assessment of aortic enlargement or dissection.

Advantages and disadvantages

The Cardiac Hemodynamic Imaging and Remodeling in Pregnancy (CHIRP) study compared CMR with transthoracic echocardiogram (TTE) evaluation, finding that CMR results were more accurate, reproducible, and had less intraobserver and interobserver variability.[62] One limitation of CMR use, especially in late pregnancy, is that patients find it difficult to remain still in a narrow tunnel for an extended time period, resulting in motion artifact.[63] Another is that uterine compression of the inferior vena cava after approximately 20 weeks' gestation may affect hemodynamic assessment unless the imaging is performed in the left lateral decubitus position.[64] These changes may be more prominent in women who are of normal weight than in obese women.[64] For women who require serial CMR during pregnancy, imaging should be performed from a consistent position.[65]

CMR imaging is considered safe in pregnancy.[66,67] However, gadolinium-based contrast agents traverse the placental barrier, resulting in possible accumulation in amniotic fluid. This finding has raised concerns of gadolinium deposition in fetal cutaneous tissues (nephrogenic systemic fibrosis) or on the brain surface.[68] The American College of Obstetricians and Gynecologists recommends limiting the use of gadolinium contrast with MRI, unless it significantly improves diagnostic performance and is expected to improve fetal or maternal outcome.[69] If a gadolinium-based agent is required, it is recommended to pick more stable agents, such as gadoteridol, gadobenate dimeglumine, and gadoterate meglumine.[68] Less thermodynamically stable agents such as gadodiamide, gadoversetamide, and gadopentetate should be avoided.[68] Use of superparamagnetic iron oxide contrast agent is currently contraindicated because there are no animal or human fetal studies and no data on use during pregnancy or lactation.[69] There is only minimal gadolinium-based contrast excretion into breast milk, and more minute absorption from the baby's gut, therefore lactation need not be interrupted for use of the modality postpartum.[69]

Pregnancy-related findings

The CHIRP study found general agreement in hemodynamic parameters by CMR and TTE.[62] Stewart and colleagues[70] prospectively studied CMR during pregnancy, showing substantial cardiac remodeling. Increases in LV mass were proportional to maternal size in both normal-weight and overweight women. Changes resolved by 3 months postpartum. A major advantaged of CMR is that it allows a detailed assessment of the right ventricle (RV). The CHIRP study also showed increasing RV mass without changes in RV function.[62] Postpartum CMR imaging in women with peripartum cardiomyopathy with LGE showed that fibrosis was associated with reduced myocardial recovery, but most patients do not have evidence for enhancement.[26]

TESTS THAT USE IONIZING RADIATION

Although it is preferable to avoid unnecessary exposure to ionizing radiation, this should not be a deterrent when a procedure is key to maternal diagnosis or management. Fetal risk from radiation exposure depends on gestational stage and absorbed dose. Risks are greatest during organogenesis but subsequently decrease as the pregnancy progresses. When not emergent, procedures should be delayed until after completion of organogenesis and follow the principle of maintaining exposure as low as reasonably achievable (ALARA).[9,71] To minimize fetal exposure, the maximum recommended acceptable cumulative dose of ionizing radiation in pregnancy is 50 mGy (equivalent to 50 mSv or 5 rad).[72] Many procedures can be performed at an acceptable level of exposure. Comparison of sample radiation exposures with different procedures is shown in **Table 3**.

Computed Tomography

Indications

The most common indication for computed tomography (CT) testing during pregnancy is suspected pulmonary embolism. Recent European guidelines for evaluation of pulmonary embolism in pregnancy and up to 6 weeks postpartum recommend a combination of D-dimer testing, chest radiograph, and compression proximal duplex ultrasonography if symptoms are suggestive of concomitant deep venous thrombosis (DVT).[73] MRI may be a useful adjunct in the setting of suspected pelvic vein thrombosis. If a DVT is not present and chest radiograph is abnormal, the recommendation is to proceed to CT pulmonary artery imaging (computed tomographic pulmonary angiography [CTPA]). If chest radiograph is normal, either CTPA or perfusion lung scan is acceptable.[73]

Additional indications include coronary CT angiography (CCTA) assessment for anomalous coronary artery origin, spontaneous coronary artery dissection (SCAD), and assessment of complex congenital heart disease when CMR is contraindicated. CCTA for evaluation for anomalous coronaries is both highly specific and sensitive.[74]

CCTA is an efficient tool for coronary assessment at low and intermediate risk of acute coronary syndromes outside of pregnancy.[75] Although occasionally used, efficacy has not been confirmed, nor does it exclude acute SCAD. CCTA is generally not recommended in patients with high-risk coronary syndromes as first-line assessment.[75,76] The amount of intravenous contrast dye for CCTA is greater than for diagnostic catheterization and, if subsequent interventions are required, they cannot be performed in the same setting.

Table 3 Estimated maternal and fetal effective radiation doses for various diagnostic techniques		
Procedure	**Maternal Exposure (mGy)**	**Fetal Exposure (mGy)**
Chest radiograph (PA and lateral)	0.1	<0.01
Pulmonary CTA	2–20	0.1–0.66
Low-dose perfusion scintigraphy	0.6–1.0	0.1–0.37
Ventilation-perfusion scintigraphy	1.2–6.8	0.1–0.8
Coronary CTA[a]	18–21	~3
Coronary angiography[a]	7	1.5

Abbreviations: CTA, CT angiography; PA, posteroanterior.
[a] Effective dose depends on the number and the angle of the views.
Data from Colletti PM, Lee KH, Elkayam U. Cardiovascular imaging of the pregnant patient. AJR Am J Roentgenol 2013;200(3):515-21; and Waksmonski CA. Cardiac imaging and functional assessment in pregnancy. Semin Perinatol 2014;38(5):240-4.

Use of CT imaging in pregnancy is predominantly limited by concerns about ionizing radiation. Use of CT and associated contrast agents should not be withheld if clinically indicated, but a discussion about risk and benefits should take place.[29] Fetal radiation dose during CTPE can be as low as 0.1 to 0.4 mSv when performed carefully with dose reduction protocols and results in lower fetal exposure compared with ventilation-perfusion scanning.[29,77–79] Iodinated contrast is not considered teratogenic or carcinogenic, but it does cross the human placenta and may have transient effects on the fetal thyroid.[69] Nursing mothers may continue breastfeeding uninterruptedly after iodinated contrast administration.[29]

Coronary Angiography

Indications
Diagnosis of acute coronary syndromes (ACSs; ST-elevation myocardial infarction, non–ST-elevation myocardial infarction, unstable angina unresponsive to medical therapy) is the primary indication for coronary angiography during pregnancy. In addition, angiography may be used as an adjunct to other percutaneous interventions.

Advantages and disadvantages
The causes of ACSs are more varied during pregnancy. In addition to atherosclerosis, acute coronary dissection (SCAD) and coronary thrombosis are more common causes. Normal coronary vasculature, spasm, and takotsubo causes are also reported.[80] Coronary angiography allows precise determination of causes and early invasive intervention when warranted. Standard dedicated intracoronary methods, including intravascular ultrasonography of optical coherence tomography, are sometimes required to make the diagnosis of SCAD. These techniques are not always available and have additional risks and costs.[76] In the setting of SCAD, this includes increased risk of dissection propagation.[76]

The main risks of angiography are related to vascular access and exposure to ionizing radiation. Historically, transfemoral access has been the mainstay, but the transradial approach is increasingly the access route of choice.[81] Advantages of the radial approach include lesser bleeding risk, earlier ambulation, and decreased vascular complications.[81] For pregnant patients, radiation exposure to the fetus is lower because the fetus in not in the direct x-ray beam. In addition, the patient can be positioned to avoid compression of the vena cava.[82] Exposure to patients with radial approach of ionizing radiation may be higher, but specific techniques can be used to reduce this by using low frame rates,

avoiding angulated projections, simple fluoroscopy rather than cineangiography, and lower magnification.[81,82] Ultimately, choice of vascular access is operator dependent and should depend on operator's expertise.

SUMMARY

Maternal cardiovascular morbidity and mortality reviews suggest that pregnancy-associated cardiac complications are preventable with appropriate evaluation and management. Ideally, this is performed before pregnancy in women with known disease. For women who present during pregnancy, are at significant risk of CVD, or are having symptoms of CVD, this may need to be performed during pregnancy. Twelve-lead electrocardiography, measurement of cardiac biomarkers, and echocardiography are the main standards for assessment for most patients. Additional assessment with more invasive approaches, including CMR, CT, and cardiac catheterization, is required in some patients for full diagnosis and management. These approaches can be performed with acceptable levels of risk and should not be withheld when indicated.

CLINICS CARE POINTS

1. Many pregnancy-associated complications are preventable with improved health care provider management and early recognition. Providers should maintain a high index of suspicion for underlying cardiac decompensation.
2. A broad range of cardiac disease can be diagnosed and managed with non–ionizing radiation–based modalities.
3. Echocardiography remains the mainstay for evaluation but should be supplemented with additional modalities such as CMR, CT testing, and angiography when required.
4. Advances in radiograph imaging technology allow reduced radiation exposure to the fetus, including operator-driven protocols, such as radial access, to ensure the lowest exposure possible (ALARA principle) and improved positioning of pregnant patients. Procedures requiring ionizing radiation should not be withheld when clinically indicated.

DISCLOSURE

Authors have nothing to disclose.

REFERENCES

1. CDC. Severe maternal morbidity in the United States. 2017. Available at: https://www.cdc.gov/

reproductivehealth/maternalinfanthealth/severema
ternalmorbidity.html. Accessed May 10, 2017.

2. CDC. Trends in pregnancy related mortality. Available at: http://www.cdc.gov/reproductivehealth/maternalinfanthealth/pmss.html http://www.cdc.gov/reproductivehealth/maternalinfanthealth/pmss.html. Accessed November 5, 2019.

3. Schlichting LE, Insaf TZ, Zaidi AN, et al. Maternal comorbidities and complications of delivery in pregnant women with congenital heart disease. J Am Coll Cardiol 2019;73(17):2181–91.

4. van Hagen IM, Boersma E, Johnson MR, et al. Global cardiac risk assessment in the registry of pregnancy and cardiac disease: results of a registry from the European Society of Cardiology. Eur J Heart Fail 2016;18(5):523–33.

5. Soma-Pillay P, Seabe J, Sliwa K. The importance of cardiovascular pathology contributing to maternal death: confidential Enquiry into Maternal Deaths in South Africa, 2011-2013. Cardiovasc J Afr 2016; 27(2):60–5.

6. Briller J, Koch AR, Geller SE. Maternal cardiovascular mortality in Illinois, 2002-2011. Obstet Gynecol 2017;129(5):819–26.

7. Report from nine maternal mortality review committees. 2018. Available at: http://reviewtoaction.org/Report_from_Nine_MMRCs. Accessed April 30, 2019.

8. Pfaller B, Sathananthan G, Grewal J, et al. Preventing complications in pregnant women with cardiac disease. J Am Coll Cardiol 2020;75(12):1443–52.

9. Regitz-Zagrosek V, Roos-Hesselink JW, Bauersachs J, et al. 2018 ESC Guidelines for the management of cardiovascular diseases during pregnancy. Eur Heart J 2018;39(34):3165–241.

10. Wolfe DS, Hameed AB, Taub CC, et al. Addressing maternal mortality: the pregnant cardiac patient. Am J Obstet Gynecol 2019;220(2):167.e1-8.

11. ACOG practice bulletin No. 212: pregnancy and heart disease. Obstet Gynecol 2019;133(5): e320–56.

12. Hameed AB, Chan K, Ghamsary M, et al. Longitudinal changes in the B-type natriuretic peptide levels in normal pregnancy and postpartum. Clin Cardiol 2009;32(8):E60–2.

13. Kansal M, Hibbard JU, Briller J. Diastolic function in pregnant patients with cardiac symptoms. Hypertens Pregnancy 2012;31(3):367–74.

14. Resnik JL, Hong C, Resnik R, et al. Evaluation of B-type natriuretic peptide (BNP) levels in normal and preeclamptic women. Am J Obstet Gynecol 2005;193(2):450–4.

15. Kampman MA, Balci A, van Veldhuisen DJ, et al. N-terminal pro-B-type natriuretic peptide predicts cardiovascular complications in pregnant women with congenital heart disease. Eur Heart J 2014;35(11): 708–15.

16. Daniels LB, Clopton P, Bhalla V, et al. How obesity affects the cut-points for B-type natriuretic peptide in the diagnosis of acute heart failure. Results from the Breathing Not Properly Multinational Study. Am Heart J 2006;151(5):999–1005.

17. Ravichandran J, Woon SY, Quek YS, et al. High-sensitivity cardiac troponin I levels in normal and hypertensive pregnancy. Am J Med 2019;132(3): 362–6.

18. Korff S, Katus HA, Giannitsis E. Differential diagnosis of elevated troponins. Heart 2006;92(7): 987–93.

19. Schlant RC, Adolph RJ, DiMarco JP, et al. Guidelines for electrocardiography. A report of the American College of Cardiology/American Heart Association Task Force on assessment of diagnostic and therapeutic cardiovascular procedures (committee on electrocardiography). J Am Coll Cardiol 1992;19(3):473–81.

20. Honigberg MC, Elkayam U, Rajagopalan N, et al. Electrocardiographic findings in peripartum cardiomyopathy. Clin Cardiol 2019;42(5):524–9.

21. Carruth JE, Mivis SB, Brogan DR, et al. The electrocardiogram in normal pregnancy. Am Heart J 1981; 102(6 Pt 1):1075–8.

22. Bett GC. Hormones and sex differences: changes in cardiac electrophysiology with pregnancy. Clin Sci 2016;130(10):747–59.

23. Oram S, Holt M. Innocent depression of the S-T segment and flattening of the T-wave during pregnancy. J Obstet Gynaecol Br Emp 1961;68: 765–70.

24. Tanindi A, Akgun N, Pabuccu EG, et al. Electrocardiographic P-wave duration, QT interval, T peak to end interval and Tp-e/QT ratio in pregnancy with respect to trimesters. Ann Noninvasive Electrocardiol 2016;21(2):169–74.

25. American College of Cardiology Foundation Appropriate Use Criteria Task Force, American Society of Echocardiography, American Heart Association, et al. ACCF/ASE/AHA/ASNC/HFSA/HRS/SCAI/SCCM/SCCT/SCMR 2011 appropriate use criteria for echocardiography. A report of the American College of Cardiology Foundation Appropriate Use Criteria Task Force, American Society of Echocardiography, American Heart Association, American Society of Nuclear Cardiology, Heart Failure Society of America, Heart Rhythm Society, Society for Cardiovascular Angiography and Interventions, Society of Critical Care Medicine, Society of Cardiovascular Computed Tomography, Society for Cardiovascular Magnetic Resonance American College of Chest Physicians. J Am Soc Echocardiogr 2011;24(3): 229–67.

26. Davis MB, Arany Z, McNamara DM, et al. Peripartum cardiomyopathy: JACC state-of-the-art review. J Am Coll Cardiol 2020;75(2):207–21.

27. Elkayam U, Goland S, Pieper PG, et al. High-risk cardiac disease in pregnancy: Part II. J Am Coll Cardiol 2016;68(5):502–16.

28. Pieper PG, Walker F. Pregnancy in women with hypertrophic cardiomyopathy. Neth Heart J 2013; 21(1):14–8.

29. Jain C. ACOG committee opinion No. 723: guidelines for diagnostic imaging during pregnancy and lactation. Obstet Gynecol 2019;133(1):186.

30. Colletti PM, Lee KH, Elkayam U. Cardiovascular imaging of the pregnant patient. AJR Am J Roentgenol 2013;200(3):515–21.

31. Canobbio MM, Warnes CA, Aboulhosn J, et al. Management of pregnancy in patients with complex congenital heart disease: a scientific statement for healthcare professionals from the American Heart Association. Circulation 2017;135(8):e50–87.

32. Lindheimer MD, Katz AI. Sodium and diuretics in pregnancy. N Engl J Med 1973;288(17):891–4.

33. Robson SC, Hunter S, Boys RJ, et al. Serial study of factors influencing changes in cardiac output during human pregnancy. Am J Physiol 1989;256(4 Pt 2): H1060–5.

34. Savu O, Jurcut R, Giusca S, et al. Morphological and functional adaptation of the maternal heart during pregnancy. Circ Cardiovasc Imaging 2012;5(3): 289–97.

35. Desai DK, Moodley J, Naidoo DP. Echocardiographic assessment of cardiovascular hemodynamics in normal pregnancy. Obstet Gynecol 2004;104(1):20–9.

36. Liu S, Elkayam U, Naqvi TZ. Echocardiography in pregnancy: Part 1. Curr Cardiol Rep 2016;18(9):92.

37. Adeyeye VO, Balogun MO, Adebayo RA, et al. Echocardiographic assessment of cardiac changes during normal pregnancy among Nigerians. Clin Med Insights Cardiol 2016;10:157–62.

38. Bamfo JE, Kametas NA, Nicolaides KH, et al. Maternal left ventricular diastolic and systolic long-axis function during normal pregnancy. Eur J Echocardiogr 2007;8(5):360–8.

39. Melchiorre K, Sharma R, Khalil A, et al. Maternal cardiovascular function in normal pregnancy: evidence of maladaptation to chronic volume overload. Hypertension 2016;67(4):754–62.

40. Estensen ME, Beitnes JO, Grindheim G, et al. Altered maternal left ventricular contractility and function during normal pregnancy. Ultrasound Obstet Gynecol 2013;41(6):659–66.

41. Cong J, Fan T, Yang X, et al. Maternal cardiac remodeling and dysfunction in preeclampsia: a three-dimensional speckle-tracking echocardiography study. Int J Cardiovasc Imaging 2015;31(7):1361–8.

42. Fok WY, Chan LY, Wong JT, et al. Left ventricular diastolic function during normal pregnancy: assessment by spectral tissue Doppler imaging. Ultrasound Obstet Gynecol 2006;28(6):789–93.

43. Mesa A, Jessurun C, Hernandez A, et al. Left ventricular diastolic function in normal human pregnancy. Circulation 1999;99(4):511–7.

44. Kametas NA, McAuliffe F, Hancock J, et al. Maternal left ventricular mass and diastolic function during pregnancy. Ultrasound Obstet Gynecol 2001;18(5): 460–6.

45. Valensise H, Novelli GP, Vasapollo B, et al. Maternal cardiac systolic and diastolic function: relationship with uteroplacental resistances. A Doppler and echocardiographic longitudinal study. Ultrasound Obstet Gynecol 2000;15(6):487–97.

46. Campos O. Doppler echocardiography during pregnancy: physiological and abnormal findings. Echocardiography 1996;13(2):135–46.

47. Campos O, Andrade JL, Bocanegra J, et al. Physiologic multivalvular regurgitation during pregnancy: a longitudinal Doppler echocardiographic study. Int J Cardiol 1993;40(3):265–72.

48. Penning S, Robinson KD, Major CA, et al. A comparison of echocardiography and pulmonary artery catheterization for evaluation of pulmonary artery pressures in pregnant patients with suspected pulmonary hypertension. Am J Obstet Gynecol 2001;184(7):1568–70.

49. Castleman JS, Ganapathy R, Taki F, et al. Echocardiographic structure and function in hypertensive disorders of pregnancy: a systematic review. Circ Cardiovasc Imaging 2016;9(9):e004888.

50. Cong J, Fan T, Yang X, et al. Structural and functional changes in maternal left ventricle during pregnancy: a three-dimensional speckle-tracking echocardiography study. Cardiovasc Ultrasound 2015;13:6.

51. Sugahara M, Kagiyama N, Hasselberg NE, et al. Global left ventricular strain at presentation is associated with subsequent recovery in patients with peripartum cardiomyopathy. J Am Soc Echocardiogr 2019;32(12):1565–73.

52. Tzemos N, Silversides CK, Carasso S, et al. Effect of pregnancy on left ventricular motion (twist) in women with aortic stenosis. Am J Cardiol 2008;101(6):870–3.

53. Dennis AT. Transthoracic echocardiography in obstetric anaesthesia and obstetric critical illness. Int J Obstet Anesth 2011;20(2):160–8.

54. Neuman G, Koren G. Safety of procedural sedation in pregnancy. J Obstet Gynaecol Can 2013;35(2): 168–73.

55. Fett JD, Fristoe KL, Welsh SN. Risk of heart failure relapse in subsequent pregnancy among peripartum cardiomyopathy mothers. Int J Gynaecol Obstet 2010;109(1):34–6.

56. MacPhail A, Davies GA, Victory R, et al. Maximal exercise testing in late gestation: fetal responses. Obstet Gynecol 2000;96(4):565–70.

57. Heenan AP, Wolfe LA, Davies GA. Maximal exercise testing in late gestation: maternal responses. Obstet Gynecol 2001;97(1):127–34.

58. Szymanski LM, Satin AJ. Exercise during pregnancy: fetal responses to current public health guidelines. Obstet Gynecol 2012;119(3):603–10.

59. Szymanski LM, Satin AJ. Strenuous exercise during pregnancy: is there a limit? Am J Obstet Gynecol 2012;207(3):179.e1–179.e6.

60. Franklin BA, Whaley MH, Howley ET, et al. ACSM's guidelines for exercise testing and prescription. Sixth edition. Philadelphia: Lippincott Williams & Wilkins; 2000.

61. Myers J, Arena R, Franklin B, et al. Recommendations for clinical exercise laboratories: a scientific statement from the american heart association. Circulation 2009;119(24):3144–61.

62. Ducas RA, Elliott JE, Melnyk SF, et al. Cardiovascular magnetic resonance in pregnancy: insights from the cardiac hemodynamic imaging and remodeling in pregnancy (CHIRP) study. J Cardiovasc Magn Reson 2014;16:1.

63. Bijl RC, Valensise H, Novelli GP, et al. Methods and considerations concerning cardiac output measurement in pregnant women: recommendations of the International Working Group on Maternal Hemodynamics. Ultrasound Obstet Gynecol 2019;54(1): 35–50.

64. Nelson DB, Stewart RD, Matulevicius SA, et al. The effects of maternal position and habitus on maternal cardiovascular parameters as measured by cardiac magnetic resonance. Am J Perinatol 2015;32(14): 1318–23.

65. Rossi A, Cornette J, Johnson MR, et al. Quantitative cardiovascular magnetic resonance in pregnant women: cross-sectional analysis of physiological parameters throughout pregnancy and the impact of the supine position. J Cardiovasc Magn Reson 2011;13:31.

66. ACOG Committee Opinion #299: Guidelines for Diagnostic Imaging During Pregnancy. Obstet Gynecol 2004;104(3):647. Available at: http://ovidsp.ovid.com/ovidweb.cgi?T=JS&PAGE=reference&D=ovftg&NEWS=N&AN=00006250-200409000-00053. Accessed October 26, 2020.

67. Kanal E, Barkovich AJ, Bell C, et al. ACR guidance document for safe MR practices: 2007. AJR Am J Roentgenol 2007;188(6):1447–74.

68. Elkayam U. Cardiac problems in pregnancy. fourth edition. John Wiley & Sons; 2019.

69. Committee on Obstetric P. Committee opinion No. 723: guidelines for diagnostic imaging during pregnancy and lactation. Obstet Gynecol 2017;130(4): e210–6.

70. Stewart RD, Nelson DB, Matulevicius SA, et al. Cardiac magnetic resonance imaging to assess the impact of maternal habitus on cardiac remodeling during pregnancy. Am J Obstet Gynecol 2016; 214(5):640.e1–640.e6.

71. Waksmonski CA. Cardiac imaging and functional assessment in pregnancy. Semin Perinatol 2014; 38(5):240–4.

72. Brent RL. The effect of embryonic and fetal exposure to x-ray, microwaves, and ultrasound: counseling the pregnant and nonpregnant patient about these risks. Semin Oncol 1989;16(5):347–68.

73. Konstantinides SV, Meyer G, Becattini C, et al. 2019 ESC Guidelines for the diagnosis and management of acute pulmonary embolism developed in collaboration with the European Respiratory Society (ERS). Eur Heart J 2020;41(4):543–603.

74. Budoff MJ, Ahmed V, Gul KM, et al. Coronary anomalies by cardiac computed tomographic angiography. Clin Cardiol 2006;29(11):489–93.

75. Rybicki FJ, Udelson JE, Peacock WF, et al. 2015 ACR/ACC/AHA/AATS/ACEP/ASNC/NASCI/SAEM/SCCT/SCMR/SCPC/SNMMI/STR/STS appropriate utilization of cardiovascular imaging in Emergency Department patients with chest pain: a joint document of the American College of Radiology Appropriateness Criteria Committee and the American College of Cardiology appropriate use criteria task force. J Am Coll Cardiol 2016;67(7):853–79.

76. Hayes SN, Kim ESH, Saw J, et al. Spontaneous coronary artery dissection: current state of the science: a scientific statement from the American heart Association. Circulation 2018;137(19):e523–57.

77. Winer-Muram HT, Boone JM, Brown HL, et al. Pulmonary embolism in pregnant patients: fetal radiation dose with helical CT. Radiology 2002;224(2):487–92.

78. Pierce T, Hovnanian M, Hedgire S, et al. Imaging of cardiovascular disease in pregnancy and the peripartum period. Curr Treat Options Cardiovasc Med 2017;19(12):94.

79. Patel SJ, Reede DL, Katz DS, et al. Imaging the pregnant patient for nonobstetric conditions: algorithms and radiation dose considerations. Radiographics 2007;27(6):1705–22.

80. Elkayam U, Jalnapurkar S, Barakkat MN, et al. Pregnancy-associated acute myocardial infarction: a review of contemporary experience in 150 cases between 2006 and 2011. Circulation 2014;129(16): 1695–702.

81. Mason PJ, Shah B, Tamis-Holland JE, et al. An update on radial artery access and best practices for transradial coronary angiography and intervention in acute coronary syndrome: a scientific statement from the American Heart Association. Circ Cardiovasc Interv 2018;11(9):e000035.

82. Vidovich MI, Gilchrist IC. Minimizing radiological exposure to pregnant women from invasive procedures. Interv Cardiol 2013;5:345–57.

Cardiovascular Medications in Pregnancy
A Primer

Karen L. Florio, DO[a,b,*], Christopher DeZorzi, MD[b,c], Emily Williams, MD[b], Kathleen Swearingen, MSN, APRN, FNP-C[a], Anthony Magalski, MD, FHFSA[b,c]

KEYWORDS

- Cardio-obstetrics • Cardiac medications • Pregnancy • Medication safety
- Heart disease in pregnancy

KEY POINTS

- Pregnancy induces dramatic physiologic and anatomic changes in the cardiovascular system beginning in the first trimester and continuing through the postpartum period.
- Maternal cardiac arrhythmias during pregnancy are a common occurrence and treatment should be considered from both obstetric and electrophysiologic standpoints.
- Anticoagulation and antiplatelet medications are prescribed commonly in both cardiology and obstetrics for various reasons.

INTRODUCTION

Cardiovascular disease and its related disorders are the leading causes of maternal morbidity and mortality in the United States.[1,2] The increasing age at first pregnancy coupled with the rising rates of obesity likely contribute to this trend. More women are desiring delayed fertility, which results in higher rates of hypertensive disorders during gestation.[3] Increases in women with repaired congenital cardiovascular disease becoming pregnant also add to this patient population. As a result, the use of cardiovascular medications during pregnancy also is increasing. It has been reported that up to 94% of women take at least 1 medication while pregnant and approximately 70% are taking medication during fetal organogenesis.[4] The ROPAC trial reported as many as 28% of women with underlying cardiovascular conditions were taking medication, a number that is likely higher in the United States because the burden of disease is significantly greater.[5] As

such, clinicians need to have a breadth of fundamental knowledge regarding the safety profiles of medication use during pregnancy. Many different factors need to be balanced when deciding on medications during pregnancy, including gestational age, reported teratogenicity, placental transport, altered pharmacokinetics, route of administration, and dosing. Safety profiles are limited because reports of teratogenic effects are from observational trials or registries due to the ethical dilemma of research on this vulnerable population.[4] The purpose of this review is to guide clinical decisions for both obstetricians and cardiologists when confronted with a pregnant woman affected by cardiovascular disease requiring treatment. This is not meant to be an all-encompassing review of every medication utilized during pregnancy but rather an overview of the more commonly used cardiovascular medications (**Table 1**) from preconception through postpartum and lactation.

[a] Heart Disease in Pregnancy Program, Saint Luke's Hospital of Kansas City, 4401 Wornall Road PEET Center, Kansas City, MO 64111, USA; [b] University of Missouri-Kansas City School of Medicine, 4401 Wornall Road PEET Center, Kansas City, MO 64111, USA; [c] Saint Luke's Mid America Heart Institute, Kansas City, MO, USA
* Corresponding author. Heart Disease in Pregnancy Program, Saint Luke's Hospital of Kansas City, 4401 Wornall Road PEET Center, Kansas City, MO 64111.
E-mail address: kflorio@saint-lukes.org

Cardiol Clin 39 (2021) 33–54
https://doi.org/10.1016/j.ccl.2020.09.011

Table 1
Classification of cardiac medications used during pregnancy

Drug	Mechanism of Action	Onset of Action	Metabolism	Side Effects	Teratogenicity	Lactation/ Breastfeeding
Abciximab	Monoclonal antibody, binds to glycoprotein IIb/IIIa, inhibits platelet aggregation	Half-life: 30 min Onset: 10 min	Opsonization by way of reticuloendothelial system (when bound to platelets)	Bleeding, chest pain, hypotension, nausea, vomiting, abdominal pain, thrombocytopenia, anaphylaxis	No mutagenicity in animal models; limited human data without evidence of teratogenicity; crosses placenta	No reports of use in literature; unlikely crosses into breast milk (large molecule)
Acebutolol	Cardioselective β_1-blockade	Half-life: 3–4 h	Extensive first-pass metabolism	Bronchospasm, bradycardia, heart block, fatigue, dizziness, diarrhea, nausea, vomiting	No increased teratogenicity, some reports of neonatal hypotension	AAP recommends giving "with caution." plasma ratio in milk higher than other β-blockers
Adenosine	Slows AV node conduction, activation of cell-surface A_1 and A_2 adenosine receptors	Half-life: 10 s	Phosphorylation intracellularly to adenosine monophosphate	Flushing, dyspnea, chest discomfort, headaches, nausea	No reported teratogenicity (rapid degradation by placenta); no effect on fetal heart rate	Paucity of data—likely safe due to short half life
Alteplase	Binds to fibrin and converts plasminogen to plasmin	Half-life: initial 5 min with terminal half-life of 72 min	Hepatic metabolism	Hemorrhage, angioedema, anaphylaxis, fever	No mutagenicity in animal models (minimal placental passage)	No data available
Amiloride	Potassium-sparing diuretic, inhibits sodium absorption in the renal tubules	Half-life: 6–9 h	Excreted unchanged in kidneys	Headache, weakness, nausea, vomiting, muscle cramps, hyperkalemia, aplastic anemia, neutropenia	No mutagenicity in animal models. Limited human data (1 case report with skeletal anomalies)	No data available

Drug	Mechanism	Half-life	Metabolism	Side effects	Fetal/pregnancy effects	Breastfeeding
Amiod-arone	Benzofuran derivative; relaxes vascular smooth muscle; acts as an antiarrhythmic (prolongs QRS and QT intervals)	Half-life: depends on patient but varies from 15–142 d (active metabolite 14–75 d) Plasma half-life 3.2–79.7 h.	CYP34 A and CYP2C8 in liver	Nausea, vomiting, visual disturbances, hypothyroidism, skin discoloration, AV block, QT prolongation	Fetal goiter, fetal thyroid dysfunction, possible association with IUGR, congenital heart defects, neurodevelopmental delay; crosses term placenta in higher concentration than maternal serum	Avoid use during breastfeeding
Amlod-ipine	Calcium channel blocker: blocks calcium entry into cells causing smooth muscle relaxation	Half-life: 30–50 h	90% metabolized in liver, 10% excreted unchanged in urine	Peripheral edema, fatigue, palpitations, flushing, nausea, hypotension	No mutagenicity in animal models; limited human data but small case series with increased fetal loss and limb defects	Limited data—probably compatible
Argat-roban	Inhibits thrombin-catalyzed or induced reactions; activates factors V, VIII, and XIII; enhances platelet aggregation	39–51 min	Hydroxylation and aromatization in the liver	Chest pain, hypotension, cough, hypersensitivity reaction, fever, ventricular arrhythmias, bleeding, bradycardia	Minimal animal data (no teratogenic effects at dose 0.3× human doses); minimal human data available (likely maternal benefit outweighs fetal toxicity)	No data available
Aspirin	Blocks prostaglandin synthesis (nonselective COX-1 and COX-2 inhibitor)	13–19 min	Hydrolyzed in plasma to salicylic acid, metabolized in liver	Bleeding, dyspepsia, vomiting, thrombocytopenia, nausea	At large doses, teratogenic to animal models; no increased risk of human teratogenesis with normal dosing	WHO Working Group on Human Lactation classified as unsafe

(continued on next page)

Table 1
(continued)

Drug	Mechanism of Action	Onset of Action	Metabolism	Side Effects	Teratogenicity	Lactation/ Breastfeeding
Atenolol	Cardioselective β_1-blockade	6–7 h	Minimal metabolism in liver, most is excreted unchanged in the urine	Bradycardia, hypotension, bronchospasm, diarrhea, fatigue, nausea, SLE-like reaction	Decreased fetal weight in animal models; crosses placenta, not associated with birth defects but with FGR	Excreted in breast milk in higher amounts than maternal plasma, WHO recommends caution with breastfeeding
Carvedilol	Combined α_1/β-adrenergic blocker	7–10 h	Hydroxylated by CYP system in liver; also undergoes glucuronidation; 98% protein bound	Bradycardia, hyperglycemia, nausea, headache, BUN elevation, AST/ALT elevation, pulmonary edema	Animal models with decreased fetal weight and pregnancy loss; no increased teratogenicity but increase neonatal hypoglycemia	Limited human data—probably compatible
Cholesty-ramine	Forms resin that acts as a bile acid sequestrant and limits absorption of bile	6 min	No modification or absorption in gut, excreted bound to bile acids	Constipation, flatulence, nausea, vomiting, steatorrhea	No mutagenicity in animal models; no fetal teratogenicity but some cases of abnormal fetal heart tracings and meconium	Limited human data—probably compatible
Clonidine	α_2-Adrenergic agonist	6–23 h	Hydroxylation by CYP enzymes in liver (but is poorly understood)	Somnolence, headaches, nightmares, emotional lability, hypotension, reflex HTN with withdrawal	No mutagenicity in therapeutic doses in animal models, increased fetal loss in higher doses in animal models; some case reports of teratogenicity with first trimester use	Excreted in breast milk in higher concentrations than maternal plasma; neonatal hypotension. Likely compatible

Clopidogrel	Platelet inhibitor that binds to P2Y$_{12}$ADP receptors on platelets preventing aggregation	6 h; active metabolite is 30 min	85%–90% metabolized by liver by CYP system	Bleeding, pruritis, agranulocytosis, pancytopenia	No mutagenicity in animal models; limited human data with 1 report of PFO (likely compatible)	Limited data but likely compatible
Dalteparin	Potentiates activity of ATIII, inhibiting factor Xa and thrombin	IV: half-life 2 h Subcutaneous: 3–5 h	Liver and reticuloendothelial system biotransformation (disulphation and depolymerization)	Bleeding, thrombocytopenia, hematuria, ALT/AST elevation, rash, pruritis	No mutagenicity in animal models; no increased teratogenicity in human fetuses	Not transferred in breast milk; compatible
Diltiazem	Calcium channel blocker: blocks calcium entry into cells causing smooth muscle relaxation	Immediate release: 3–4.5 h Delayed-release: 6–9 h	Extensive first-pass metabolism in CYP3A4 system	Headaches, dizziness, hypotension, bradycardia, first-degree AV block, AST/ALT elevations, syncope	Increase in limb and tail malformations in animal models; small increase in fetal loss in first trimester in humans, no increase in birth defects	Limited human data—likely compatible
Digoxin	Hemodynamic, electrophysiologic and neurohormonal effects; stimulates parasympathetic nervous system via vagus nerve, reversibly inhibits sodium-potassium ATPase enzyme	1.5–2 d	Only approximately 13% is metabolized (skeletal muscle), 25% protein bound	Dizziness, headaches, nausea, vomiting, anorexia, bradycardia, palpitations, gynecomastia, depression, AV block, delirium	No mutagenicity in animal models; no increased risk of birth defects when used in first trimester (utilized in pregnancy for fetal SVT)	AAP classifies as compatible with breastfeeding
Enoxaparin	Inhibition of factor Xa, binds to and accelerates ATIII	4.5 h	Desulphation and polymerization in liver; 80% protein bound	Hemorrhage, fever, ALT/AST elevations, nausea, thrombocytopenia, osteoporosis (long-term use)	No mutagenicity in animal models; does not cross human placenta, no increased fetal risks	Compatible

(continued on next page)

Table 1
(continued)

Drug	Mechanism of Action	Onset of Action	Metabolism	Side Effects	Teratogenicity	Lactation/ Breastfeeding
Enalapril	RAAS activated angiotensin II enzyme inhibitor	11–14 h	Hydrolyzed by de-esterification by hepatic enzymes; <50% protein bound	Dizziness, hypotension, fatigue, cough, hyperkalemia, Cr elevations, photosensitivity, angioedema, neutropenia	No mutagenicity in animal models with doses much higher than used in humans, some studies with fetal wastage and nephrotoxicity; human data suggests outcomes similar to lisinopril	Compatible
Esmolol	Cardioselective β_1-blockade	2 min	Rapid hydrolysis of ester linkage in RBCs; 55% protein bound	Hypotension, nausea, dizziness, somnolence, agitation, headaches, bradycardia	No mutagenicity in animal models; no increased risk of human birth defects but neonatal effects include apnea and hypoglycemia	Limited human data—probably compatible
Ezetimibe	Selectively inhibits absorption of cholesterol and phytosterol (targets Niemann-Pick C1-like protein)	22 h	Rapidly and extensively metabolized by phase II glucuronidation in liver	Upper respiratory infections, diarrhea, myalgias, fatigue, back pain, hypersensitivity, hepatitis	No mutagenicity at therapeutic dosing (associated with skeletal changes at doses $10\times$ human dose) in animal models; no human data	No human data—animal models suggest risk
Flecainide	Blocks fast inward sodium channels, shortens action potential of Purkinje fibers	13 h	Metabolized by CYP2D6 and CYP1A2 in liver	Dizziness, headaches, fatigue, palpitations, chest pain, tremors, abdominal pain, dyspnea, heart block, QT prolongation	In high-dose models, increased clubbed feet and skeletal defects; no increased teratogenicity in humans but in neonates, increased bilirubin and abnormal EKGs	Limited human data—probably compatible

Drug	Mechanism	Half-life	Metabolism	Adverse effects	Pregnancy data	Lactation
Fondaparinux	ATIII-mediated selective inhibition of factor Xa	17–21 h	Not metabolized, 94% protein bound	Bleeding, AST/ALT elevations, anemia	No mutagenicity in animal models; does not cross placenta (1 case report documenting neonatal exposure), no teratogenicity	No human data—probably compatible
Furosemide	Blocks tubular absorption of sodium and chloride in proximal and distal tubules	4–4.5 h	Kidneys clear 85%, 40% biotransformation in the liver	Hypokalemia, AST/ALT elevation, hyperuricemia, hyperglycemia, hypotension, muscle cramps, weakness, metabolic acidosis, ototoxicity	Skeletal anomalies in animal models in high doses; can cross the human placenta and increase fetal urine production, possible increase in PDA, neonatal sensorineural hearing loss	Limited human data—probably compatible
Gemfibrozil	Activates peroxisome proliferator-activated receptors, which alter lipid metabolism	1.5 h	Hydroxylation at the 5′methyl and 4′ positions in the CYP2C8 enzymatic system	Dyspepsia, abdominal pain, diarrhea, nausea, vomiting, AST/ALT elevations	No mutagenicity in animal models; limited human data, some case reports of brain and facial defects	No human data—potential toxicity
Heparin	Inhibition of factor Xa	1.5 h	Biotransformation in the liver and reticuloendothelial system	Bleeding, thrombocytopenia, prolonged clotting time, fever, AST/ALT elevations, HIT	No mutagenicity in animal models; does not cross human placenta	Compatible
Hydrochlorothiazide	Inhibits sodium and chloride in proximal renal tubules and reduces absorption of water	5.6–14.8 h	Not metabolized	Electrolyte imbalances, hypercalcemia, dizziness, anorexia, muscle cramps	No mutagenicity in animal models; no increase teratogenicity but associated with neonatal thrombocytopenia, bleeding, electrolyte imbalances	Compatible (may decrease milk production in first month)

(continued on next page)

Table 1
(continued)

Drug	Mechanism of Action	Onset of Action	Metabolism	Side Effects	Teratogenicity	Lactation/ Breastfeeding
Hydralazine	Interferes with calcium transport, also competes with protocollagen prolyl hydroxylase (preventing degradation of HIF-α1)	2.2–7.8 h	Hydroxylation and glucuronidation in liver	Headache, hypotension, palpitations, nausea, vomiting, diarrhea, neutropenia, lupus-like reaction	Abnormal embryo development in animal models likely due to uteroplacental hypoperfusion; no reports of teratogenicity in limited human data	Limited human data— probably compatible
Labetalol	Nonselectively antagonizes β_1/β_2-receptors, α_1-agonist	1.7–.1 h	Metabolized to glucuronide metabolites in liver	Hypotension, dizziness, headaches, fatigue, edema, BUN/Cr elevation, bronchospasm, Raynaud disease, bradycardia, syncope	No mutagenicity in animal models but decreased birth weights; some reports associated with hypospadias, low birth weight	Limited human data— probably compatible
Lisinopril	Angiotensin II enzyme inhibitor	12.6 h	Excreted unchanged in the urine; no protein binding	Dizziness, hypotension, Cr elevations, cough, fatigue, photosensitivity, angioedema, neutropenia	Abnormal/birth defects in animal models; human data in first trimester limited to conclude teratogenicity but does increased risk of malformations and death in second/third trimester	Not compatible
Methyl-ldopa	Stimulates central inhibitory α-adrenergic receptors	105 min	Extensively metabolized in the liver	Sedation, angina, weakness, bradycardia, diarrhea, vomiting, myocarditis, hypotension	No mutagenicity in animal models; single study in humans showing malformations	Compatible

Drug	Mechanism	Half-life	Metabolism	Adverse effects	Studies	Compatibility
Metoprolol	β_1-adrenergic receptor inhibitor	3–7 h	Extensive first pass metabolism through CYP2D6 enzymatic system	Bradycardia, influenza-like symptoms, fatigue, headache, rash, hyperuricemia, sleep disturbances, heart block	No mutagenicity in animal models; some small case studies with fetal malformations, associated with low birth weight	Compatible
Milrinone	Inhibits erythrocyte phosphodiesterase in myocardium and vascular smooth muscle, leading to increased cAMP in red cells	2.3 h	O-glucuronidation in liver, 80% protein bound	Ventricular arrhythmias, ectopy, tachycardia, hypotension, headache, anaphylaxis	No mutagenicity in animal studies; no teratogenicity in human studies	No human data— probably compatible
Nadolol	Nonselective β-adrenergic blocker	20–24 h	Excreted unchanged in the kidney	Bradycardia, fatigue, dizziness, nausea, vomiting, constipation, Raynaud disease, bronchospasm	No mutagenicity in animal studies; no increased risk of teratogenicity but is associated with low birth weight	Compatible
Nicardipine	Calcium channel blocker: blocks calcium entry into cells causing smooth muscle relaxation	8.6 h	Metabolized extensively in liver; 95% protein bound	Headache, dizziness, hypotension, nausea, vomiting, tachycardia, palpitations	May interfere with embryo development in small animal studies; no increased teratogenicity in small studies	Probably compatible
Nifedipine	Inhibits L-type voltage-gated calcium channels	2 h	Metabolized by CYP3A4 enzymatic system in liver; 92%–98% protein bound	Headaches, fatigue, nausea, flushing, vomiting, palpitations, hypotension, bradycardia	May interfere with embryo development in small animal studies; no increased teratogenicity in small studies	Compatible

(continued on next page)

Table 1
(continued)

Drug	Mechanism of Action	Onset of Action	Metabolism	Side Effects	Teratogenicity	Lactation/ Breastfeeding
Propafenone	Class 1C antiarrhythmic (reduction in upstroke of action potential); reduces fast inward sodium ions	2–10 h	Extensively metabolized in liver; 97% protein bound	Dizziness, nausea, edema, taste changes, vomiting, blurred vision, ecchymosis, ventricular arrhythmias, QT prolongation	Embryotoxic in animals at doses 3–6× maximum human dose; limited human data but appears to have no increased teratogenicity, is associated in small case series with fetal loss	Limited human data— probably compatible
Propranolol	Nonselective β-adrenergic antagonist	8 h	Side chain oxidation (to metabolites) or glucuronidation in liver; 85%–96% protein bound	Fatigue, dizziness, bradycardia, hypotension, nausea, vomiting, purpura, disorientation, depression, heart block	No mutagenicity in animal models; no increased teratogenicity but is associated with decreased birth weights	Compatible
Rivaroxaban	Inhibits factor Xa	5–9 h	Metabolized by CYP enzymatic system in liver; 92%–95% protein bound	Bleeding, back pain, pruritis, dizziness, thrombocytopenia, agranulocytosis	No mutagenicity in animal models; minimal human data with only 1 case report of teratogenicity, does cross placenta and cause neonatal bleeding risk	Limited human data— caution recommended
Spirono-lactone	Inhibits aldosterone-dependent sodium exchange channels in distal convoluted tubules	1.4 h	Deacetylation and excretion in the urine; >90% protein bound	Electrolyte imbalances, nausea, vomiting, dizziness, lethargy, menstrual irregularities, GI bleeding, gastritis, gynecomastia	Antiandrogenic effect in animal data with adverse effects on male genitalia, this was not seen in human data, some case reports with ambiguous genitalia	Compatible

Drug	Class/Mechanism	Half-life	Metabolism	Side effects	Animal/teratogenicity data	Breastfeeding
Sotalol	β_1-adrenergic antagonist, rapid potassium channel inhibitor	10–20 h	Not metabolized and not protein bound	Fatigue, dizziness, bradycardia, palpitations, headaches, insomnia, heart block, QT prolongation	No mutagenicity in animal models but 1 case of fetal death secondary to arrhythmia; no teratogenicity	Considered unsafe (excreted in breast milk in large quantities)
Timolol	β_1/β_2-adrenergic antagonist	2.9 h	Metabolized by P450 2D6 system in liver; 10% protein bound	Bradycardia, fatigue, dizziness, nightmares, headaches, heart block, ocular irritation	No mutagenicity in animal models; no teratogenicity but is associated with low birth weight	Compatible
Verapamil	Calcium channel blocker: blocks calcium entry into cells causing smooth muscle relaxation	2.8–7.4 h	Extensively metabolized by P450 system in liver	Dizziness, nausea, hypotension, headaches, fatigue, hypotension, bradycardia, hepatotoxicity	Possible cardiac and CNS malformations in animal models; some case reports of teratogenicity and is associated with low birth weight	Compatible
Warfarin	VKA	37–89 h	Oxidation in liver by CYP system, limited conjugation	Bleeding, ecchymosis, abdominal pain, lethargy, taste changes, paresthesia, skin necrosis, calciphylaxis	Mutagenicity in animal models; associated with structural malformations in dose-dependent manner in human data, neonatal bleeding	Compatible

Abbreviations: AAP, American Academy of Pediatrics; ALT, alanine aminotransferase; AST, aspartate aminotransferase; ATIII, antithrombin III deficiency; AV, atrioventricular; BUN, blood urea nitrogen; cAMP, cyclic adenosine monophosphate; CNS, central nervous system; COX, cyclo-oxygenase; CR, creatinine; CYP, cytochrome P450; GI, gastrointestinal; HIF, hypoxia-inducible factor; HIT, heparin-induced thrombocytopenia; HTN, hypertension; IUGR, intrauterine growth restriction; PDA, patent ductus arteriosus; P2Y12ADP, chemo receptor for adenine diphosphate; PFO, patent foramen ovale; RAAS, renin angiotensin system; RBC, red blood cell; SLE, systemic lupus; WHO, World Health Organization.

PHYSIOLOGIC CHANGES IN PREGNANCY
Cardiovascular Changes

Pregnancy induces dramatic physiologic and anatomic changes in the cardiovascular system beginning in the first trimester and continuing through the postpartum period. These coordinated changes function to supply the growing fetus with oxygen and nutrients throughout pregnancy. Prior to conception, only approximately 2% to 3% of total cardiac output flows through the uterine arteries compared with 25% at term.[6,7] This shift in cardiac output begins very early on, peaking at term, and returning to normal at 3 months to 6 months.[6]

The heart undergoes progressive adaptive remodeling and structural alterations, including displacement into the thoracic cavity that is upward and forward.[8] This creates a barrel shape to the maternal chest, giving the appearance of cardiomegaly on chest imaging and left axis deviation on electrocardiogram (EKG) recordings.[9,10] Left ventricular wall mass and right ventricular wall mass increase, by 52% and 40%, respectively.[11–14] This likely is due to a combination of increased blood volume and signaling from progesterone and vascular endothelial growth factors, leading to hypertrophy of the cardiac myocytes and increased angiogenesis.[15,16] Placental lactogen enhances erythropoietin production, leading to an increase in red blood cell mass by 30%.[17,18] Total body water and plasma volume increase by a larger proportion, creating a physiologic anemia.[19,20] Increased estrogen activates the renin-angiotensin-aldosterone system, increasing sodium resorption and thereby water uptake. Estrogen also mediates the release of vasopressin from the hypothalamus, lowering the maternal osmostat and decreasing the thirst threshold. This leads to a decrease in colloid osmotic pressure, which contributes to dependent edema and an increased risk for pulmonary edema.[21] This physiologic dependent edema can be difficult to discern from edema secondary to cardiac failure.

To accommodate for the increasing volume, there is a compensatory increase in venous and arterial distensibility and a softening of the intimal lining of the arterial vessels.[14,22,23] Nitric oxide, relaxin, and progesterone mediate smooth muscle relaxation and a drop in systemic vascular resistance (SVR).[24,25] This drop in SVR is offset by the increase in preload and subsequently cardiac output, which leads to minimal change in the mean arterial pressure. This 25% to 30% drop in blood pressure reaches it's nadir in mid–second trimester and returns to normal prepregnancy values by the third trimester.[26,27] Dimensions of all cardiac chambers increase to compensate for the continued increase in plasma volume, resulting in trivial regurgitation in the mitral, tricuspid, and pulmonary valves.[28] Cardiac myocyte hypertrophy coupled with increased myocyte stretch leads to higher contractility without an increase in left ventricular strain or a change in overall ejection fraction.[8,13] There is a sharp increase in cardiac output in the first trimester and again in the third trimester, driven by the drop in SVR and increased maternal blood volume.[6] By 24 weeks, there is a 45% increase in cardiac output over baseline, and this rises to between 60% and 80% within the hour after delivery secondary to increased venous return and maternal autotransfusion. Cardiac output does not drop to normal prepregnancy values until 3 months to 6 months postdelivery.[11,26,29] Increased sympathetic tone increases maternal heart rate by 10 beats per minute (bpm) to 20 bpm, but stroke volume is the driving force behind the rise in cardiac output.[30–32]

Respiratory Changes

Much like the cardiovascular system, the respiratory system undergoes dramatic changes in order to efficiently transport oxygen to and offload carbon dioxide from the fetal-placental unit. Fetal offloading of carbon dioxide is dependent on a diffusion differential from the fetal umbilical arteries to the maternal venous system. In order for this to be accomplished, the respiratory physiology alters to create a state of alkalosis mediated by a drop in arterial P_{CO_2} and by compensatory excretion of bicarbonate by the kidneys.[33,34] There is an approximate 20% increase in oxygen consumption, which is accomplished by increasing both tidal volume and resting minute volume.[35] The functional residual capacity decreases by 20% due to a decrease in both expiratory reserve and residual volume, which puts pregnant women at risk for hypoxia due to lower oxygen reserves.[6,36] Perceived hyperventilation is driven by progesterone and can lead to the sensation of dyspnea in up to 70% of women by 30 weeks' gestation.[6] Most importantly, from a drug metabolism standpoint, is the reduced buffering capacity of the system and the shift in the oxygen-dissociation curve to the right to ensure offloading to the fetoplacental unit.[35,36]

Gastrointestinal and Hepatic Changes

From a pharmacologic standpoint, the important changes in the gastrointestinal system that potentially could alter absorption, distribution, and excretion include a decrease in serum albumin secondary to hemodilution (and some renal excretion), altering drug binding. As each organ system receives an incremental increase in the proportion of cardiac output, so too does the liver, which either can increase or decrease drug clearance depending on the medication involved.[37] The cytochrome P450 enzymes are up-regulated, which changes the metabolic clearance of many drugs, including some cardiovascular medications.[37,38] Gastric acidity also is increased due to increased placental production of gastrin.[6,39] This coupled with decreased sphincter tone leads to increased rates of reflux. In and of itself this does not interfere with drug metabolism and absorption but the treatment—antacids—can decrease bioavailability of many cardiac medications.[40] Altered α_1-acid glycoprotein along with an increase in fatty acids and lipids can displace bound drugs and increase the unbound drug fraction.[41]

Renal Changes

The drop in SVR affects the renal vasculature with a concomitant dilatation of the renal arterial system as the result of rising progesterone levels. Progesterone likewise mediates resistance to certain angiogenic factors, such as angiotensin II, ensuring the vasodilatory effects are not mitigated.[42] Relaxin stimulates formation of endothelin, which in turn mediates vasodilation of the renal arteries via nitric oxide synthesis.[23,43] This hormonally driven drop in blood pressure coupled with increasing blood volume creates a state of underfilling that is unique to pregnancy, signaling the osmostat to increase water absorption despite a continued rise total body water.[44] Decreased SVR despite rising plasma volumes is only physiologically possible because 80% of the volume increase is within the maternal venous system.[42] With the increasing cardiac output to the renal arteries, there is an increase in glomerular filtration by 50% by the end of the first trimester.[45] As a result, creatinine clearance increases and serum creatinine levels fall, both of which can significantly affect the metabolism and clearance of many cardiac medications.[44] Drug clearance also can be affected by the increasing albumin excretion as the result of increased glomerular permeability.[46] Despite an increase in fractional excretion of albumin, the normal concentration in the urine should not exceed 300 mg/d.[47]

MATERNAL PHARMACOKINETIC ALTERATIONS DURING PREGNANCY

All of the aforementioned physiologic changes contribute to altered drug distribution and their clinical effect during pregnancy. Delayed gastric emptying and increased gastrin production can lead to altered drug absorption and lowered tissue distribution. For example, prolonged gut transit can decrease the absorption of metoprolol or verapamil, and drugs that require an acidic environment may have higher bioavailability leading to toxicity.[48] Pregnant women tend to have more gastric reflux, which can lead to higher consumption of chelators, such as antacids, inadvertently altering cardiac drug metabolism.[49] Higher serum albumin levels lead to higher levels of bound drugs, decreasing the metabolically active free-form and subsequent decreased mechanism of action on the target tissue.[50] Increased glomerular filtration rate (GFR) and renal clearance also can lead to lower drug concentrations, as discussed previously. The increased blood flow to the liver with increased hepatic enzyme activity can alter the doses of certain cardiac medications leading to a change in dosing requirements in order to have the desired effects.[51,52]

PLACENTAL CONTRIBUTION TO PHARMACOKINETICS

The placenta was long held to be a senescent organ, functioning as both a barrier to toxic substances and a transport mediator for nutrients to the growing fetus. In vivo studies, however, have found that the placenta is active in both transport and metabolism of many xenobiotics in the maternal circulation, and these factors should be considered when dosing maternal medications.[53] Other important considerations include the solubility and lipophilic nature of the drug being given, because many drugs easily cross the placental barrier by diffusion and become trapped in the fetal compartment as a result of the lower pH in both the amniotic fluid and fetal blood.[37,53,54] This leads to ionization and accumulation of basic drugs within the fetal system and studies of cord blood analysis at birth have shown that certain medications concentrate in the fetal blood stream compared with the maternal system. In general, uncharged, unionized molecules with high lipid solubility and lower molecular weights readily can cross the placental barrier.[53,55] Solute levels also play a key role in maternal and fetal concentrations, which can change dramatically with the previously described changes within the maternal cardiovascular system. Active transport is accomplished through several different membrane-bound transporters and, although they do not play a significant role in the movement of nutrients and wastes, they can be targets for transplacental drug transfer. During the first trimester, a member of the adenosine triphosphate–binding cassette superfamily (ABC) plays a critical role in eliminating medications from the fetal compartment, and many cardiac medications, such as verapamil, can inhibit its function.[55,56] The placenta possesses metabolizing enzymes for both phase I (drug oxidation, reduction, and hydrolysis) and phase II (conjugation) reactions that can substantially alter drug levels and transport across the placenta.[53,56]

CLASSIFICATION OF CARDIOVASCULAR MEDICATIONS

Most of the fetal organs fully developed have by the end of the first trimester, which is the epoch in pregnancy referred to as organogenesis.[57] This is the time frame wherein the fetus is most susceptible to teratogens. Most medications are not teratogenic when used in therapeutic doses, but, again, due to the rapidly changing physiology of pregnancy, medication levels can inadvertently rise causing unwanted side effects. The baseline risk for congenital malformations is 1% to 3%.[58] Of these, up to 10% can be attributed to medication use during pregnancy.[58] The US Food and Drug Administration previously had categorized medication risk in pregnancy according to letters (A, B, C, D, and X) with category A medications posing no substantial risk to the fetus and category X medications contraindicated due to the high risk of teratogenicity.[59] Due to the ambiguity of such classification, however, a newer risk stratification model was adopted entitled the Pregnancy and Lactation Labeling Rule, whereby drug applications submitted after June 2015 were categorized according to this new model.[59] The newer labeling removed the dichotomization of the antepartum and labor and delivery time frames and has a new subsection for persons of reproductive potential.[60] The newer labeling is meant to provide more general information, including medication (pregnancy) registries, fetal risks, and the likelihood of developmental abnormalities. In addition, clinical considerations regarding timing, dose, and duration of exposure with both animal and human data are included. It no longer is recommended to use the previous letter classification for clinical decision making.[61] Use of medications during pregnancy is not without some level of risk, and discussing the potential outcomes should be part of the counseling of women with cardiovascular disease who desire to become or who already are pregnant.

The following sections delineate the most commonly used medications in pregnancy and their safety profiles.

ANTIARRHYTHMIC THERAPIES

Maternal cardiac arrhythmias during pregnancy are a common occurrence and treatment should be considered thoughtfully from both obstetric and electrophysiologic standpoints. Ventricular arrhythmias, although rare, represent an emergency, and unstable patients should be treated immediately with electrical cardioversion. Atrial arrhythmias, however, are more common and likely are due to the overall increase in cardiac output and blood volume.[62] Medications frequently are indicated in these patients more so for symptom control rather than for an acute emergency. Pregnant women at risk for arrhythmias include those with prior structural heart disease and those who have had prior cardiac surgery due to congenitally corrected lesions. A careful history should be obtained prior to initiating any antiarrhythmic drugs, because some medications, such as sotalol or flecainide, can cause unwanted maternal drug-drug interactions or side effects. Physicians must consider both adverse maternal and fetal side effects. Patients with underlying preexcitation on EKG should avoid the use of verapamil and digoxin to avoid promoting conduction down an accessory pathway. Careful consideration in the pregnant patient should be taken with digoxin because it has reduced drug effect on the mother during pregnancy due to increased drug clearance and increased unbound fraction of digoxin.[63,64] Due to a digoxin-like substance reported in the maternal serum, digoxin serum levels are not as reliable as in the nonpregnant population.[65] In addition, digoxin is cleared renally and, due to the 50% increase in renal blood flow during pregnancy, may require dosage adjustments. Adenosine also may require increased dosages in pregnancy.

The fetal effects of antiarrhythmic drugs are important to understand and more frequent monitoring may be necessary. Flecainide has an overall good safety profile and is used widely throughout gestation.[66–69] There are some small case reports, however, of flecainide associated with neonatal prolonged QT and heart failure at toxic levels and decreased fetal heart rate variability on external fetal cardiac monitoring.[52] Adenosine does not cross the placenta and has a short half-life and, therefore, is thought to pose minimal risk.[52] Significant fetal effects have been reported after the use of amiodarone, including hypothyroidism and neurodevelopmental complications, making it a last resort in the treatment of arrhythmias.[61] β-Blockers are a commonly used medication for rate control (discussed later). As a class, they usually are considered safe without an increase in congenital cardiac abnormalities, and first trimester use has not been found to be associated with a higher risk of any specific congenital anomalies.[70–73] There are numerous studies looking at fetal growth restriction (FGR) and β-blockers, including 1 study showing FGR in a group of patients taking propranolol, metoprolol, atenolol, or bisoprolol compared with control.[74,75] Atenolol was associated most strongly with FGR and, therefore, should be avoided in pregnancy.[76]

Use of these medications while breastfeeding is an important consideration when discussing medication options in the postpartum period. Some medications, although contraindicated during pregnancy, can be used safely during breastfeeding and lactation. Most antiarrhythmic medications, including β-blockers, calcium channel blockers, digoxin, flecainide, lidocaine, mexiletine, procainamide, propafenone, quinidine, and sotalol, are compatible with breastfeeding because they have little transfer into the breast milk.[77] It is unknown if adenosine transfers to the breast milk. Amiodarone is a bit more controversial and requires a conversation with the patient prior to initiation. If a patient is on amiodarone and wishes to breastfeed, the infant's pediatrician should be alerted so that neonatal plasma levels can to be monitored because breast milk and infant serum levels are somewhat unpredictable, likely due to the long half-life.[78]

ANTICOAGULATION AND ANTIPLATELET THERAPY
Maternal Issues

Anticoagulation and antiplatelet medications are prescribed commonly in both cardiology and obstetrics for various reasons. An understanding of the hypercoagulable state of pregnancy is paramount because it may change the indication, dosing, and frequency of certain medications. Although anticoagulation commonly is used in the obstetrics realm for thrombophilia or prophylaxis after surgery, a pregnant patient with a mechanical valve is an uncommon situation, which may involve multidisciplinary discussion regarding use and safety. Due to the thrombogenic propensity of pregnancy, these people are at increased risk for valve thrombosis.[79] As well, the changing volume of distribution creates significant challenges in regard to therapeutic windows, putting them at risk for a venous thrombus embolism or hemorrhage, and these women should be monitored more regularly.[61] The risk of valve thrombosis depends on the type and position of the mechanical valve with lower pressure positions (mitral valve) being at higher risk for thrombosis.[79] The risks of fetal teratogenesis with warfarin need to be weighed against the relatively high risk of valve thrombosis with the use of first-trimester heparin, and which modality to use should be a joint discussion between the patient, the obstetrician and the cardiologist. The use of low-molecular-weight heparin (LMWH) is associated with less risk of valve thrombosis than unfractionated heparin but still higher than with vitamin K antagonists (VKAs).[79] The higher risk of valve thrombosis with heparin use likely is secondary to its increased excretion in the maternal kidneys as a result of the higher GFR in pregnancy, because heparin is known to be excreted renally. Meticulous monitoring of anti-Xa levels (rather than partial thromboplastin time) should be employed and followed by an experienced cardiologist or maternal-fetal medicine specialist because these patients are at increased risk for both subtherapeutic and supratherapeutic levels due to these physiologic changes. According to the European Society of Cardiology 2018 guidelines, the use of VKAs throughout pregnancy, under strict international normalized ratio control, is the safest regimen to prevent valve thrombosis.[61] Concomitant aspirin use for valve thromboprophylaxis is recommended by the American College of Cardiology (ACC) and the American Heart Association (AHA) and has been shown to be safe for both mom and fetus alike.[52] It also is used widely in the high-risk obstetrics population to mitigate the risk for preeclampsia.[80] Studies have shown there is no evidence that low-dose aspirin alone increases maternal or fetal bleeding risks, risk of placental abruption, or complications at the time of neuraxial anesthesia during delivery. The risk of bleeding, however, when combined with other anticoagulants has led the ESC guidelines, in contrast to the AHA/ACC guidelines, to not recommend use of low-dose aspirin for mechanical valves.[61,81–83]

Fetal Issues

Warfarin embryopathy is a significant morbidity associated with VKAs.[84] First-trimester transplacental passage increases the risk for fetal warfarin syndrome or Di Sala syndrome.[85] The most common teratogenic findings include facial dysmorphisms, such as nasal hypoplasia, skeletal abnormalities (limb hypoplasia and stippled epiphyses), central nervous system abnormalities (ventral and dorsal midline dysplasia), and cardiac defects.[84–88] In the second and third trimesters, there is a 0.7% to 2% risk of ocular/central nervous system abnormalities and intracranial hemorrhage with VKAs.[61] There are higher rates of miscarriage and stillbirth reported when daily doses exceed 5 mg.[89] Current guidelines recommend women who are taking this dose or higher during the first trimester to be transitioned to

LMWH or unfractionated heparin by the end of the sixth week of gestation to decrease the risk of fetal malformations.[83] In women on warfarin who present in labor, the recommendation is to consider cesarean delivery to avoid neonatal intracranial hemorrhage.[90] During the last week of gestation, it is not unreasonable to admit patients and have them on a heparin drip in either anticipation of spontaneous labor or for a planned induction. Heparin and LMWH both are large molecules and do not cross the placenta. Given the changing volume of distribution in pregnancy along with increase excretion of these medications through higher GFR, both peak and trough levels should be monitored throughout pregnancy. A meta-analysis of maternal and fetal outcomes in more than 800 women with mechanical heart valves utilizing different anticoagulant strategies found that VKAs were associated with the lowest risk of adverse maternal outcomes, whereas the use of LMWH was associated with the lowest risk of adverse fetal outcomes.[79]

There are minimal human data on the teratogenic effects of aspirin use in the first trimester.[77] Case-control studies of children with congenital heart defects found no association between these abnormalities and maternal use of aspirin.[91,92] A meta-analysis did not find an increased risk of congenital defects associated with first trimester use of aspirin and a prospective study of more than 50,000 pregnancies did not report aspirin-associated malformations, altered birth weight, or perinatal deaths.[93,94] High-dose aspirin and near-term use of aspirin and other prostaglandin synthase inhibitors may result in closure or constriction of the fetal ductus arteriosus with resultant pulmonary hypertension.[95]

There are several case reports of clopidogrel used during pregnancy without documented congenital defects although sufficient data to determine absolute safety are lacking.[96–98] There are insufficient data to recommend direct oral anticoagulants for women in pregnancy and few data in regard to prasugrel, ticagrelor, abciximab, or eptifibatide; therefore, their use is not recommended.[52]

Breastfeeding and Lactation

Although there are variations in the ability of these medications to transfer to breast milk, there are few absolute contraindications to their use. Aspirin is excreted in the breast milk and likely is safe at a lower doses.[77] Prasugrel and ticagrelor have been shown to transfer in rat studies but, overall, as with clopidogrel, their effect largely is unknown.[99] Warfarin has only minimal transfer and generally

is considered safe.[77,89] Unfractionated heparin and enoxaparin largely are considered safe but the amount that crosses into breast milk is unknown.[77]

HYPERTENSIVE DISORDERS AND PREECLAMPSIA: RECOMMENDED TREATMENT

Hypertensive disorders of pregnancy (HDPs) affect up to 10% of all pregnancies in the United States and the rates continue to climb.[100] Due to the rising rates of obesity, women entering pregnancy with comorbid chronic hypertension also are on the rise. Chronic hypertension, or elevated blood pressure, either prior to pregnancy or as a new diagnosis, defined by 2 blood pressures of 140 mm Hg systolic or higher and/or 90 mm Hg diastolic or higher separated by 4 hours prior to 20 weeks, complicates 3% of all pregnancies and, therefore, makes up a large portion of the morbidity associated with adverse pregnancy outcomes.[100,101] Definitions are important because they dictate management, timing of delivery, and treatment recommendations. As well, outcomes for different HDPs are varied, with more severe events occurring in women with higher recorded blood pressures. For instance, women with gestational hypertension (new-onset elevated blood pressures as defined by a systolic pressure of 140 mm Hg or higher and/or a diastolic pressure of 90 mm Hg or higher on 2 occasions separated by 4 hours without proteinuria or any other signs of end-organ damage) have lower rates of adverse outcomes including small for gestational age infants and maternal stroke as well as lower rates of recurrence of HDPs in any future pregnancies.[100,102–104] As well, the American College of Obstetricians and Gynecologists does not recommend that women with gestational hypertension receive antihypertensive treatment because studies have not shown an improvement in outcomes with treatment and, because up to 50% of women with gestational hypertension progress to preeclampsia, treatment would be masking any worsening disease.[104] Severe disease should be treated, however, once a diagnosis has been established. Preeclampsia has been redefined and now women with new-onset elevated blood pressures of 140 mm Hg systolic and/or 90 mm Hg on 2 occasions separated by 4 hours after 20 weeks' gestation with proteinuria now are reclassified as preeclamptics without severe features.[104] Preeclampsia with severe features has numerous laboratory and clinical inclusion criteria. For the treating cardiologist, the most important change is that preeclampsia with severe features (previously known as severe preeclampsia) can be defined by blood pressures alone, despite being aproteinuric.[101,104] Any new-onset severe range blood pressures, defined by systolic of 160 mm Hg or greater and/or diastolic readings of 110 mm Hg or greater separated within minutes, can qualify as pr-eclampsia with severe features.[104] Although women with gestational hypertension or preeclampsia without severe features are managed without antihypertensive therapy on an outpatient basis, it is recommended that women with preeclampsia with severe features remain in the hospital until delivery and receive antihypertensive therapy to prevent adverse maternal outcomes, such as worsening hypertension and stroke.[3,104,105]

Usually, a cardiologist is asked to become involved to manage chronic hypertension prior to 20 weeks or during the postpartum period when fluid shifts and autotransfusion after delivery can exacerbate HDPs. It, therefore, is important to have knowledge regarding the safety profiles of the most commonly used antihypertensives for both pregnancy and lactation.

Treatment of hypertensive Disorders of Pregnancy: Recommended Antihypertensive Medications

Although β-blockers are considered fourth-line therapy outside of pregnancy, due to their fetal and neonatal safety profile, labetalol is the first-line agent recommended for the treatment of both chronic hypertension and acute hypertensive emergencies throughout gestation.[100,104–106] Labetalol is a nonselective α_1-, β_1-, and β_2-adrenergic blocker, which lowers blood pressure by peripheral vasodilation and has not been shown to have teratogenic effects when used in the first trimester despite its ability to cross the placenta.[107] It has been associated with maternal hypotension, fetal bradycardia, perinatal jaundice, and neonatal hypoglycemia.[70,108,109] There is the association of low birth weight with the use of labetalol; however, this likely is independent of drug use and rather a manifestation of the hypertension itself.[110] Although it has been found in the maternal breast milk, it generally is considered safe for the neonate.[111] Labetalol is recommended as first-line therapy for women with chronic hypertension planning a pregnancy and for the acute treatment of severe hypertension secondary to either chronic hypertension exacerbation or preeclampsia with severe features (intravenous dosing only).[100,104] Due to the increased volume of distribution, labetalol may require 3-times daily dosing during pregnancy. Metoprolol has a similar safety profile to labetalol but a longer onset of action, which is not ideal for acute hypertensive emergencies in pregnancy. Women treated for underlying chronic hypertension on metoprolol can continue with their current medication regimen, however, keeping in mind that metoprolol has a higher clearance rate in the second and third trimesters and may require aggressive adjustments in dosing/frequency in order to maintain a therapeutic window.[112] Both have long-term follow-up studies in children exposed in utero with no associated adverse health outcomes.[113,114]

Hydralazine is a potent arterial vasodilator that is recommended as a second-line alternative to labetalol for the treatment of acute hypertensive urgencies during pregnancy.[104,105] Hydralazine does, however, have a higher risk for hypotension compared with oral nifedipine or intravenous labetalol and should be taken into consideration when administering due to the risk for uterine hypoperfusion and subsequent non-reassuring fetal status.[115] There are no associated risks for birth defects when used in the first trimester and it is considered safe for breastfeeding mothers.[107,116]

Calcium channel blockers are categorized as either dihydropyridines or nondihydropyridines. Nifedipine, a dihydropyridine, is used widely in pregnancy for control of chronic hypertension, acute hypertensive emergencies, and uterine tocolysis.[100,104,117] It has been shown more effective at lowering and maintaining blood pressure in an acute hypertensive crisis than hydralazine and its rapid onset of action makes it ideal for women without intravenous access or with contraindications to β-blockade.[104,115,118] Nifedipine is considered safe during the first trimester and does not pose an increase in teratogenic risk.[119]

Methyldopa is an α_2-receptor agonist with a long track record of safety in pregnancy. Although previously the first-line agent, its longer onset of action precludes it from being used in hypertensive urgencies.[120] Women with chronic hypertension who come into pregnancy well-controlled on methyldopa may continue using it but again should be aware that due to the increased volume of distribution may require more frequent and/or increased dosing.[121] It has not been associated with any fetal, neonatal, or maternal adverse outcomes.[122]

Antihypertensive Medications To Be Used with Caution

Amlodipine, another dihydropyridine, has not been used widely in pregnancy and, therefore, there are minimal safety data reported. There are some case series, however, reporting an increase in seizure activity in neonates exposed in utero and variable reports on birth defects and neurodevelopmental outcomes.[123] Although not contraindicated, amlodipine should be considered only in refractory cases or when contraindications to other, safer options are present.

Diuretics are utilized judiciously outside of pregnancy for the control of hypertension through reduced preload and plasma volume. The normal physiology of pregnancy dictates that plasma volume and, thereby, uterine artery blood flow increase in order to transfer nutrients to the growing fetus, which is counterintuitive to the mechanism of action for diuretics. Thiazide diuretics can cross the placenta and have been associated with neonatal jaundice, thrombocytopenia, hyponatremia, and fetal bradycardia.[65] Hydrochlorothiazide and furosemide are not associated with birth defects but, due to the risk for uterine hypoperfusion, should not be initiated during pregnancy for the treatment of hypertension; women who enter into pregnancy with underlying heart failure on these medications do have the option of continuation.[65] The development of preeclampsia—an intravascularly volume deplete disease state—and concomitant use of diuretics should be approached with extreme caution because this will further decreases end-organ perfusion.

Diltiazem commonly is used in women with underlying renal dysfunction due to its purported renal-protective properties and has minimal transfer across the placental barrier.[124] There are some reports of increased fetal loss; therefore, it should not be started as a first-line agent in the first trimester.[119]

SUMMATION

Reducing maternal morbidity and mortality is an essential public health initiative that requires partnerships across all medical specialties. Because cardiologists and obstetricians collaborate in the care of women with congenital and acquired heart disease, a significant shift toward improved outcomes undoubtedly will be seen. Possessing a basic knowledge of safe medication use in the care of this population aids the practitioner in providing safe guidance to women throughout the puerperium. The lack of randomized control trials will continue to present a challenge in pharmaceutical guidelines for pregnancy, but registries, case studies, and retrospective analyses may assist in filling this knowledge gap.

DISCLOSURE

The authors have nothing to disclose.

REFERENCES

1. Carroll AE. Why is US maternal mortality rising? JAMA 2017;318(4):321.
2. Callaghan WM. Overview of maternal mortality in the United States. Semin Perinatol 2012;36(1):2–6.
3. Lo JO, Mission JF, Caughey AB. Hypertensive disease of pregnancy and maternal mortality. Curr Opin Obstet Gynecol 2013;25(2):124–32.
4. Mitchell AA, Gilboa SM, Werler MM, et al. Medication use during pregnancy, with particular focus on prescription drugs: 1976-2008. Am J Obstet Gynecol 2011;205(1):51.e1–8.
5. Ruys TPE, Maggioni A, Johnson MR, et al. Cardiac medication during pregnancy, data from the ROPAC. Int J Cardiol 2014;177(1):124–8.
6. Tan EK, Tan EL. Alterations in physiology and anatomy during pregnancy. Best Pract Res Clin Obstet Gynaecol 2013;27(6):791–802.
7. Thaler I, Manor D, Itskovitz J, et al. Changes in uterine blood flow during human pregnancy. Am J Obstet Gynecol 1990;162(1):121–5.
8. Savu O, Jurcuţ R, Giuşcă S, et al. Morphological and functional adaptation of the maternal heart during pregnancy. Circ Cardiovasc Imaging 2012; 5(3):289–97.
9. Izci B, Vennelle M, Liston WA, et al. Sleep-disordered breathing and upper airway size in pregnancy and post-partum. Eur Respir J 2006;27(2): 321–7.
10. Akinwusi PO, Oboro VO, Adebayo RA, et al. Cardiovascular and electrocardiographic changes in Nigerians with a normal pregnancy. Cardiovasc J Afr 2011;22(2):71–5.
11. Robson SC, Dunlop W. When do cardiovascular parameters return to their preconception values? Am J Obstet Gynecol 1992;167(5):1479.
12. Robson SC, Dunlop W, Hunter S. Haemodynamic changes during the early puerperium. Br Med J Clin Res Ed 1987;294(6579):1065.
13. Ducas RA, Elliott JE, Melnyk SF, et al. Cardiovascular magnetic resonance in pregnancy: insights from the cardiac hemodynamic imaging and remodeling in pregnancy (CHIRP) study. J Cardiovasc Magn Reson 2014;16:1.
14. Sanghavi M, Rutherford JD. Cardiovascular physiology of pregnancy. Circulation 2014;130(12): 1003–8.
15. Umar S, Nadadur R, Iorga A, et al. Cardiac structural and hemodynamic changes associated with physiological heart hypertrophy of pregnancy are reversed postpartum. J Appl Physiol (1985) 2012; 113(8):1253–9.
16. Goldstein J, Sites CK, Toth MJ. Progesterone stimulates cardiac muscle protein synthesis via receptor-dependent pathway. Fertil Steril 2004; 82(2):430–6.

17. Cavill I. Iron and erythropoiesis in normal subjects and in pregnancy. J Perinat Med 1995;23(1–2): 47–50.

18. Nakada D, Oguro H, Levi BP, et al. Oestrogen increases haematopoietic stem-cell self-renewal in females and during pregnancy. Nature 2014; 505(7484):555–8.

19. Chesley LC. Plasma and red cell volumes during pregnancy. Am J Obstet Gynecol 1972;112(3): 440–50.

20. Pritchard JA. Changes in the blood volume during pregnancy and delivery. Anesthesiology 1965;26: 393–9.

21. Wu PY, Udani V, Chan L, et al. Colloid osmotic pressure: variations in normal pregnancy. J Perinat Med 1983;11(4):193–9.

22. Henry F, Quatresooz P, Valverde-Lopez JC, et al. Blood vessel changes during pregnancy: a review. Am J Clin Dermatol 2006;7(1):65–9.

23. Jelinic M, Marshall SA, Leo CH, et al. From pregnancy to cardiovascular disease: lessons from relaxin-deficient animals to understand relaxin actions in the vascular system. Microcirculation 2019;26(2):e12464.

24. Carbillon L, Uzan M, Uzan S. Pregnancy, vascular tone, and maternal hemodynamics: a crucial adaptation. Obstet Gynecol Surv 2000;55(9):574–81.

25. Pears S, Makris A, Hennessy A. The chronobiology of blood pressure in pregnancy. Pregnancy Hypertens 2018;12:104–9.

26. Mahendru AA, Everett TR, Wilkinson IB, et al. A longitudinal study of maternal cardiovascular function from preconception to the postpartum period. J Hypertens 2014;32(4):849–56.

27. Soma-Pillay P, Nelson-Piercy C, Tolppanen H, et al. Physiological changes in pregnancy. Cardiovasc J Afr 2016;27(2):89–94.

28. Campos O, Andrade JL, Bocanegra J, et al. Physiologic multivalvular regurgitation during pregnancy: a longitudinal Doppler echocardiographic study. Int J Cardiol 1993;40(3):265–72.

29. Ling HZ, Guy GP, Bisquera A, et al. Maternal hemodynamics in screen-positive and screen-negative women of the ASPRE trial. Ultrasound Obstet Gynecol 2019;54(1):51–7.

30. Ekholm EM, Erkkola RU. Autonomic cardiovascular control in pregnancy. Eur J Obstet Gynecol Reprod Biol 1996;64(1):29–36.

31. Herrera S, Kuhlmann-Capek MJ, Rogan SC, et al. Stroke volume recruitability during the third trimester of pregnancy. Am J Perinatol 2018; 35(8):737–40.

32. Vinayagam D, Thilaganathan B, Stirrup O, et al. Maternal hemodynamics in normal pregnancy: reference ranges and role of maternal characteristics. Ultrasound Obstet Gynecol 2018;51(5): 665–71.

33. Pardi G, Marconi AM, Cetin I, et al. Fetal oxygenation and acid base balance during pregnancy. J Perinat Med 1991;19(Suppl 1):139–44.

34. Blechner JN. Maternal-fetal acid-base physiology. Clin Obstet Gynecol 1993;36(1):3–12.

35. Elkus R, Popovich J. Respiratory physiology in pregnancy. Clin Chest Med 1992;13(4):555–65.

36. Hegewald MJ, Crapo RO. Respiratory physiology in pregnancy. Clin Chest Med 2011;32(1):1–13.

37. Feghali M, Venkataramanan R, Caritis S. Pharmacokinetics of drugs in pregnancy. Semin Perinatol 2015;39(7):512–9.

38. Tracy TS, Venkataramanan R, Glover DD, et al, National Institute for Child Health and Human Development Network of Maternal-Fetal-Medicine Units. Temporal changes in drug metabolism (CYP1A2, CYP2D6 and CYP3A Activity) during pregnancy. Am J Obstet Gynecol 2005;192(2):633–9.

39. Ouzounian JG, Elkayam U. Physiologic changes during normal pregnancy and delivery. Cardiol Clin 2012;30(3):317–29.

40. Sadowski DC. Drug interactions with antacids. Mechanisms and clinical significance. Drug Saf 1994;11(6):395–407.

41. Larsson A, Palm M, Hansson L-O, et al. Reference values for alpha1-acid glycoprotein, alpha1-antitrypsin, albumin, haptoglobin, C-reactive protein, IgA, IgG and IgM during pregnancy. Acta Obstet Gynecol Scand 2008;87(10):1084–8.

42. Belzile M, Pouliot A, Cumyn A, et al. Renal physiology and fluid and electrolyte disorders in pregnancy. Best Pract Res Clin Obstet Gynaecol 2019;57:1–14.

43. Conrad KP. Maternal vasodilation in pregnancy: the emerging role of relaxin. Am J Physiol Regul Integr Comp Physiol 2011;301(2):R267–75.

44. Lopes van Balen VA, van Gansewinkel TAG, de Haas S, et al. Maternal kidney function during pregnancy: systematic review and meta-analysis. Ultrasound Obstet Gynecol 2019;54(3):297–307.

45. Lindheimer MD, Davison JM, Katz AI. The kidney and hypertension in pregnancy: twenty exciting years. Semin Nephrol 2001;21(2):173–89.

46. Cheung KL, Lafayette RA. Renal physiology of pregnancy. Adv Chronic Kidney Dis 2013;20(3): 209–14.

47. Higby K, Suiter CR, Phelps JY, et al. Normal values of urinary albumin and total protein excretion during pregnancy. Am J Obstet Gynecol 1994; 171(4):984–9.

48. Tamargo J, Rosano G, Walther T, et al. Gender differences in the effects of cardiovascular drugs. Eur Heart J Cardiovasc Pharmacother 2017;3(3): 163–82.

49. Gugler R, Allgayer H. Effects of antacids on the clinical pharmacokinetics of drugs. An update. Clin Pharmacokinet 1990;18(3):210–9.

50. Isoherranen N, Thummel KE. Drug metabolism and transport during pregnancy: how does drug disposition change during pregnancy and what are the mechanisms that cause such changes? Drug Metab Dispos 2013;41(2):256–62.

51. Qasqas SA, McPherson C, Frishman WH, et al. Cardiovascular pharmacotherapeutic considerations during pregnancy and lactation. Cardiol Rev 2004;12(4):201–21.

52. Halpern DG, Weinberg CR, Pinnelas R, et al. Use of medication for cardiovascular disease during pregnancy: JACC state-of-the-art review. J Am Coll Cardiol 2019;73(4):457–76.

53. Koren G, Ornoy A. The role of the placenta in drug transport and fetal drug exposure. Expert Rev Clin Pharmacol 2018;11(4):373–85.

54. Mitani GM, Steinberg I, Lien EJ, et al. The pharmacokinetics of antiarrhythmic agents in pregnancy and lactation. Clin Pharmacokinet 1987;12(4): 253–91.

55. Young AM, Allen CE, Audus KL. Efflux transporters of the human placenta. Adv Drug Deliv Rev 2003; 55(1):125–32.

56. Tetro N, Moushaev S, Rubinchik-Stern M, et al. The placental barrier: the gate and the fate in drug distribution. Pharm Res 2018;35(4):71.

57. Thelander HE. Interference with organogenesis and fetal development. Tex Rep Biol Med 1973; 31(4):791–861.

58. Koren G, Pastuszak A, Ito S. Drugs in pregnancy. N Engl J Med 1998;338(16):1128–37.

59. Federal register, Part 201 (21 CFR Part 201). Available at: https://www.govinfo.gov/content/pkg/FR-2014-12-04/pdf/2014-28241.pdf. Accessed June 27, 2020.

60. Pregnancy and lactation labeling final Rule. Published online March 23, 2018. Available at: https://www.fda.gov/vaccines-blood-biologics/biologics-rules/pregnancy-and-lactation-labeling-final-rule. Accessed June 27, 2020.

61. Regitz-Zagrosek V, Roos-Hesselink JW, Bauersachs J, et al. 2018 ESC guidelines for the management of cardiovascular diseases during pregnancy. Kardiol Pol 2019;77(3): 245–326.

62. Enriquez AD, Economy KE, Tedrow UB. Contemporary management of arrhythmias during pregnancy. Circ Arrhythm Electrophysiol 2014;7(5): 961–7.

63. Gonser M, Stoll P, Kahle P. Clearance prediction and drug dosage in pregnancy: a clinical study on metildigoxin, and application to other drugs with predominant renal elimination. Clin Drug Investig 1995;9(4):197–205.

64. Hebert MF, Easterling TR, Kirby B, et al. Effects of pregnancy on CYP3A and P-glycoprotein activities as measured by disposition of midazolam and digoxin: a University of Washington specialized center of research study. Clin Pharmacol Ther 2008;84(2):248–53.

65. Elkayam U. Cardiac problems in pregnancy. 4th edition. Hoboken (NJ): Wiley Blackwell; 2020.

66. Wagner X, Jouglard J, Moulin M, et al. Coadministration of flecainide acetate and sotalol during pregnancy: lack of teratogenic effects, passage across the placenta, and excretion in human breast milk. Am Heart J 1990;119(3 Pt 1):700–2.

67. Villanova C, Muriago M, Nava F. Arrhythmogenic right ventricular dysplasia: pregnancy under flecainide treatment. G Ital Cardiol 1998;28(6): 691–3.

68. Chauveau S, Le Vavasseur O, Morel E, et al. Flecainide is a safe and effective treatment for pre-excited atrial fibrillation rapidly conducted to the ventricle in pregnant women: a case series. Eur Heart J Case Rep 2019;3(2). https://doi.org/10.1093/ehjcr/ytz066.

69. Ahmed K, Issawi I, Peddireddy R. Use of flecainide for refractory atrial tachycardia of pregnancy. Am J Crit Care 1996;5(4):306–8.

70. Bateman BT, Patorno E, Desai RJ, et al. Late pregnancy β blocker exposure and risks of neonatal hypoglycemia and bradycardia. Pediatrics 2016; 138(3). https://doi.org/10.1542/peds.2016-0731.

71. Bateman BT, Heide-Jørgensen U, Einarsdóttir K, et al. β-Blocker use in pregnancy and the risk for congenital malformations: an International Cohort Study. Ann Intern Med 2018;169(10):665–73.

72. Bergman JEH, Lutke LR, Gans ROB, et al. Beta-blocker use in pregnancy and risk of specific congenital anomalies: a european case-malformed control study. Drug Saf 2018;41(4): 415–27.

73. Duan L, Ng A, Chen W, et al. β-blocker exposure in pregnancy and risk of fetal cardiac anomalies. JAMA Intern Med 2017;177(6):885–7.

74. Tanaka K, Tanaka H, Kamiya C, et al. Beta-blockers and fetal growth restriction in pregnant women with cardiovascular disease. Circ J 2016;80(10): 2221–6.

75. Grewal J, Siu SC, Lee T, et al. Impact of beta-blockers on birth weight in a high-risk cohort of pregnant women with CVD. J Am Coll Cardiol 2020;75(21):2751–2.

76. Lip GY, Beevers M, Churchill D, et al. Effect of atenolol on birth weight. Am J Cardiol 1997;79(10): 1436–8.

77. Briggs G, Freeman R, Yaffe S. Drugs in pregnancy and lactation: a reference guide to fetal and neonatal risk. 9th edition. Lippincott: Williams and Wilkins; 2012.

78. Khurana R, Bin Jardan YA, Wilkie J, et al. Breast milk concentrations of amiodarone, desethylamiodarone, and bisoprolol following short-term drug

exposure: two case reports. J Clin Pharmacol 2014;54(7):828–31.

79. Steinberg ZL, Dominguez-Islas CP, Otto CM, et al. Maternal and fetal outcomes of anticoagulation in pregnant women with mechanical heart valves. J Am Coll Cardiol 2017;69(22):2681–91.

80. Poon LC, Wright D, Rolnik DL, et al. Aspirin for Evidence-Based Preeclampsia Prevention trial: effect of aspirin in prevention of preterm preeclampsia in subgroups of women according to their characteristics and medical and obstetrical history. Am J Obstet Gynecol 2017;217(5):585.e1–5.

81. Askie LM, Duley L, Henderson-Smart DJ, et al, PARIS Collaborative Group. Antiplatelet agents for prevention of pre-eclampsia: a meta-analysis of individual patient data. Lancet 2007;369(9575): 1791–8.

82. CLASP: a randomised trial of low-dose aspirin for the prevention and treatment of pre-eclampsia among 9364 pregnant women. CLASP (Collaborative Low-dose Aspirin Study in Pregnancy) Collaborative Group. Lancet 1994;343(8898):619–29.

83. Nishimura RA, Otto CM, Bonow RO, et al. 2014 AHA/ACC guideline for the management of patients with valvular heart disease: a report of the American College of Cardiology/American Heart Association Task Force on practice guidelines. J Am Coll Cardiol 2014;63(22):e57–185.

84. Holzgreve W, Carey JC, Hall BD. Warfarin-induced fetal abnormalities. Lancet 1976;2(7991):914–5.

85. Kumar M, Bhasker SK, Singh R, et al. Di Sala syndrome. BMJ Case Rep 2012;2012.

86. Dilli D, Oğuz S, Dilmen U. A case of congenital warfarin syndrome due to maternal drug administration during the pregnancy. Genet Couns Geneva Switz 2011;22(2):221–6.

87. Stevenson RE, Burton OM, Ferlauto GJ, et al. Hazards of oral anticoagulants during pregnancy. JAMA 1980;243(15):1549–51.

88. Harrod MJ, Sherrod PS. Warfarin embryopathy in siblings. Obstet Gynecol 1981;57(5):673–6.

89. Vitale N, De Feo M, De Santo LS, et al. Dose-dependent fetal complications of warfarin in pregnant women with mechanical heart valves. J Am Coll Cardiol 1999;33(6):1637–41.

90. Barbour LA. Current concepts of anticoagulant therapy in pregnancy. Obstet Gynecol Clin North Am 1997;24(3):499–521.

91. Werler MM, Mitchell AA, Shapiro S. The relation of aspirin use during the first trimester of pregnancy to congenital cardiac defects. N Engl J Med 1989;321(24):1639–42.

92. Marsh CA, Cragan JD, Alverson CJ, et al. Case-control analysis of maternal prenatal analgesic use and cardiovascular malformations: Baltimore–Washington Infant Study. Am J Obstet Gynecol 2014;211(4):404.e1–9.

93. Slone D, Siskind V, Heinonen OP, et al. Aspirin and congenital malformations. Lancet 1976;1(7974): 1373–5.

94. Kozer E, Nikfar S, Costei A, et al. Aspirin consumption during the first trimester of pregnancy and congenital anomalies: a meta-analysis. Am J Obstet Gynecol 2002;187(6):1623–30.

95. Moise KJ, Huhta JC, Sharif DS, et al. Indomethacin in the treatment of premature labor. Effects on the fetal ductus arteriosus. N Engl J Med 1988; 319(6):327–31.

96. Myers GR, Hoffman MK, Marshall ES. Clopidogrel use throughout pregnancy in a patient with a drug-eluting coronary stent. Obstet Gynecol 2011;118(2 Pt 2):432–3.

97. Al-Aqeedi RF, Al-Nabti AD. Drug-eluting stent implantation for acute myocardial infarction during pregnancy with use of glycoprotein IIb/IIIa inhibitor, aspirin and clopidogrel. J Invasive Cardiol 2008; 20(5):E146–9.

98. Klinzing P, Markert UR, Liesaus K, et al. Case report: successful pregnancy and delivery after myocardial infarction and essential thrombocythemia treated with clopidrogel. Clin Exp Obstet Gynecol 2001;28(4):215–6.

99. De Santis M, De Luca C, Mappa I, et al. Clopidogrel treatment during pregnancy: a case report and a review of literature. Intern Med Tokyo Jpn 2011; 50(16):1769–73.

100. American College of Obstetricians and Gynecologists' Committee on Practice Bulletins—Obstetrics. ACOG practice bulletin No. 203: chronic hypertension in pregnancy. Obstet Gynecol 2019;133(1): e26–50.

101. Vest AR, Cho LS. Hypertension in pregnancy. Curr Atheroscler Rep 2014;16(3):395.

102. van Oostwaard MF, Langenveld J, Schuit E, et al. Recurrence of hypertensive disorders of pregnancy: an individual patient data metaanalysis. Am J Obstet Gynecol 2015;212(5):624.e1-7.

103. Ebbing C, Rasmussen S, Skjaerven R, et al. Risk factors for recurrence of hypertensive disorders of pregnancy, a population-based cohort study. Acta Obstet Gynecol Scand 2017;96(2):243–50.

104. ACOG practice bulletin No. 202: gestational hypertension and preeclampsia. Obstet Gynecol 2019; 133(1):e1–25.

105. American College of Obstetricians and Gynecologists; Task Force on Hypertension in Pregnancy. Hypertension in pregnancy. Report of the American College of Obstetricians and Gynecologists' Task Force on Hypertension in Pregnancy. Obstet Gynecol 2013;122(5):1122–31.

106. National Clinical Guideline Centre (UK). Hypertension: The Clinical Management of Primary Hypertension in Adults: Update of Clinical Guidelines 18 and 34. Royal College of Physicians (UK). 2011.

Available at: http://www.ncbi.nlm.nih.gov/books/NBK83274/. Accessed June 28, 2020.

107. Fisher SC, Van Zutphen AR, Werler MM, et al. Maternal antihypertensive medication use and selected birth defects in the National Birth Defects Prevention Study. Birth Defects Res 2018;110(19):1433–42.

108. Davis RL, Eastman D, McPhillips H, et al. Risks of congenital malformations and perinatal events among infants exposed to calcium channel and beta-blockers during pregnancy. Pharmacoepidemiol Drug Saf 2011;20(2):138–45.

109. Fitton CA, Steiner MFC, Aucott L, et al. In-utero exposure to antihypertensive medication and neonatal and child health outcomes: a systematic review. J Hypertens 2017;35(11):2123–37.

110. Orbach H, Matok I, Gorodischer R, et al. Hypertension and antihypertensive drugs in pregnancy and perinatal outcomes. Am J Obstet Gynecol 2013;208(4):301.e1–6.

111. Lunell NO, Kulas J, Rane A. Transfer of labetalol into amniotic fluid and breast milk in lactating women. Eur J Clin Pharmacol 1985;28(5):597–9.

112. Ryu RJ, Eyal S, Easterling TR, et al. Pharmacokinetics of metoprolol during pregnancy and lactation. J Clin Pharmacol 2016;56(5):581–9.

113. Pasker-de Jong PCM, Zielhuis GA, van Gelder MMHJ, et al. Antihypertensive treatment during pregnancy and functional development at primary school age in a historical cohort study. BJOG 2010;117(9):1080–6.

114. Chan WS, Koren G, Barrera M, et al. Neurocognitive development of children following in-utero exposure to labetalol for maternal hypertension: a cohort study using a prospectively collected database. Hypertens Pregnancy 2010;29(3):271–83.

115. Alavifard S, Chase R, Janoudi G, et al. First-line antihypertensive treatment for severe hypertension in pregnancy: a systematic review and network meta-analysis. Pregnancy Hypertens 2019;18:179–87.

116. Heinonen OP, Sloan D, Shapiro S. Birth Defects and Drugs in Pregnancy. Publishing Science Groups, Inc. 1977. Available at: http://hdl.handle.net/2027.42/38133. Accessed June 28, 2020.

117. American College of Obstetricians and Gynecologists, Committee on Practice Bulletins—Obstetrics. ACOG practice bulletin no. 127: management of preterm labor. Obstet Gynecol 2012;119(6):1308–17.

118. Duley L, Meher S, Jones L. Drugs for treatment of very high blood pressure during pregnancy. Cochrane Database Syst Rev 2013;7:CD001449.

119. Magee LA, Schick B, Donnenfeld AE, et al. The safety of calcium channel blockers in human pregnancy: a prospective, multicenter cohort study. Am J Obstet Gynecol 1996;174(3):823–8.

120. Molvi SN, Mir S, Rana VS, et al. Role of antihypertensive therapy in mild to moderate pregnancy-induced hypertension: a prospective randomized study comparing labetalol with alpha methyldopa. Arch Gynecol Obstet 2012;285(6):1553–62.

121. Tamargo J, Caballero R, Delpón E. Pharmacotherapy for hypertension in pregnant patients: special considerations. Expert Opin Pharmacother 2019;20(8):963–82.

122. Easterling T, Mundle S, Bracken H, et al. Oral antihypertensive regimens (nifedipine retard, labetalol, and methyldopa) for management of severe hypertension in pregnancy: an open-label, randomised controlled trial. Lancet Lond Engl 2019;394(10203):1011–21.

123. Ahn HK, Nava-Ocampo AA, Han JY, et al. Exposure to amlodipine in the first trimester of pregnancy and during breastfeeding. Hypertens Pregnancy 2007;26(2):179–87.

124. Khandelwal M, Kumanova M, Gaughan JP, et al. Role of diltiazem in pregnant women with chronic renal disease. J Matern-fetal Neonatal Med 2002;12(6):408–12.

Pregnancy in Women with Adult Congenital Heart Disease

Katherine B. Salciccioli, MD[a], Timothy B. Cotts, MD[a,b],*

KEYWORDS

- Pregnancy • Congenital heart disease • Tetralogy of Fallot • Transposition of the great arteries
- Fontan

KEY POINTS

- Preconception counseling should include discussions about cardiac optimization, medication changes needed before pregnancy, genetic transmission of congenital heart disease, and patient-specific maternal and fetal risks.
- Multidisciplinary care throughout pregnancy should include adult congenital cardiology, obstetrics, and anesthesia, most especially for higher-risk patients.
- Lesion-specific hemodynamic considerations and risk stratification should drive management decisions during pregnancy, labor, and delivery.
- With rare exceptions, vaginal delivery is the preferred mode of delivery.

INTRODUCTION

As medical and surgical advances in the care of congenital heart disease (CHD) have allowed most children born with heart defects to survive into adulthood, pregnancy in women with repaired or palliated CHD is becoming increasingly common.[1–5] Women with CHD are responsible for less than 0.1% of pregnancies in the United States, and this percentage is increasing.[6] Although maternal mortality remains low, women with CHD have much higher rates of serious cardiac events than the general population: up to 2.8% in a recent multicenter study.[7] However, there is evidence that nearly half of these complications are preventable, suggesting that better understanding of the underlying physiology and expectant management will help improve both maternal and fetal outcomes in this growing population.[7]

To accomplish this goal, multidisciplinary care involving obstetrics, anesthesia, and congenital cardiology is critical. Ideally, pregnancy in a mother with CHD is a planned event with preconception optimization and medication adjustment. Realistically, however, pregnancy may be a time when women with CHD who have been lost to cardiology follow-up return to care and, as such, serves as a key time for reconnecting them for future follow-up.[8]

PRECONCEPTION COUNSELING

Preconception counseling should begin during adolescence with discussions about contraception and pregnancy as a planned event.[9]

[a] Adult Congenital Heart Disease, Department of Internal Medicine, University of Michigan, University of Michigan Congenital Heart Center, C.S. Mott Children's Hospital, 1540 East Hospital Drive, Ann Arbor, MI 48109-4204, USA; [b] Adult Congenital Heart Disease, Department of Pediatrics, University of Michigan, University of Michigan Congenital Heart Center, C.S. Mott Children's Hospital, 1540 East Hospital Drive, Ann Arbor, MI 48109-4204, USA
* Corresponding author. Department of Internal Medicine, University of Michigan, 1540 East Hospital Drive, Ann Arbor, MI 48109-4204.
E-mail address: cottstim@med.umich.edu

Cardiol Clin 39 (2021) 55–65
https://doi.org/10.1016/j.ccl.2020.09.004
0733-8651/21/© 2020 Elsevier Inc. All rights reserved.

Discussions regarding individual anatomy, functional status, and risk factors should be continued longitudinally. Historically, many women with CHD were told they should never become pregnant, but, in the current era, there are very few lesions that are considered true contraindications to pregnancy.[10]

The 2018 American Heart Association (AHA)/American College of Cardiology (ACC) Guideline for the Management of Adults with Congenital Heart Disease outlines a framework for preconception counseling. All women with CHD should have prepregnancy counseling discussing maternal cardiac and obstetric risks as well as fetal risks, including the potential for transmission of CHD to the fetus.[10] Individual assessment should include the new adult CHD? complexity classification, which accounts for both underlying CHD complexity and current physiologic/functional status.[10] Ideally, a woman's cardiac status should be optimized before pursuing pregnancy. For example, patients meeting criteria for valve replacement should undergo the procedure before conception, allowing for full recovery and return to a new baseline before adding the hemodynamic stresses of pregnancy.

Medications should be carefully reviewed to assess for teratogenic potential before conception. Commonly used medications with known adverse fetal effects include angiotensin-converting enzyme inhibitors, endothelin receptor antagonists, and amiodarone. Highly effective contraception is required when using such medications, with pregnancy planning important to reduce the risk of fetal teratogenicity. Special consideration should be given to discussions of anticoagulation given recent advances in the understanding of the risk of warfarin embryopathy compared with other options as well as the intricacies of laboratory monitoring throughout pregnancy.[11]

Multiple risk-stratification scores have been created to predict adverse maternal and fetal outcomes in women with CHD. The most commonly used scoring systems are the Cardiac Disease in Pregnancy (CARPREG and CARPREG2) scores, the original and modified World Health Organization (WHO) classification scores, and the ZAHARA (acronym based on Dutch translation) score.[12–17] The CARPREG systems use generic risk factors such as functional classification and severity of valve disease, whereas the WHO classification is primarily based on underlying congenital cardiac condition. Although subsequent analysis and comparison of these scoring systems has shown that they often overestimate adverse events, they have overall been useful in identifying specific factors that increase the risk of complications (eg, depressed ventricular function, left heart obstruction).[18] Of the available risk-stratification scores, the modified WHO classification system for maternal cardiovascular risk is currently favored by both ACC/AHA and European Society of Cardiology (ESC) guidelines for cardiac care in pregnancy.[10,15,18–20]

In addition to determining a patient's anatomic and physiologic classification and using existing risk-stratification scoring systems, cardiopulmonary exercise testing (CPET) can be helpful in objectively predicting maternal tolerance of the hemodynamic changes of pregnancy. Abnormal heart rate responses to prepregnancy CPET are strongly associated with maternal cardiac and neonatal complications, possibly because the impaired ability to augment heart rate during exercise suggests that cardiac output will not be adequately increased during pregnancy.[21,22]

After thoroughly discussing maternal cardiac risks associated with pregnancy, attention should be turned to discussing fetal risks. Risk of transmission of CHD to future children is a common question and is variable depending on maternal CHD type, presence of a syndrome, and multiple other factors but overall is in the range of 3% to 7%, and slightly higher when the affected parent is the mother.[23–25] Although most CHD is not associated with a defined syndrome (eg, trisomy 21) or definitive single-gene mendelian inheritance (eg, Holt-Oram syndrome), care should be taken to obtain careful personal and family histories of both cardiac and extracardiac manifestations to help identify more subtle syndromes, such as Noonan syndrome or DiGeorge syndrome, which may have well-defined inheritance patterns.[24] Given the expanding knowledge of the genetic causes of CHD and the increasing number of genetic testing options, involving a genetic counselor before conception is ideal to facilitate discussion of risks as well as arranging appropriate testing.

In addition to the risk of genetic transmission, neonatal complications are more common than in the general population and are highly correlated with baseline maternal cardiac status (poor functional status, cyanosis, mechanical valves, and so forth) and maternal pregnancy complications.[14] Additional maternal comorbidities such as obesity, diabetes, and smoking confer additional, likely additive, risks and should be addressed before conception as much as possible.

PRENATAL CARE

Multidisciplinary management of pregnancy for women with CHD is extremely important in optimizing coordination of care, setting appropriate expectations, and minimizing complications. Key topics that should be discussed early in pregnancy and documented in the electronic medical record for future caregivers to see should include medication plans, especially for anticoagulants; planned schedule of cardiac evaluation and testing during pregnancy and in the peripartum time period; recommended location of delivery; ideal mode of delivery; and any notable peripartum considerations. In addition, fetal echocardiography should be offered to all mothers with CHD.

Prenatal Maternal Monitoring

In general, frequency of maternal cardiac evaluation during pregnancy is related to a woman's cardiac status and risk. Most women should have routine echocardiography screening performed in the early third trimester, when volume load and cardiac output are the highest. Most women should also have an echocardiogram performed in the first trimester unless it has been recently performed. Evaluation of valve and ventricular function as well as any other particular areas of interest, such as aortic size, can help tailor the delivery plan.

Routine screening with brain natriuretic peptide (BNP) levels or N-terminal-proBNP levels is becoming increasing common to help predict peripartum complications. When measured at 20 weeks' gestation, proBNP levels less than 128 pg/dL had a 95% negative predictive value for adverse cardiac events.[26]

LABOR AND DELIVERY

Given the significant hemodynamic changes associated with labor and delivery, it is a stressful time for both mothers with CHD and their care teams. Careful planning before presentation in labor is critical in optimizing labor and delivery for both maternal and fetal outcomes. Based on the degree of monitoring and interdisciplinary care anticipated around the time of delivery, the ideal hospital for delivery can be identified, taking into consideration the balance of proximity to patient home and need for subspecialty care.

Mode of Delivery

Although many women with CHD have historically been told the cesarean delivery is the safer mode of delivery for women with heart disease, it is now widely accepted that vaginal delivery is preferred in the absence of obstetric and/or fetal reasons for cesarean delivery.[27] With early epidural placement and assisted second stage of labor, the overall risk of complications is lower for vaginal versus cesarean delivery. Although overall safe, a cesarean section is a major abdominal surgery with significant blood volume shifts. Most higher-risk mothers are safe for a trial of labor with excellent anesthesia and pain management. The list of indications for primary cesarean section is short and in general consists of patients who would most likely have been counseled to avoid pregnancy, such as those with severe pulmonary hypertension, aortopathy with dilated aortas, severe left heart obstruction, and severe ventricular dysfunction.

Anesthesia Considerations and Monitoring

Early epidural placement with careful titration is important in allowing appropriate pain management and a more controlled stage 2 of labor while minimizing significant fluctuations in blood pressure as much as possible. This approach also allows for easier transition should cesarean delivery become necessary, minimizing the risk of needing to convert to general anesthesia.

Maternal monitoring should be agreed on by the anesthesia, obstetric, and cardiology teams on an individual basis. Although many patients need routine perinatal monitoring, those at high risk of arrhythmias may benefit from telemetry monitoring. Invasive monitoring with arterial lines or pulmonary artery catheters is rarely indicated.

Endocarditis Prophylaxis

The 2007 AHA guidelines for endocarditis prophylaxis state that procedures involving the genitourinary systems do not require antibiotic prophylaxis, regardless of the underlying heart disease or patient history.[28] In a meta-analysis reviewing all reported cases of prenatal and peripartum endocarditis, only 11 cases of CHD-related endocarditis were published from 1988 to 2012.[29] Furthermore, only 28% of all reported cases (n = 25), regardless of CHD, occurred in the postpartum period,[29] suggesting that peripartum endocarditis prophylaxis would have an exceptionally high number needed to treat.

POSTPARTUM CARE AND FOLLOW-UP

Although labor and delivery require significant hemodynamic changes, the risk of serious cardiac events is higher in the postpartum period.[7] It takes several weeks for hemodynamics to gradually return to baseline, and this occurs during a time when new mothers have many infant-related concerns that may detract from focus on their own well-being. Individualized plans for in-hospital postpartum monitoring, timing of discharge from the hospital, counseling on concerning signs and symptoms after discharge home, and outpatient cardiology follow-up, usually no later than 6 weeks postpartum with repeat echocardiogram, are extremely important in avoiding preventable complications.

SPECIFIC LESIONS
Repaired Simple Lesions

In general, women with repaired simple disease such as atrial septal defect (ASD), ventricular septal defect, and patent ductus arteriosus are appropriate for routine obstetric care if they are clinically well without other ongoing cardiac complications such as arrhythmias, valvular disease, or ventricular dysfunction. For example, repaired ASDs were shown to have no increased risk of complications compared with a control group of women without CHD in a national registry study in Belgium.[30] These women can often be followed by general obstetric teams after being evaluated by a CHD cardiologist early in pregnancy to confirm stable physiologic status.

Shunts
Atrial septal defects and partial anomalous pulmonary venous return

Unrepaired shunting lesions occurring upstream from the tricuspid valve are often asymptomatic or minimally symptomatic for many years and frequently diagnosed during pregnancy because of increased cardiac output. Low-pressure left-to-right shunting leads to right heart volume overload and eventual dilatation if there is sufficient flow. If the lesion is thought to be hemodynamically significant before pregnancy, as shown by right heart dilatation or arrhythmias, repair before conception should be considered.

Maternal risks There is an increased risk of arrhythmias caused by right atrial dilatation, although most are well tolerated. Even in patients with all left-to-right shunting across an ASD at baseline, there is a theoretic risk of paradoxic embolus during the hypercoagulable state of pregnancy and the postpartum period.[23,30] In addition, there is increased risk of preeclampsia (~7%, odds ratio 3.5 in 1 study).[31]

Fetal risks There is increased risk of small-for-gestational-age infants.[30]

Management considerations Echocardiography should be performed early in pregnancy to evaluate for pulmonary hypertension. Evaluation for

arrhythmia is reasonable for complaints of palpitations. Counseling about the risk of thromboembolic disease with prompt evaluation for concerning symptoms should be performed. Meticulous attention to the prevention of deep vein thrombus is required in the peripartum period. The use of intravenous filters should be considered during labor and delivery to reduce the risk for paradoxic embolism. The use of aspirin or prophylactic anticoagulation with low-molecular-weight heparin should be considered in high-risk patients. Routine screening for preeclampsia and intrauterine growth restriction is appropriate.

Ventricular septal defect and patent ductus arteriosus

Small unrepaired shunting lesions occurring downstream from the tricuspid valve are usually asymptomatic, although significant murmurs may be present. If the lesions are hemodynamically significant enough to cause left heart dilatation, careful evaluation for pulmonary hypertension should be performed.

Maternal risks Overall, small posttricuspid shunts are well tolerated during pregnancy.

Fetal risks There is increased risk of small-for-gestational-age infants.[32]

Management considerations Echocardiography should be performed early in pregnancy to evaluate for pulmonary hypertension. Routine screening for preeclampsia and intrauterine growth restriction is appropriate.

Atrioventricular septal defects

Care for women with atrioventricular septal defects (AVSDs) during pregnancy depends on the type of lesions that are present either before repair or as residua from previous surgery. Determination of atrial-level and ventricular-level shunting, atrioventricular valve regurgitation, left ventricular outflow tract obstruction, and pulmonary hypertension should be performed early in pregnancy, with management considerations determined by the predominant lesions.

Eisenmenger syndrome

Patients with unrepaired shunting lesions, especially large posttricuspid shunts, may develop pulmonary hypertension caused by increased pulmonary blood flow, ultimately leading to right-to-left shunting through the defect. Given extremely high historical maternal mortality of up to 50%, it has previously been considered a contraindication to pregnancy.[33] However, with careful monitoring and management, contemporary mortality is significantly lower, although morbidity remains high.[34–38]

Maternal risks A recent review including 30 pregnant women with Eisenmenger syndrome described mortality of 16.5% with morbidity and/or complications in nearly all patients, including clinical heart failure, thromboembolic disease, arrhythmia, preeclampsia, HELLP (hemolysis, elevated liver enzymes, and low platelet count) syndrome, and postpartum hemorrhage.[35]

Fetal risks Fetal complications are closely linked with maternal status, including maternal oxygen saturation. Most babies are delivered preterm and in addition many are small for gestational age.[34,35,38,39]

Management considerations Given the significant maternal and fetal risks, termination of pregnancy is recommended. If pregnancy is continued, close follow-up with both cardiology and obstetric teams should be continued throughout pregnancy at an experienced center. Consideration of anticoagulation given the risks of thromboembolic disease is reasonable, although this must be balanced with the risks of bleeding, including hemoptysis. Given the risk of worsened right-to-left shunting with systemic vasodilatation, general anesthesia should be avoided if possible and epidural and spinal anesthetics should be titrated with caution. If available, filters for intravenous lines may decrease the risk of paradoxic air emboli.

Ebstein Anomaly

Ebstein anomaly of the tricuspid valve can range from a mildly abnormal valve with minimal tricuspid regurgitation to a very abnormal and dysfunctional valve and right ventricle. Regardless of the degree of tricuspid regurgitation, pregnancy is usually well tolerated in women with Ebstein anomaly without baseline cyanosis or heart failure symptoms.[40] If they meet criteria for tricuspid valve repair before becoming pregnant, surgical repair should be performed before conception.[10]

Maternal risks
Although most women do well, those with abnormal right ventricular function are at slightly increased risk for heart failure symptoms. Patients with residual atrial-level shunts can develop right-to-left shunting with cyanosis and the potential risk of paradoxic emboli, especially in patient with severe tricuspid regurgitation and impaired right ventricular compliance. Given the often dilated right atrium as well as the frequency of associated Wolff-Parkinson-White syndrome, atrial

arrhythmias are more common in this group than in the general population.[41]

Fetal risks
Fetal loss is increased for mothers with Ebstein anomaly. In successful pregnancies, infants are at increased risk of prematurity.[42]

Management considerations
Monitoring for arrhythmias is reasonable in patients with palpitations or other symptoms. Heart failure symptoms may be exacerbated by fluid retention during pregnancy and should be managed medically.

Tetralogy of Fallot

In women with repaired tetralogy of Fallot, the most common residual lesion is pulmonary regurgitation, which tends to be well tolerated for many years. However, severe pulmonary regurgitation with right ventricular dysfunction have been associated with adverse cardiac events during pregnancy, as have left ventricular dysfunction, pulmonary hypertension, and maternal cardiac medication use.[43–45] As with previous lesions, patients who meet criteria for pulmonary valve replacement or other intervention should ideally undergo repair before conceiving.

Maternal risks
Women with tetralogy of Fallot are at increased risk of supraventricular arrhythmias and progressive right ventricular dilatation during pregnancy, with variable amounts of time needed to recover following delivery.[43–45] Other potential complications include symptomatic heart failure, thromboembolic disease, progressive aortic root dilatation, and preeclampsia.

Fetal risks
The risk of fetal loss is increased, with reports of spontaneous abortion in up to 24% of pregnancies.[43,45,46] One study reported a rate of premature birth of 18% of pregnancies, as well as a higher perinatal mortality (6%) than previously reported, but these data have not been reproduced.[43] The risk of fetal CHD in mothers with tetralogy of Fallot has been reported to be anywhere from 3% to 7%, with the slightly higher than average transmission potentially caused by undiagnosed DiGeorge syndrome.[43,45,47] In addition, the rate of noncardiac congenital anomalies is up to twice the national average (6% vs 3%).[45]

Management considerations
Careful medical management of arrhythmias and volume status are keys to decreasing maternal complications. Given the relationship between

tetralogy of Fallot and DiGeorge syndrome, prenatal or perinatal genetic counseling as well as maternal genetic testing may be of increased importance in this population.

Coarctation of the Aorta

Coarctation of the aorta is a narrowing of the thoracic aortic, usually in the region of the patent ductus arteriosus. Women of childbearing age may have undergone a surgical repair, percutaneous intervention, or have undergone no intervention. Angiography of a young woman before and after stenting of aortic coarctation is shown in **Fig. 1**. Most women with coarctation of the aorta tolerate pregnancy well, although overall they are at increased risk for cesarean delivery and longer hospital stay than women with normal aortas.[48,49] Prenatal MRI may be helpful in risk stratification, because women with smaller aortic dimensions have increased risks of complications.[50] Even in the absence of a residual gradient, these women are at higher risk for baseline or exercise-induced hypertension, which should be controlled before conception. Many women have increased aortic gradients during pregnancy caused by increased flow, but these often return to baseline after pregnancy. If there is a family history of cerebral aneurysms, screening should be performed before pregnancy.[10]

Maternal risks
Miscarriage risk is higher for women with coarctation of the aorta, regardless of repair status.[48,49,51] The most significant maternal risks are related to hypertensive disorders of pregnancy, ranging from gestational hypertension to preeclampsia to HELLP syndrome.[48,49] There is also a risk of aortic dissection at the repair site or in other aortic locations, especially the ascending aorta, if the coarctation is associated with a bicuspid aortic valve.

Fetal risks
Infants are more likely to be small for gestational age, especially in women who develop hypertensive disorders of pregnancy.

Management considerations
Left-sided obstructive lesions can amplify in children of affected mothers; this should be included in prenatal or early pregnancy counseling, and fetal echocardiography should be performed in the second trimester. Strict blood pressure monitoring and control should be maintained throughout pregnancy; home monitoring may be helpful, and more frequent clinic follow-up may be needed for women with medication requirements. Women with abnormal aortic dimensions should have careful delivery planning with plans for an epidural and assisted stage II to minimize excessive blood pressure increases.

Transposition of the Great Arteries

Atrial switch procedure
Atrial switch procedures involve baffling systemic venous blood to the left ventricle and the pulmonary venous blood to the right ventricle; this allows for appropriate physiologic blood flow through the body and lungs but leaves the tricuspid valve and right ventricle in the systemic circulation. The Mustard and Senning procedures have been almost entirely replaced by the arterial switch procedure for D-transposition of the great arteries. Although women often begin to experience

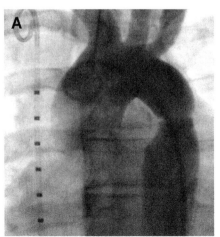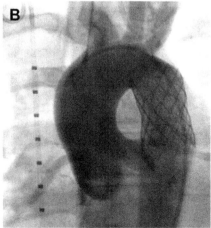

Fig. 1. (*A*) Aortogram in a woman with coarctation of the aortic showing a discrete narrowing in the proximal descending aorta. (*B*) Aortogram after stent placement showing increase in dimension at the coarctation site.

cardiac complications in their childbearing years, these issues are likely to occur with or without pregnancy.[52] Preconception systemic right ventricular function and overall functional status are important factors in counseling. If hemodynamically significant, baffle leaks and/or valvular disease should be addressed before conception.

Maternal risks Historically, women with systemic right ventricles were thought to have significantly increased risk of peripartum mortality, but the contemporary risk remains low overall for women following atrial switch.[53] Although not more common than in matched patients with atrial switch procedures who were not pregnant, atrial arrhythmias, baffle leaks, and thromboembolic events occur in more than half of this population during pregnancy.[52] Pregnancy leads to worsening ventricular function and/or worsening systemic tricuspid regurgitation in about one-quarter of women, which may not resolve after delivery.[52,54]

Fetal risks Many infants are premature and small for gestational age.[52,55]

Management considerations Careful attention should be given to control of atrial arrhythmias, optimization of volume status, and blood pressure control to minimize additional afterload on the systemic right ventricle. Although most women deliver safely vaginally, many require induction or either maternal or fetal indications.[52]

Arterial switch procedure

The arterial switch operation for D-transposition of the great arteries establishes normal ventricular-arterial relationships so the left ventricle delivers oxygenated blood to the systemic circulation and the right ventricle delivers deoxygenated blood to the pulmonary circulation. The coronary arteries are translocated during the procedure in infancy, but coronary complications are often found during childhood. Residual lesions are often related to pulmonary artery stenosis or semilunar valvular disease.

Maternal risks Data are limited because the first generations of patients who underwent arterial switches are becoming pregnant, but several case series showed excellent outcomes without neoaortic dilatation or other complications.[56–60]

Fetal risks Overall, there does not seem to be increased risk for fetal complications compared with baseline other than for transmission of CHD.

Management consideration Alterations in routine management are determined by the presence of residual lesions.

Congenitally corrected transposition of the great arteries

When not associated with other cardiac lesions, corrected transposition of the great arteries (ccTGA) is frequently undiagnosed until the hemodynamic changes of pregnancy highlight the limitations of the systemic right ventricle. It is a rare lesion in which blood flows in appropriate sequence to the lungs and body, but via the morphologic left ventricle in the subpulmonary position and the morphologic right ventricle in the systemic position. As with patients following the atrial switch, systemic right ventricles are often less able to tolerate the increased volume and cardiac output needed during pregnancy. Additional risks may be present because of cyanosis or other associated lesions.

Maternal risks Women with ccTGA are at increased risk of atrial arrhythmias and worsened systemic right ventricular function during pregnancy.[61,62] One small study of longer-term outcomes after pregnancy did not find any increased morbidity, complications, or hospital admissions for women with ccTGA who had completed a pregnancy compared with those who had not been pregnant.[62]

Fetal risks Fetal loss is more common in women with ccTGA, especially those with associated lesions.[63]

Management considerations As with women with systemic right ventricles following atrial switch, control of atrial arrhythmias, optimization of volume status, and blood pressure control to minimize additional afterload on the systemic right ventricle are important throughout pregnancy.

Fontan Circulation

The Fontan procedure is the ultimate palliative procedure for a variety of complex congenital heart lesions. In general, these lesions are single-ventricle lesions with atresia or severe hypoplasia of an atrioventricular valve or ventricle. Although there are a variety of anatomic variations of the procedure, the common result is an anastomosis between the systemic venous return and the pulmonary arteries (**Fig. 2**). This condition results in passive blood flow through the lungs, with increased systemic venous pressures. This passive blood flow to the lungs is also the preload for the single ventricle, with any decrease in venous return leading to a decrease in cardiac output. These hemodynamic derangements lead to unique responses during the increased blood volume and increased necessary cardiac output

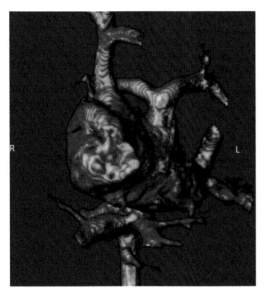

Fig. 2. Three-dimensional cardiac MRI in a patient after an atriopulmonary Fontan procedure showing an anastomosis between the right atrial appendage and the pulmonary arteries.

during pregnancy. In particular, the placenta is uniformly abnormal in Fontan physiology; this may account for the high rates of fetal loss and other complications.[64]

Although maternal mortality for women with Fontan physiology is low, pregnancy-related complications are extremely common. Even without the added hemodynamic stress of pregnancy, the third and fourth decades of life bring complications such as valvular disease, ventricular dysfunction, atrial arrhythmias, and thromboembolic disease; by the time patients with a Fontan are 40 years old, they have the life expectancy of an otherwise healthy 75-year-old.[65–67] Because of these increased complications and decreased baseline maternal longevity, as well as the unclear long-term cardiac effects of pregnancy on the single ventricle, preconception counseling beginning in adolescence is of utmost importance.[68] Medication adjustments; medical and surgical optimization of residual lesions, including right-to-left shunts; and anticipatory guidance about risk stratification and likely complications during pregnancy should be routinely discussed with all women of childbearing age.

Maternal risks

The most frequent maternal complications in patients with a single ventricle are atrial arrhythmias and worsening heart failure symptoms.[69,70] Thromboembolic complications, especially during the hypercoagulable peripartum period, are also extremely common.

Fetal risks

Up to half of all pregnancies in patients with Fontan physiology end in fetal loss.[70–72] Pregnancies that are successfully carried into the third trimester have higher rates of prematurity and small-for-gestational-age infants.[70,72,73]

Management considerations

Close follow-up with cardiology and maternal-fetal obstetrics throughout pregnancy is critical for this high-risk group of patients. Medical management for atrial arrhythmias should be prompt, because sustained tachycardia is poorly tolerated because of passive atrial filling. Medical management of heart failure symptoms such as dyspnea and edema should be addressed using medications with good fetal safety profiles. Given the increased risk of thromboembolic complications, aspirin should in general be continued throughout pregnancy, and early mobility, compression stockings, and sequential compressions devices should be used during hospitalizations and as much as possible during labor and delivery. Given the risk for thrombotic events around the time of delivery, some patients should be considered for full anticoagulation in the peripartum period.

During labor or induction, epidural titration should be slow to minimize systemic vasodilatation, which leads to decreased preload. Vaginal delivery is almost always the preferred mode of delivery because of the increased risks of bleeding and fluid shifts during cesarean delivery. Careful monitoring of respiratory status after delivery of the placenta is important because of effective fluid bolus from autotransfusion.

SUMMARY

Almost all women with CHD can safely carry pregnancies to term and deliver vaginally. Counseling regarding pregnancy risks should begin at an early age and continue through the childbearing years. Pregnant women with CHD should be managed in a multidisciplinary manner, with input from cardiology, maternal-fetal medicine, and anesthesiology. A written plan of care should be created and documented in the medical record such that it is visible to all on-call providers. Caregivers should be aware that maternal risks do not end with the delivery of the child and that continued vigilance is required in the postpartum period. Patients should have individualized counseling and care based on the anatomic diagnosis as well as the physiologic status.

CLINICS CARE POINTS

- Preconception counseling should include discussions about cardiac optimization, medication changes needed before pregnancy, genetic transmission of CHD, and patient-specific maternal and fetal risks.
- Multidisciplinary care throughout pregnancy should include adult congenital cardiology, obstetrics, and anesthesia, most especially for higher-risk patients.
- Lesion-specific hemodynamic considerations and risk stratification should drive management decisions during pregnancy, labor, and delivery.
- With rare exceptions, vaginal delivery is the preferred mode of delivery.

DISCLOSURE

The authors have nothing to disclose.

REFERENCES

1. Gilboa SM, Devine OJ, Kucik JE, et al. Congenital heart defects in the United States: estimating the magnitude of the affected population in 2010. Circulation 2016;134(2):101–9.
2. Warnes CA, Liberthson R, Danielson GK, et al. Task force 1: the changing profile of congenital heart disease in adult life. J Am Coll Cardiol 2001;37(5):1170–5.
3. Marelli AJ, Mackie AS, Ionescu-Ittu R, et al. Congenital heart disease in the general population: changing prevalence and age distribution. Circulation 2007;115(2):163–72.
4. Marelli AJ, Ionescu-Ittu R, Mackie AS, et al. Lifetime prevalence of congenital heart disease in the general population from 2000 to 2010. Circulation 2014;130(9):749–56.
5. Larsen SH, Olsen M, Emmertsen K, et al. Interventional treatment of patients with congenital heart disease: Nationwide Danish experience over 39 years. J Am Coll Cardiol 2017;69(22):2725–32.
6. Opotowsky AR, Siddiqi OK, D'Souza B, et al. Maternal cardiovascular events during childbirth among women with congenital heart disease. Heart 2012;98(2):145–51.
7. Pfaller B, Sathananthan G, Grewal J, et al. Preventing complications in pregnant women with cardiac disease. J Am Coll Cardiol 2020;75(12):1443–52.
8. Gurvitz M, Valente AM, Broberg C, et al. Prevalence and predictors of gaps in care among adult congenital heart disease patients: HEART-ACHD (The Health, Education, and Access Research Trial). J Am Coll Cardiol 2013;61(21):2180–4.
9. Canobbio MM. Health care issues facing adolescents with congenital heart disease. J Pediatr Nurs 2001;16(5):363–70.
10. Stout KK, Daniels CJ, Aboulhosn JA, et al. 2018 AHA/ACC guideline for the management of adults with congenital heart disease: executive summary: a report of the American College of cardiology/American heart association task force on clinical Practice guidelines. J Am Coll Cardiol 2019;73(12):1494–563.
11. Alshawabkeh L, Economy KE, Valente AM. Anticoagulation during pregnancy: evolving Strategies with a focus on mechanical valves. J Am Coll Cardiol 2016;68(16):1804–13.
12. Drenthen W, Boersma E, Balci A, et al. Predictors of pregnancy complications in women with congenital heart disease. Eur Heart J 2010;31(17):2124–32.
13. Siu SC, Sermer M, Colman JM, et al. Prospective multicenter study of pregnancy outcomes in women with heart disease. Circulation 2001;104(5):515–21.
14. Regitz-Zagrosek V, Blomstrom Lundqvist C, Borghi C, et al. ESC guidelines on the management of cardiovascular diseases during pregnancy: the task force on the management of cardiovascular diseases during pregnancy of the European Society of cardiology (ESC). Eur Heart J 2011;32(24):3147–97.
15. Thorne S, MacGregor A, Nelson-Piercy C. Risks of contraception and pregnancy in heart disease. Heart 2006;92(10):1520–5.
16. Suwanrath C, Thongphanang P, Pinjaroen S, et al. Validation of modified World Health Organization classification for pregnant women with heart disease in a tertiary care center in southern Thailand. Int J Womens Health 2018;10:47–53.
17. Silversides CK, Grewal J, Mason J, et al. Pregnancy outcomes in women with heart disease: the CARPREG II Study. J Am Coll Cardiol 2018;71(21):2419–30.
18. Balci A, Sollie-Szarynska KM, van der Bijl AG, et al. Prospective validation and assessment of cardiovascular and offspring risk models for pregnant women with congenital heart disease. Heart 2014;100(17):1373–81.
19. Regitz-Zagrosek V, Roos-Hesselink JW, Bauersachs J, et al. 2018 ESC Guidelines for the management of cardiovascular diseases during pregnancy. Eur Heart J 2018;39(34):3165–241.
20. Lu CW, Shih JC, Chen SY, et al. Comparison of 3 risk estimation methods for predicting cardiac outcomes in pregnant women with congenital heart disease. Circ J 2015;79(7):1609–17.
21. Lui GK, Silversides CK, Khairy P, et al. Heart rate response during exercise and pregnancy outcome in women with congenital heart disease. Circulation 2011;123(3):242–8.

22. Kampman MA, Valente MA, van Melle JP, et al. Cardiac adaption during pregnancy in women with congenital heart disease and healthy women. Heart 2016;102(16):1302–8.

23. Bhatt AB, DeFaria Yeh D. Pregnancy and adult congenital heart disease. Cardiol Clin 2015;33(4):611–23, ix.

24. De Backer J, Bondue A, Budts W, et al. Genetic counselling and testing in adults with congenital heart disease: a consensus document of the ESC Working group of Grown-up congenital heart disease, the ESC Working group on aorta and Peripheral Vascular disease and the European Society of Human genetics. Eur J Prev Cardiol 2019;27(13):1423–35.

25. Yokouchi-Konishi T, Yoshimatsu J, Sawada M, et al. Recurrent congenital heart diseases among neonates born to mothers with congenital heart diseases. Pediatr Cardiol 2019;40(4):865–70.

26. Kampman MA, Balci A, van Veldhuisen DJ, et al. N-terminal pro-B-type natriuretic peptide predicts cardiovascular complications in pregnant women with congenital heart disease. Eur Heart J 2014;35(11):708–15.

27. Asfour V, Murphy MO, Attia R. Is vaginal delivery or caesarean section the safer mode of delivery in patients with adult congenital heart disease? Interact Cardiovasc Thorac Surg 2013;17(1):144–50.

28. Wilson W, Taubert KA, Gewitz M, et al. Prevention of infective endocarditis: guidelines from the American heart association: a guideline from the American heart association Rheumatic Fever, endocarditis, and Kawasaki disease Committee, Council on cardiovascular disease in the young, and the Council on clinical cardiology, Council on cardiovascular surgery and anesthesia, and the Quality of care and outcomes Research interdisciplinary Working group. Circulation 2007;116(15):1736–54.

29. Kebed KY, Bishu K, Al Adham RI, et al. Pregnancy and postpartum infective endocarditis: a systematic review. Mayo Clin Proc 2014;89(8):1143–52.

30. Yap SC, Drenthen W, Meijboom FJ, et al. Comparison of pregnancy outcomes in women with repaired versus unrepaired atrial septal defect. BJOG 2009;116(12):1593–601.

31. Bredy C, Mongeon FP, Leduc L, et al. Pregnancy in adults with repaired/unrepaired atrial septal defect. J Thorac Dis 2018;10(Suppl 24):S2945–52.

32. Yap SC, Drenthen W, Pieper PG, et al. Pregnancy outcome in women with repaired versus unrepaired isolated ventricular septal defect. BJOG 2010;117(6):683–9.

33. Presbitero P, Somerville J, Stone S, et al. Pregnancy in cyanotic congenital heart disease. Outcome of mother and fetus. Circulation 1994;89(6):2673–6.

34. Katsurahgi S, Kamiya C, Yamanaka K, et al. Maternal and fetal outcomes in pregnancy complicated with Eisenmenger syndrome. Taiwan J Obstet Gynecol 2019;58(2):183–7.

35. Li Q, Dimopoulos K, Liu T, et al. Peripartum outcomes in a large population of women with pulmonary arterial hypertension associated with congenital heart disease. Eur J Prev Cardiol 2019;26(10):1067–76.

36. Sliwa K, Baris L, Sinning C, et al. Pregnant women with uncorrected congenital heart disease: heart failure and mortality. JACC Heart Fail 2020;8(2):100–10.

37. Yadav V, Sharma JB, Kachhawa G, et al. Successful pregnancy outcome in Eisenmenger's syndrome during pregnancy. Eur J Obstet Gynecol Reprod Biol 2018;223:146–7.

38. Yuan SM. Eisenmenger syndrome in pregnancy. Braz J Cardiovasc Surg 2016;31(4):325–9.

39. Hartopo AB, Anggrahini DW, Nurdiati DS, et al. Severe pulmonary hypertension and reduced right ventricle systolic function associated with maternal mortality in pregnant uncorrected congenital heart diseases. Pulm Circ 2019;9(4). 2045894019884516.

40. Lima FV, Koutrolou-Sotiropoulou P, Yen TY, et al. Clinical characteristics and outcomes in pregnant women with Ebstein anomaly at the time of delivery in the USA: 2003-2012. Arch Cardiovasc Dis 2016;109(6–7):390–8.

41. Franklin WJ, Gandhi M. Congenital heart disease in pregnancy. Cardiol Clin 2012;30(3):383–94.

42. Connolly HM, Warnes CA. Ebstein's anomaly: outcome of pregnancy. J Am Coll Cardiol 1994;23(5):1194–8.

43. Balci A, Drenthen W, Mulder BJ, et al. Pregnancy in women with corrected tetralogy of Fallot: occurrence and predictors of adverse events. Am Heart J 2011;161(2):307–13.

44. Uebing A, Arvanitis P, Li W, et al. Effect of pregnancy on clinical status and ventricular function in women with heart disease. Int J Cardiol 2010;139(1):50–9.

45. Veldtman GR, Connolly HM, Grogan M, et al. Outcomes of pregnancy in women with tetralogy of Fallot. J Am Coll Cardiol 2004;44(1):174–80.

46. Wang K, Xin J, Wang X, et al. Pregnancy outcomes among 31 patients with tetralogy of Fallot, a retrospective study. BMC Pregnancy Childbirth 2019;19(1):486.

47. Meijer JM, Pieper PG, Drenthen W, et al. Pregnancy, fertility, and recurrence risk in corrected tetralogy of Fallot. Heart 2005;91(6):801–5.

48. Krieger EV, Landzberg MJ, Economy KE, et al. Comparison of risk of hypertensive complications of pregnancy among women with versus without coarctation of the aorta. Am J Cardiol 2011;107(10):1529–34.

49. Vriend JW, Drenthen W, Pieper PG, et al. Outcome of pregnancy in patients after repair of aortic coarctation. Eur Heart J 2005;26(20):2173–8.

50. Jimenez-Juan L, Krieger EV, Valente AM, et al. Cardiovascular magnetic resonance imaging predictors of pregnancy outcomes in women with coarctation of the aorta. Eur Heart J Cardiovasc Imaging 2014; 15(3):299–306.

51. Siegmund AS, Kampman MAM, Bilardo CM, et al. Pregnancy in women with corrected aortic coarctation: Uteroplacental Doppler flow and pregnancy outcome. Int J Cardiol 2017;249:145–50.

52. Cataldo S, Doohan M, Rice K, et al. Pregnancy following Mustard or Senning correction of transposition of the great arteries: a retrospective study. BJOG 2016;123(5):807–13.

53. Jain VD, Moghbeli N, Webb G, et al. Pregnancy in women with congenital heart disease: the impact of a systemic right ventricle. Congenit Heart Dis 2011;6(2):147–56.

54. D'Souza R, Silversides C. Pregnancy following atrial-switch repair. BJOG 2016;123(5):814.

55. Canobbio MM, Morris CD, Graham TP, et al. Pregnancy outcomes after atrial repair for transposition of the great arteries. Am J Cardiol 2006;98(5): 668–72.

56. Fricke TA, Konstantinov IE, Grigg LE, et al. Pregnancy outcomes in women after the arterial switch operation. Heart Lung Circ 2019;29(7):1087–92.

57. Horiuchi C, Kamiya CA, Ohuchi H, et al. Pregnancy outcomes and mid-term prognosis in women after arterial switch operation for dextro-transposition of the great arteries - tertiary hospital experiences and review of literature. J Cardiol 2019;73(3): 247–54.

58. Ploeg M, Drenthen W, van Dijk A, et al. Successful pregnancy after an arterial switch procedure for complete transposition of the great arteries. BJOG 2006;113(2):243–4.

59. Stoll VM, Drury NE, Thorne S, et al. Pregnancy outcomes in women with transposition of the great arteries after an arterial switch operation. JAMA Cardiol 2018;3(11):1119–22.

60. Tobler D, Fernandes SM, Wald RM, et al. Pregnancy outcomes in women with transposition of the great arteries and arterial switch operation. Am J Cardiol 2010;106(3):417–20.

61. Connolly HM, Grogan M, Warnes CA. Pregnancy among women with congenitally corrected transposition of great arteries. J Am Coll Cardiol 1999; 33(6):1692–5.

62. Kowalik E, Klisiewicz A, Biernacka EK, et al. Pregnancy and long-term cardiovascular outcomes in women with congenitally corrected transposition of the great arteries. Int J Gynaecol Obstet 2014; 125(2):154–7.

63. Therrien J, Barnes I, Somerville J. Outcome of pregnancy in patients with congenitally corrected transposition of the great arteries. Am J Cardiol 1999; 84(7):820–4.

64. Gentles TL, De Laat MWM. Fontan pregnancy and the placenta: more information needed. Int J Cardiol 2019;289:56–7.

65. Diller GP, Kempny A, Alonso-Gonzalez R, et al. Survival Prospects and Circumstances of Death in contemporary adult congenital heart disease patients under follow-up at a large tertiary Centre. Circulation 2015;132(22):2118–25.

66. Rychik J, Atz AM, Celermajer DS, et al. Evaluation and management of the child and adult with fontan circulation: a Scientific Statement from the American heart association. Circulation 2019. https://doi.org/10.1161/CIR.0000000000000696.

67. Karsenty C, Zhao A, Marijon E, et al. Risk of thromboembolic complications in adult congenital heart disease: a literature review. Arch Cardiovasc Dis 2018;111(10):613–20.

68. Moroney E, Zannino D, Cordina R, et al. Does pregnancy impact subsequent health outcomes in the maternal Fontan circulation? Int J Cardiol 2020; 301:67–73.

69. Khan A, Kim YY. Pregnancy in complex CHD: focus on patients with Fontan circulation and patients with a systemic right ventricle. Cardiol Young 2015;25(8): 1608–14.

70. Garcia Ropero A, Baskar S, Roos Hesselink JW, et al. Pregnancy in women with a fontan circulation: a systematic review of the literature. Circ Cardiovasc Qual Outcomes 2018;11(5):e004575.

71. Cheung YF, Chow PC, So EK, et al. Circulating transforming growth factor-beta and aortic dilation in patients with repaired congenital heart disease. Sci Rep 2019;9(1):162.

72. Bonner SJ, Asghar O, Roberts A, et al. Cardiovascular, obstetric and neonatal outcomes in women with previous fontan repair. Eur J Obstet Gynecol Reprod Biol 2017;219:53–6.

73. Cauldwell M, Von Klemperer K, Uebing A, et al. A cohort study of women with a Fontan circulation undergoing preconception counselling. Heart 2016;102(7):534–40.

Arrhythmias and Pregnancy
Management of Preexisting and New-Onset Maternal Arrhythmias

Dominique S. Williams, MD[a],*, Krasimira Mikhova, MD[b],
Sandeep Sodhi, MD[c]

KEYWORDS

- Pregnancy • Maternal arrhythmias • Arrhythmias • Atrial fibrillation • Supraventricular tachycardia
- Ventricular tachycardia • Structural heart disease

KEY POINTS

- Women with preexisting arrhythmias are at high risk for recurrent arrhythmias and/or exacerbation arrhythmias with pregnancy.
- Arrhythmias may present at any time during pregnancy. Higher risk periods include the latter part of the second trimester, third trimester, and peripartum period.
- New-onset atrial fibrillation and ventricular arrhythmias should prompt evaluation for structural heart disease.

BACKGROUND

Arrhythmias are the most common cardiovascular complication of pregnancy. Hospitalizations due to arrhythmias in pregnancy have increased by 58% from 2000 to 2012, mainly due to a rise in atrial fibrillation.[1] This rise is likely due to the increase in pregnancy in women with structural heart disease. Arrhythmias may present for the first time in pregnancy, and in women with a history of arrhythmias, pregnancy may lead to an exacerbation of a previously controlled arrhythmia. Identification and appropriate management of arrhythmias are of utmost importance in order to optimize maternal and fetal health.

PATHOPHYSIOLOGY

Cardiac output increases by 30% to 50% in pregnancy, heart rate increases by 10 to 15 beats per minute, and peripheral vascular resistance declines. These changes are amplified in multiple gestation pregnancy, with cardiac output increasing by 60% to 70%.[2,3] Physiologic changes peak in the second trimester, and again in labor and delivery where cardiac output increases due to "auto transfusion" with uterine contractions. Sympathomimetic tone is also increased due multiple factors including neurohormonal changes during pregnancy, and pain and anxiety during labor and delivery.[3,4]

Cardiac myocytes have estrogen and progesterone receptors. The downstream effects of estrogen and progesterone on cardiac myocytes is not well understood, but studies have shown these hormones play a role in repolarization.[4] Temporary cardiac remodeling during pregnancy may contribute to the development of arrhythmias. Atrial enlargement and stretch may create a substrate for atrial arrythmias.[5,6]

[a] Cardiovascular Division, John T. Milliken Department of Internal Medicine, Washington University School of Medicine, 660 South Euclid Avenue, Campus Box 8086, St Louis, MO 63110, USA; [b] Cardiovascular Division, Electrophysiology, John T. Milliken Department of Internal Medicine, Washington University School of Medicine, 660 South Euclid Avenue, Campus Box 8086, St Louis, MO 63110, USA; [c] Department of Medicine, Cardiovascular Division, John T. Milliken Department of Medicine, Washington University School of Medicine, 660 South Euclid Avenue, Campus Box 8086, St Louis, MO 63110, USA
* Corresponding author.
E-mail address: dwillia1@wustl.edu

Cardiol Clin 39 (2021) 67–75
https://doi.org/10.1016/j.ccl.2020.09.013
0733-8651/21/Published by Elsevier Inc.

PREMATURE BEATS

Premature atrial and ventricular beats are common in pregnancy, occurring in ~59% of pregnancies in one study.[7] Premature beats are often benign and patient reassurance can be provided. However, in some patients, premature beats can be associated with structural heart disease and further workup and evaluation are prudent.

Premature ventricular contractions (PVC) may be an initial presentation of a cardiomyopathy or lead to the development of a cardiomyopathy. PVC burden has been shown to correlate with left ventricular function. Most cases of PVC-induced cardiomyopathy occur in patients with a PVC burden of greater than 10% in 24 hours.[8] Tong and colleagues[9] performed a prospective case control study of 53 pregnancies in 43 women with a PVC burden of greater than 1%, mean PVC burden of 13.9%, and no structural heart disease. PVCs presented more commonly in the first trimester. In 25 of 53 pregnancies, beta-blocker therapy was initiated due to symptoms and/or a high burden. Adverse cardiovascular events occurred in 11% of pregnancies and included heart failure, and sustained and nonsustained ventricular tachycardia. Pregnancies with adverse cardiovascular events all had a PVC burden of greater than 5%. Adverse fetal events occurred in 13% of pregnancies and included small for gestational age and preterm birth.[9]

Patients with significant symptoms and preserved systolic function should be reassured.[8] Medical therapy for PVCs is indicated for symptoms or in the setting of a reduced left ventricular ejection fraction. First-line therapy with non-dihydropyridine calcium channel blockers or beta-blockers, excluding atenolol, is recommended.[8]

Premature atrial contractions (PACs) have primarily been studied in the nonpregnant population. Frequent PACs (>100 beats in 24 hours) have been shown to increase the risk of new-onset atrial fibrillation, supraventricular tachycardia, and cardiovascular morbidity and mortality in healthy patients and patients with multiple comorbidities. including structural heart disease.[10,11]

SUPRAVENTRICULAR TACHYCARDIA

Supraventricular tachycardia (SVT) is the second most common arrhythmia in pregnancy, occurring in 22 per 100,000 pregnancy hospitalizations.[1] SVT may present at any stage of pregnancy, but commonly presents in the second trimester. SVT presents with sudden onset of palpitations, which may be associated with dyspnea, chest discomfort, or presyncope.

Atrioventricular nodal reentrant tachycardia (AVNRT) and atrioventricular reentrant tachycardia (AVRT) are the most common subtypes of SVT. AVNRT is characterized by dual AV node physiology allowing anterograde and retrograde conduction. In AVRT conduction may occur through the AV node or the accessory pathway. In antidromic AVRT, the tachycardia conducts anterograde down the accessory pathway and retrograde conduction through the AV node, creating a regular wide complex tachycardia. Antidromic AVRT accounts of 5% to 10% of AVRT.[12]

In patients with SVT, electrocardiograms in sinus rhythm are assessed for preexcitation, which may be asymptomatic and intermittently present on electrocardiogram. Findings of preexcitation include a short PR interval less than 120 ms, slurred upstroke of the QRS, and QRS prolongation greater than 110 ms. Concern arises in patients with preexcited atrial fibrillation that may degenerate into ventricular fibrillation. Preexcitation should be considered in patients with SVT who present with syncope or sudden cardiac death.

ATRIAL FIBRILLATION

Atrial fibrillation (AF) is the most common arrhythmia in pregnancy, accounting for 27 per 100,000 pregnancy hospitalizations for arrythmias.[1,13] In a meta-analysis of 7 studies totaling 301,638 pregnancies, AF incidence was significantly higher in women with structural heart disease compared with women without structural heart disease (0.3% vs 2.2%).[14]

Risk factors for AF in pregnancy are similar to risk factors in the nonpregnant state. Obesity and age older than 40 significantly increase risk of AF.[15] Additional risk factors for AF identified in the Registry of Pregnancy and Cardiac Disease (ROPAC) include congenital heart disease, preexisting history of AF, beta-blocker use before pregnancy, and valvular heart disease.[16]

AF in pregnancy is associated with adverse maternal and fetal outcomes. Adverse fetal outcomes include intrauterine growth restriction, respiratory distress syndrome, intraventricular hemorrhage, and higher rates of neonatal intensive care unit admissions. In addition, agents used for rate control may lead to maternal hypotension and decreased placental perfusion, increasing the risk for preterm labor. Adverse maternal outcomes include heart failure and thromboembolic events.[15–17]

Management of AF is similar to the nonpregnant state. In the nonpregnant population, trials have not shown a difference in cardiovascular outcomes and overall mortality between rate and rhythm control strategies.[18,19] There are no data available comparing maternal and fetal outcomes in a rate control versus rhythm control approach. According to the 2018 European Society of Cardiology Guidelines, a rhythm control strategy is preferred for management of AF in pregnancy.[20] Rhythm control allows for lower doses of rate controlling medications, such as beta-blockers, which can associated with hypotension, intrauterine growth restriction, and infant hypoglycemia. Rhythm control can be accomplished with cardioversion and/or antiarrhythmic therapy. Cardioversion is safe in pregnancy and should be considered if AF does not terminate within 24 hours of onset.[21,22] Cardioversion within 48 hours of AF onset does not negate the need for therapeutic anticoagulation.[23] Cardioversion results in atrial stunning and activation prothrombotic factors.[24] Thromboembolic events are highest the first month following cardioversion; thus, anticoagulation should be continued for a minimum of 4 weeks following cardioversion. Extended or long-term anticoagulation should be based on the patients' risk factors for thromboembolic events.[23,25,26] If the onset of AF cannot be determined with accuracy, transesophageal echocardiogram should be performed before cardioversion.

In nonpregnant women, the CHADS2 VASC Score (congestive heart failure, hypertension, age $\geq$ 75 years, diabetes mellitus, stroke or transient ischemic attack, vascular disease, age 65 to 74 years, sex category) guides anticoagulation management in AF. Therapeutic anticoagulation in recommended in patients with a nonsex CHADS2VASC score greater than 1.[23] The CHADS2VASc score is often used in AF in pregnancy; however, it has not been validated in pregnant women. There are case reports of left atrial appendage thrombus in pregnancy with persistent AF and structurally normal hearts.[27] Aspirin, therapeutic anticoagulation, and prophylactic enoxaparin have been reported in the literature. Antithrombotic therapy for AF in pregnancies varies. Use of aspirin, therapeutic anticoagulation, prophylactic enoxaparin and no therapy have all been reported.[27] If aspirin is prescribed for AF in pregnancy, the dose should not exceed 162 mg. Full-dose aspirin increases the risk of premature closure of the ductus arteriosus.

INAPPROPRIATE SINUS TACHYCARDIA

Inappropriate sinus tachycardia (IST) may present during pregnancy and can be difficult to distinguish from postural orthostatic tachycardia syndrome as well as the physiologic increase in heart rate with pregnancy. During pregnancy, the heart rate increases by 10 to 20 beats per minute but the resting heart rate rarely exceeds greater than 95 beats per minute.[28] IST is characterized by an elevated resting heart rate greater than 100 beats per minute or an average heart rate of greater than 90 beats per minute over 24 hours in the absence of secondary causes. Symptoms of IST include palpitations, fatigue, chest discomfort, dizziness, and poor exercise tolerance due to exaggerated rise in heart rate. In published case reports, IST appears to be well tolerated without adverse of maternal or fetal outcomes.[29,30]

VENTRICULAR TACHYCARDIA

Ventricular arrhythmias (VA) pose a significant risk to maternal and fetal morbidity and mortality. VAs most commonly occur in the setting of structural heart disease, ischemia, inherited arrhythmia syndromes, or QT prolongation due to drugs or electrolyte abnormalities. In an ROPAC study of 2966 pregnancies (56% congenital heart disease, 32% valvular heart disease), VAs occurred in 1.4%. Predictors of VAs included New York Heart Association Class greater than 1 before pregnancy and moderate/severe left ventricular dysfunction. There was a trend toward higher mortality in women with VAs (2.4% vs 0.3%, $P = .15$).[31] VAs are more likely to occur in women with a prior history of VAs.

Arrhythmogenic Right Ventricular Cardiomyopathy

Arrhythmogenic right ventricular cardiomyopathy (ARVC) is characterized by fibrofatty displacement and thinning of the myocardium leading to ventricular enlargement and dysfunction. ARVC predominantly affects the right ventricle but left ventricular dysfunction may also occur. The degree of ventricular dysfunction correlates with outcome. ARVC may be symptomatic or present with PVCs, ventricular tachycardia or sudden cardiac death. VAs often present before ventricular dysfunction. In patients with ARVC, VAs are often triggered by increased adrenergic activity, such as exercise.[32] Adverse cardiovascular events are not uncommon during pregnancy in women with ARVC. Wu and colleagues[33] reviewed 224 pregnancies in 120 women with ARVC. Ninety-one (76%) women had pregnancies before the diagnosis of ARVC. Adverse events occurred in 12 pregnancies and included VAs and heart failure. Women at highest risk of adverse outcomes had earlier onset of symptoms and left ventricular dysfunction (50% vs 60%, $P = .004$). In the women who became pregnant after being diagnosed with ARVC, there was no significant change in ventricular remodeling or function 1 year postpartum.[33] In a study by Hodes and colleagues[34] of 26 women with ARVC and 39 pregnancies, 5% developed heart failure and 13% developed VAs.

Hypertrophic Cardiomyopathy

Hypertrophic cardiomyopathy (HCM) is due to mutations in genes encoding sarcomere proteins, leading to increased left ventricular wall thickness and mass in the absence of secondary causes. It is inherited in an autosomal dominant manner and may occur with or without LVOT obstruction. Heart failure, arrhythmias, stroke, and sudden cardiac death account for most cardiovascular morbidity and mortality in HCM. In the ROPAC registry, VAs occurred in 22% of women with HCM with implantable cardioverter-defibrillators. There was no significant increase in VAs in women with HCM and no implantable cardioverter defibrillator.[31] In a pooled cohort of 9 studies with 207 women with HCM and 408 pregnancies, maternal mortality was less than 1% and 30% of pregnancies were associated with worsening symptoms or arrythmias. Adverse fetal outcomes included spontaneous abortion, stillbirth, and premature birth. Maternal deaths were due to sudden cardiac death.[35] Validated risk factors of sudden cardiac death in HCM should be considered when counseling women on adverse cardiovascular outcomes with pregnancy.

Inherited Arrhythmia Syndromes

Inherited arrhythmia syndromes (IAS) include congenital long QT syndrome (LQTS), catecholaminergic polymorphic ventricular tachycardia (CPVT), Brugada syndrome, short QT syndrome, idiopathic ventricular fibrillation, and early repolarization syndrome. Data on IAS and pregnancy outcomes is limited as few studies specify types of IAS. IAS is not an absolute contraindication to pregnancy. LQTS is the most common channelopathy, occurring in 1 in 2000. QTc greater than 500 ms and severe genotype (LQT2 or LQT3) is associated with high risk of torsades de pointes.[36,37] In a study of 136 pregnancies in 76 women with LQTS and mean QTc 515 ms, 10.3% of pregnancies were associated with VAs. The increased risk of VAs persisted 9 months postpartum. Beta-blocker therapy was protective of VAs during pregnancy and postpartum.[38] Beta-blockers are a Class I indication in LQTS and should be continued in pregnancy and postpartum.[39]

Catecholaminergic Polymorphic Ventricular Tachycardia

CPVT is a rare inherited arrhythmia syndrome that often presents as syncope, VAs, or sudden death in the setting of exercise or an emotional stressor in the absence of structural heart disease or prolonged QT interval. Polymorphic VT, bidirectional VT and ventricular fibrillation are characteristic of CPVT. CPVT mimics LQT1 and is not uncommonly misdiagnosed as LQT1 despite a normal QTc interval. Medical therapy for CVPT includes nonselective beta-blockers and flecainide. Nadolol is the preferred beta-blocker in CPVT.[39]

BRADYARRHYTHMIAS

Bradyarrhythmias are uncommon in pregnancy. If present, they are often due to chronotropic incompetence or high-degree atrioventricular block, which is often present before pregnancy. Women with repaired congenital heart disease or prior cardiac surgery are at an increased risk for bradyarrhythmias. In a study of 25 pregnancies in 18 women, those with untreated atrioventricular block were more likely to have progression in conduction disease with pregnancy. Women with new-onset atrioventricular block were more likely to require intervention compared with women with stable atrioventricular block before pregnancy.[40]

DIAGNOSIS AND MANAGEMENT

Clinical evaluation should be performed in a stepwise approach starting with a detailed clinical history, obstetric history, family history and physical examination. Red flags include exertional syncope, syncope triggered by emotional stress and/or auditory stimuli, palpitations associated with anginal chest pain or syncope, and a family history of sudden cardiac death.

An electrocardiogram should be obtained in all patients with specific attention to signs of preexcitation, pathologic q waves, ventricular hypertrophy, and conduction delays and intervals. Mobile cardiac telemetry or Holter monitoring should be considered based on the frequency of symptoms. Use of implantable loop recorders in pregnancy have been reported. In a study of 40 pregnant women, implantable loop recorders increased detection of arrhythmias and led to changes in management.[41] Identification of arrhythmias or frequent premature ventricular should prompt assessment of structural heart disease. Identification of structural heart disease affects risk of cardiovascular complications with pregnancy and medical therapy. Transthoracic echocardiogram is readily available and can be performed with contrast enhancement in pregnancy. Exercise stress testing or advanced imaging should be considered based on the clinical scenario (**Table 1**).

PHARMACOTHERAPY

There are no randomized trials regarding use of cardiovascular disease medication in pregnancy. Most drugs are Food and Drug Administration (FDA) class C or D. Class C drugs have limited data in human pregnancy but have been studied in animal reproduction and shown to have adverse fetal effects. Class D drugs have shown adverse fetal effects when given in pregnancy in humans. Given limited data on pharmacotherapy in pregnancy, risk versus benefit must be considered. Triggers to arrhythmias should be considered before implementation of long-term medical therapy. Triggers include severe electrolytes abnormalities, illicit drug use, supplements, and certain obstetric medications such as terbutaline and magnesium sulfate. Severe hypermagnesemia may lead to cardiac and respiratory arrest. The PR interval and QRS duration increase with plasma levels of 5 mg/dL to 10 mg/dL. Conduction defect and cardiac arrest may occur with plasma levels greater than 10 mg/dL. It is important to remember that to improve fetal and maternal outcomes, maternal health must be prioritized.

Beta-Blockers (Food and Drug Administration Class C)

Beta-blockers increase the risk of intrauterine growth restriction (IUGR), preterm birth, and neonatal hypoglycemia, bradycardia and hypotension. In a cohort study of 18,477 women with hypertension in pregnancy, beta-blocker use in the first trimester was not independently associated with an increased risk of overall malformations or cardiac malformations.[42] Variation in risk of congenital malformation with beta-blocker dose in the first trimester has not been studied.

β1 selective beta-blockers are preferred in pregnancy due to lower rates of IUGR and decreased effects on uterine activity and peripheral vasodilation. Nonselective beta-blockers are associated with higher rates of IUGR. Atenolol is the only beta-blocker listed as FDA Class D due to increased risk of congenital malformations. Use of atenolol is not recommended in pregnancy.[43]

A recent study by Grewal and colleagues analyzed the determinants of birth weight to discern the relative impact of beta-blockers.[44] Of 1757 pregnancies, 404 women were treated with beta-blockers, most commonly metoprolol (72%). Beta-blockers significantly reduced birth weight less than 200 g; however, this is unlikely to be clinically consequential. Metoprolol was associated with the smallest reduction in birth weight by 119 g. Atenolol was associated with the largest reduction in birthweight by 466 g and is not recommended for use in pregnancy.[44]

Calcium Channel Blockers (Food and Drug Administration Class C)

Calcium channel blockers (CCBs) have not been associated with increased risk of congenital malformation. Due to the mechanism of action, CCBs may cause hypotension and tocolysis. Prior studies suggested an increased risk of neonatal seizures with CCB use in the third trimester; however, this was not shown in recent large cohort study with 22,908 pregnancies.[45] Diltiazem has been associated with teratogenicity in animals but this has not been studied in pregnancy. Verapamil is considered safe in pregnancy and breastfeeding.[20]

Digoxin (Food and Drug Administration Class C)

Digoxin predominantly affects the resting heart rate and is often used as an adjunct for rate control in patients treated with beta-blockers or CCBs. Digoxin may also be used in heart failure with reduced ejection fraction. Serum levels of digoxin are not reliable in pregnancy due to an increase in unbound digoxin and an increase in renal clearance.[46] Clinical signs and symptoms should be used in addition with serum levels to assess for digoxin toxicity.

Adenosine (Food and Drug Administration Class C)

Adenosine is safe for use in pregnancy and has not been shown to have adverse fetal effects. Adenosine has a very short half-life, which prevents delivery to the fetus. It is recommended as first-line therapy for acute termination of supraventricular tachycardia in pregnancy if vagal maneuvers fail.[46] An intravenous line should be placed in the antecubital fossa or more proximal, given the short half-life. It is given as a bolus of 6 mg followed by rapid saline flush. Two subsequent doses of 12 mg can be given.[12]

Flecainide (Food and Drug Administration Class C)

Flecainide is a sodium channel blocker used in the treatment of supraventricular tachycardia, atrial arrhythmias and CPVT. Flecainide crosses the

Table 1
Diagnosis and management of arrhythmias in pregnancy

Arrhythmia	Diagnostic Testing	Treatment	Clinical Pearls
Supraventricular tachycardia	Assess for structural heart disease with echocardiography before antiarrhythmic therapy	Vagal maneuvers β-blockers Non-dihydropyridine calcium channel blockers Flecainide Sotalol Adenosine DCCV Catheter ablation	Consider antidromic SVT in differential for a regular wide complex tachycardia
Atrial fibrillation and flutter	Assess for structural heart disease with echocardiography and/or advanced cardiac imaging	β-blockers Non-dihydropyridine calcium channel blockers Digoxin Flecainide Sotalol Dofetilide Amiodarone[a] DCCV Catheter ablation	Consider DCCV for hemodynamically stable AF>24 h Aspirin <162 mg daily Therapeutic anticoagulation in high risk patients (coumadin, LMWH) Preexcited AF: Procainamide, catheter ablation
Sinus tachycardia	Distinguish physiologic tachycardia from inappropriate sinus tachycardia and postural orthostatic tachycardia syndrome	Encourage adequate hydration Compression stockings β-blockers Non-dihydropyridine calcium channel blockers	Avoidance of precipitating factors (eg, alcohol, caffeine)
Premature ventricular contractions	Quantitate PVC burden with Holter monitor Consider assessment for structural heart disease with echocardiography and/or advanced cardiac imaging	Correct electrolyte abnormalities β-blockers Non-dihydropyridine calcium channel blockers Sotalol Dofetilide Amiodarone[a] Catheter ablation	Risk of PVC-induced cardiomyopathy with higher PVC burden
Ventricular tachycardia	Assess for structural heart disease with echocardiography and/or advanced cardiac imaging Consider inherited channelopathies and ischemia	Cardioversion Correct electrolyte abnormalities β-blockers Non-dihydropyridine calcium channel blockers Sotalol Dofetilide Amiodarone[a] Catheter ablation	Avoid QT-prolonging agents Consider antidromic SVT with a regular wide complex tachycardia Consider preexcited AF with an irregular wide complex tachycardia ICD implantation (transvenous or subcutaneous) during pregnancy in qualifying patients

Abbreviations: AF, atrial fibrillation; DCCV, direct current cardioversion; ICD, implantable cardioverter defibrillator; LMWH, low molecular weight heparin; PVC, premature ventricular contractions; SVC, supraventricular tachycardia
[a] Avoid amiodarone use, Food and Drug Administration Class D.

placenta and is present in breast milk. It is used in the treatment of both maternal and fetal arrhythmias. Coadministration of atrioventricular (AV) nodal blockers are recommended in patients with AF and flutter treated with flecainide as there is potential for one-to-one atrioventricular conduction. Flecainide should not be used in patients with coronary artery disease or structural heart disease.[47]

Sotalol (Food and Drug Administration Class B)

Sotalol is a potassium channel blocker with beta-blocker properties. Due to its QT-prolonging effects, there is risk of torsade de pointes. Sotalol exhibits reverse-use dependence on the action potential. As a result, QT-prolonging effects are highest at reduced heart rates. Drug efficacy is reduced at higher heart rates.

Dofetilide (Food and Drug Administration Class C)

Dofetilide is a potassium channel blocker with reverse-use dependence. The QT prolonging of effects are greater when compared with sotalol. Dofetilide must be initiated in an inpatient setting with close monitoring of the electrocardiogram.[47] Providers should pay close attention to drug interactions and avoid coadministration of QT-prolonging agents.

Amiodarone (Food and Drug Administration Class D)

Amiodarone is reserved for refractory and/or life-threatening arrhythmias due to its adverse fetal effects which are independent of dose and duration. Adverse fetal effects include congenital goiter, hypothyroidism, neurodevelopmental abnormalities, and preterm birth. Neonatal hypothyroidism is often transient and has been reported in 23% of neonates exposed to amiodarone.[48] Use of amiodarone is not recommended in women breastfeeding.

DIRECT CURRENT CARDIOVERSION

Cardioversion is safe and effective in pregnancy and should be performed immediately in patients with hemodynamic instability.[21,22] Continuous fetal monitoring and coordination of care with maternal fetal medicine and pediatric is recommended in viable pregnancies. If anticoagulation is indicated, consideration of gestational age and potential need for emergency delivery should play a role in choosing the appropriate agent.

ELECTROPHYSIOLOGY PROCEDURES

Catheter ablation has been performed safely in pregnancy. Catheter ablation is considered in patients with refractory and/or life-threatening arrhythmias that cannot be managed with medical therapy.[20,49] If possible, catheter ablations should be performed in the second trimester with use of echocardiographic guidance to minimize or eliminate radiation exposure. Placement of implantable cardiac-defibrillators (ICD) and pacemakers are safe in pregnancy. ICD shocks have not been associated with adverse fetal effects.[50]

SUMMARY

Arrhythmias, new-onset or exacerbation of preexisting arrhythmias, are the most common cardiovascular complication in pregnancy. A detailed evaluation should be performed in patients with arrhythmias and management should be in place outlining antepartum, intrapartum, and postpartum care. A multidisciplinary approach with cardiology, maternal fetal medicine, pediatrics, and anesthesia is of utmost importance to optimize maternal and fetal outcomes.

CLINICS CARE POINTS

- Arrhythmias are the most common cardiovascular complication of pregnancy, occurring in 68 per 100,000 pregnancies.
- Women with a prior history of arrhythmias are at high risk of recurrence (30%–50%) with pregnancy.
- There are no validated risk models to assess risk of thromboembolic events in nonvalvular AF in pregnancy. The CHA2DS2-VASc score has not been validated in pregnancy. High-dose aspirin increases the risk of premature closure of the ductus arteriosus.
- Ventricular tachycardia should prompt evaluation for structural heart disease, ischemia (eg, pregnancy associated myocardial infarction, coronary spasm), use of QT-prolonging agents, and inherited channelopathies.
- Amiodarone is associated with adverse fetal effects and should be reserved for refractory and life-threatening arrhythmias.
- Cardioversion, catheter ablation, and implantation of cardioverter-defibrillators are safe in pregnancy.

DISCLOSURE

The authors have nothing to disclose.

REFERENCES

1. Vaidya VR, Arora S, Patel N, et al. Burden of arrhythmia in pregnancy. Circulation 2017;135(6): 619–21.
2. Abbas AE, Lester SJ, Connolly H. Pregnancy and the cardiovascular system. Int J Cardiol 2005; 98(2):179–89.
3. Sanghavi M, Rutherford JD. Cardiovascular physiology of pregnancy. Circulation 2014;130(12): 1003–8.
4. Ekholm EM, Erkkola RU. Autonomic cardiovascular control in pregnancy. Eur J Obstet Gynecol Reprod Biol 1996;64(1):29–36.
5. Anneken L, Baumann S, Vigneault P, et al. Estradiol regulates human QT-interval: acceleration of cardiac repolarization by enhanced KCNH2 membrane trafficking. Eur Heart J 2016;37(7):640–50.
6. Goette A, Kalman JM, Aguinaga L, et al. EHRA/HRS/APHRS/SOLAECE expert consensus on atrial cardiomyopathies: definition, characterization, and clinical implication. Heart Rhythm 2017;14(1):e3–40.
7. Shotan A, Ostrzega E, Mehra A, et al. Incidence of arrhythmias in normal pregnancy and relation to palpitations, dizziness, and syncope. Am J Cardiol 1997;79(8):1061–4.
8. Marcus GM. Evaluation and management of premature ventricular complexes. Circulation 2020; 141(17):1404–18.
9. Tong C, Kiess M, Deyell MW, et al. Impact of frequent premature ventricular contractions on pregnancy outcomes. Heart 2018;104(16):1370–5.
10. Chong BH, Pong V, Lam KF, et al. Frequent premature atrial complexes predict new occurrence of atrial fibrillation and adverse cardiovascular events. Europace 2012;14(7):942–7.
11. Lin CY, Lin YJ, Chen YY, et al. Prognostic significance of premature atrial complexes burden in prediction of long-term outcome. J Am Heart Assoc 2015;4(9):e002192.
12. Page RL, Joglar JA, Caldwell MA, et al. 2015 ACC/AHA/HRS Guideline for the management of adult patients with supraventricular tachycardia: a report of the American college of cardiology/American heart association task force on clinical practice guidelines and the heart rhythm society. J Am Coll Cardiol 2016;67(13):e27–115.
13. Katsi V, Georgiopoulos G, Marketou M, et al. Atrial fibrillation in pregnancy: a growing challenge. Curr Med Res Opin 2017;33(8):1497–504.
14. Chokesuwattanaskul R, Thongprayoon C, Bathini T, et al. Incidence of atrial fibrillation in pregnancy and clinical significance: a meta-analysis. Adv Med Sci 2019;64(2):415–22.
15. Lee MS, Chen W, Zhang Z, et al. Atrial fibrillation and atrial flutter in pregnant women-a population-based study. J Am Heart Assoc 2016;5(4):e003182.
16. Salam AM, Ertekin E, van Hagen IM, et al. Atrial fibrillation or flutter during pregnancy in patients with structural heart disease: data from the ROPAC (Registry on pregnancy and cardiac disease). JACC Clin Electrophysiol 2015;1(4):284–92.
17. Henry D, Gonzalez JM, Harris IS, et al. Maternal arrhythmia and perinatal outcomes. J Perinatol 2016;36(10):823–7.
18. Noheria A, Shrader P, Piccini JP, et al. Rhythm Control versus rate control and clinical outcomes in patients with atrial fibrillation: results from the ORBIT-AF registry. JACC Clin Electrophysiol 2016;2(2): 221–9.
19. Wyse DG, Waldo AL, DiMarco JP, et al. A comparison of rate control and rhythm control in patients with atrial fibrillation. N Engl J Med 2002; 347(23):1825–33.
20. Regitz-Zagrosek V, Roos-Hesselink JW, Bauersachs J, et al. 2018 ESC Guidelines for the management of cardiovascular diseases during pregnancy. Eur Heart J 2018;39(34):3165–241.
21. Tromp CH, Nanne AC, Pernet PJ, et al. Electrical cardioversion during pregnancy: safe or not? Neth Heart J 2011;19(3):134–6.
22. Wang YC, Chen CH, Su HY, et al. The impact of maternal cardioversion on fetal haemodynamics. Eur J Obstet Gynecol Reprod Biol 2006;126(2):268–9.
23. Lip GYH, Banerjee A, Boriani G, et al. Antithrombotic therapy for atrial fibrillation: CHEST guideline and expert panel report. Chest 2018;154(5):1121–201.
24. Harada M, Van Wagoner DR, Nattel S. Role of inflammation in atrial fibrillation pathophysiology and management. Circ J 2015;79(3):495–502.
25. Nuotio I, Hartikainen JE, Grönberg T, et al. Time to cardioversion for acute atrial fibrillation and thromboembolic complications. JAMA 2014;312(6): 647–9.
26. Hellman T, Kiviniemi T, Nuotio I, et al. Intensity of anticoagulation and risk of thromboembolism after elective cardioversion of atrial fibrillation. Thromb Res 2017;156:163–7.
27. Sauvé N, Rey É, Cumyn A. Atrial fibrillation in a structurally normal heart during pregnancy: a review of cases from a registry and from the literature. J Obstet Gynaecol Can 2017;39(1):18–24.
28. Loerup L, Pullon RM, Birks J, et al. Trends of blood pressure and heart rate in normal pregnancies: a systematic review and meta-analysis. BMC Med 2019;17(1):167.
29. Belham M, Patient C, Pickett J. Inappropriate sinus tachycardia in pregnancy: a benign phenomena? BMJ Case Rep 2017;2017. https://doi.org/10.1136/bcr-2016-217026.
30. Shabtaie SA, Witt CM, Asirvatham SJ. Natural history and clinical outcomes of inappropriate sinus tachycardia. J Cardiovasc Electrophysiol 2020;31(1): 137–43.

31. Ertekin E, van Hagen IM, Salam AM, et al. Ventricular tachyarrhythmia during pregnancy in women with heart disease: data from the ROPAC, a registry from the European society of cardiology. Int J Cardiol 2016;220:131–6.
32. Haugaa KH, Haland TF, Leren IS, et al. Arrhythmogenic right ventricular cardiomyopathy, clinical manifestations, and diagnosis. Europace 2016;18(7):965–72.
33. Wu L, Liang E, Fan S, et al. Effect of pregnancy in arrhythmogenic right ventricular cardiomyopathy. Am J Cardiol 2020;125(4):613–7.
34. Hodes AR, Tichnell C, Te Riele AS, et al. Pregnancy course and outcomes in women with arrhythmogenic right ventricular cardiomyopathy. Heart 2016;102(4):303–12.
35. Schinkel AF. Pregnancy in women with hypertrophic cardiomyopathy. Cardiol Rev 2014;22(5):217–22.
36. Mazzanti A, Maragna R, Vacanti G, et al. Interplay between genetic substrate, QTc Duration, and arrhythmia risk in patients with long QT syndrome. J Am Coll Cardiol 2018;71(15):1663–71.
37. Priori SG, Schwartz PJ, Napolitano C, et al. Risk stratification in the long-QT syndrome. N Engl J Med 2003;348(19):1866–74.
38. Ishibashi K, Aiba T, Kamiya C, et al. Arrhythmia risk and β-blocker therapy in pregnant women with long QT syndrome. Heart 2017;103(17):1374–9.
39. Al-Khatib SM, Stevenson WG, Ackerman MJ, et al. 2017 AHA/ACC/HRS Guideline for management of patients with ventricular arrhythmias and the prevention of sudden cardiac death: executive summary: a report of the American college of cardiology/American heart association task force on clinical practice guidelines and the heart rhythm society. Circulation 2018;138(13):e210–71.
40. Thaman R, Curtis S, Faganello G, et al. Cardiac outcome of pregnancy in women with a pacemaker and women with untreated atrioventricular conduction block. Europace 2011;13(6):859–63.
41. Sliwa K, Azibani F, Johnson MR, et al. Effectiveness of implanted cardiac rhythm recorders with electrocardiographic monitoring for detecting arrhythmias in pregnant women with symptomatic arrhythmia and/or structural heart disease: a randomized clinical trial. JAMA Cardiol 2020. https://doi.org/10.1001/jamacardio.2019.5963.
42. Bateman BT, Heide-Jørgensen U, Einarsdóttir K, et al. β-Blocker use in pregnancy and the risk for congenital malformations: an international cohort study. Ann Intern Med 2018;169(10):665–73.
43. Tanaka K, Tanaka H, Kamiya C, et al. Beta-blockers and fetal growth restriction in pregnant women with cardiovascular disease. Circ J 2016;80(10):2221–6.
44. Grewal J, Siu SC, Lee T, et al. Impact of beta-blockers on birth weight in a high-risk cohort of pregnant women with CVD. J Am Coll Cardiol 2020;75(21):2751–2.
45. Bateman BT, Huybrechts KF, Maeda A, et al. Calcium channel blocker exposure in late pregnancy and the risk of neonatal seizures. Obstet Gynecol 2015;126(2):271–8.
46. Costantine MM. Physiologic and pharmacokinetic changes in pregnancy. Front Pharmacol 2014;5:65.
47. January CT, Wann LS, Alpert JS, et al. 2014 AHA/ACC/HRS guideline for the management of patients with atrial fibrillation: executive summary: a report of the American College of Cardiology/American heart association task force on practice guidelines and the heart rhythm society. Circulation 2014;130(23):2071–104.
48. Lomenick JP, Jackson WA, Backeljauw PF. Amiodarone-induced neonatal hypothyroidism: a unique form of transient early-onset hypothyroidism. J Perinatol 2004;24(6):397–9.
49. Driver K, Chisholm CA, Darby AE, et al. Catheter ablation of arrhythmia during pregnancy. J Cardiovasc Electrophysiol 2015;26:698–702.
50. Miyoshi T, Kamiya CA, Katsuragi S, et al. Safety and efficacy of implantable cardioverter-defibrillator during pregnancy and after delivery. Circ J 2013;77(5):1166–70.

Hypertensive Disorders of Pregnancy

Apurva M. Khedagi, MS[a], Natalie A. Bello, MD, MPH[b],*

KEYWORDS

- Hypertensive disorders of pregnancy • Blood pressure • Hemodynamics • Preeclampsia
- Antihypertensive medications • Maternal mortality

KEY POINTS

- Hypertensive disorders of pregnancy (HDPs) include chronic hypertension, gestational hypertension, preeclampsia, and chronic hypertension with superimposed preeclampsia.
- American College of Obstetricians and Gynecologists (ACOG) defines hypertension in pregnant women as clinic systolic and diastolic blood pressure greater than or equal to 140 and/or 90 mm Hg. Severe-range hypertension, a medical emergency, is defined as blood pressure greater than or equal to 160 and/or 110 mm Hg.
- Labetalol and extended-release nifedipine are first-line agents for the outpatient management of hypertension in pregnancy. First-line agents for treatment of severe-range hypertension include intravenous labetalol and hydralazine, and oral immediate-release nifedipine.
- Both ACOG and the United States Preventive Services Task Force (USPSTF) recommend the use of low-dose aspirin between 12 and 28 weeks of gestation for women at increased risk of preeclampsia.
- The fourth trimester is a vulnerable time period when postpartum women are at risk for adverse outcomes, and in many states lose access to health care. Expanded fourth-trimester Medicaid coverage has the potential to reduce disparities in care and improve maternal outcomes.

BACKGROUND AND EPIDEMIOLOGY

Hypertension is the most common medical disorder occurring during pregnancy, complicating 5% to 10% of all pregnancies.[1] It is also the leading cause of maternal mortality in industrialized countries, and its prevalence is increasing.[2] From 1998 to 2006, the prevalence of hypertension during delivery hospitalizations increased from 67.2 to 81.4 per 1000 deliveries.[3] This increase may in part be caused by the increasing prevalence of cardiometabolic disease in women of childbearing age.[1] Maternal age more than 40 years, prepregnancy obesity, excess weight gain during pregnancy, and gestational diabetes are all associated with increased risks of maternal hypertension.[4]

An often-overlooked epidemiologic aspect of hypertensive disorders of pregnancy (HDPs) (**Box 1**) is that their prevalence and associated mortalities vary by race and ethnicity (**Fig. 1A**).[4,5] A study of the 2014 to 2015 US birth cohort data noted significant racial disparities in the prevalence of hypertension, with the highest burden in non-Hispanic black women (9.8%) followed by American Indian/Alaska Native (AIAN) (8.9%), and Filipino (7.74%) women compared with 7.2% in white women. Rates of eclampsia follow similar trends (**Fig. 1B**).[4] From 2011 to 2015, in the United States, the overall pregnancy-related mortality was 17.2 per 100,000 live births. Non-Hispanic black women and AIAN women had the highest

a Columbia University Vagelos College of Physicians & Surgeons, 622 West 168th Street, PH 3-342, New York, NY 10032, USA; b Department of Medicine, Division of Cardiology, Vagelos College of Physicians and Surgeons, Columbia University Irving Medical Center, 622 West 168th Street, PH 3-342, New York, NY 10032, USA
* Corresponding author.
E-mail address: nb338@cumc.columbia.edu
Twitter: @nataliebello9 (N.A.B.)

Cardiol Clin 39 (2021) 77–90
https://doi.org/10.1016/j.ccl.2020.09.005
0733-8651/21/© 2020 Elsevier Inc. All rights reserved.

Box 1
Hypertensive disorders of pregnancy

- Chronic hypertension
- Gestational hypertension
- Preeclampsia/eclampsia
- Chronic hypertension with superimposed preeclampsia/eclampsia

mortalities at 42.8 and 32.5 per 100,000 live births respectively.[5] Furthermore, non-Hispanic black women and Hispanic white women with HDPs have a 2-fold greater risk of stroke during delivery admission. Among women with chronic hypertension, the highest risk of stroke was seen among Asian and Pacific Islander women.[6] These variations in hypertension-associated maternal morbidity and mortality likely reflect underlying systemic disparities in access to care and differences in social determinants of health, rather than an underlying physiologic difference between women.

NORMAL PHYSIOLOGIC RESPONSE TO PREGNANCY

Pregnancy is a dynamic process during which there is a marked increase in metabolic demand and hemodynamic adaptations that vary by trimester and regress toward normal during the postpartum period (**Fig. 2**).[7] The major maternal hemodynamic adaptations during pregnancy include increased cardiac output and plasma volume along with a concurrent reduction in systemic vascular resistance. In light of these rapid and

dynamic changes, pregnancy is often considered a physiologic stress test, because insufficient adaptations result in maternal and fetal morbidity and mortality.

The first trimester, from conception to 13 weeks and 6 days of gestation, is associated with an overall decrease in blood pressure of approximately 10%. Significant vasodilation of the peripheral vasculature begins at approximately 5 weeks of gestation, partially caused by increases in estrogen and progesterone levels. In addition, serum concentration of relaxin increases and peaks at the end of the first trimester. Relaxin is a peptide hormone that has an endothelium-dependent vasodilatory effect that results in enhanced nitric oxide production.[8] These changes result in a significant decrease in systemic vascular resistance and blood pressure, and a 50% increase in renal flow and glomerular filtration rates by the end of the first trimester. To maintain adequate blood pressure in this setting, additional maternal hemodynamic adaptations take place. There is an increased sympathetic and as well as maternal baroreceptor sensitivity. In addition, the renin-angiotensin-aldosterone system is activated, counteracting the salt and water loss secondary to renal vasodilatation and leading to an increase in heart rate and cardiac output.[9]

During the second trimester, which is defined as 14 to 27 weeks and 6 days of gestation, there is a plateau in the reduction in systemic vascular resistance, as relaxin decreases to an intermediate value once the uteroplacental circulation is formed, resulting in a sink of low vascular resistance. In addition, arterial pressures reach a nadir during the second trimester, whereas cardiac output continues to increase to 45% above

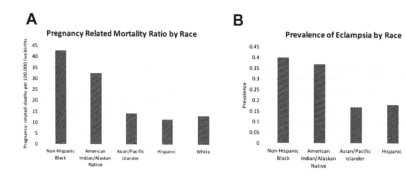

Adapted from Peterson and Singh[5,6]

Fig. 1. Racial disparities in morbidity and mortality associated with hypertensive disorders. (*Adapted from* Singh GK, Siahpush M, Liu L, Allender M. Racial/Ethnic, Nativity, and Sociodemographic Disparities in Maternal Hypertension in the United States, 2014-2015. Int J Hypertens. 2018;2018:7897189 and Petersen EE DN, Goodman D, et al. Vital Signs: Pregnancy-Related Deaths, United States, 2011–2015, and Strategies for Prevention, 13 States, 2013–2017. MMWR Morb Mortal Wkly Rep 2019. 2019;68:423–429.)

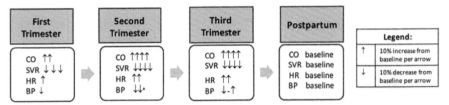

Fig. 2. Hemodynamic changes associated with pregnancy. [a] Blood pressure nadir reached at 18.6 weeks. BP, blood pressure; CO, cardiac output; HR, heart rate; SVR, systemic vascular resistance.

baseline by 24 weeks. Excessive sympathetic activity after 20 weeks of gestation is thought to be associated with gestational hypertension or preeclampsia.

The third trimester lasts from 28 weeks and 0 days of gestation through delivery. There is a peak in cardiac output in the early third trimester and blood pressure begins to increase back to baseline levels. In addition, the ratio between plasma volume and red cell mass peaks at 30 to 34 weeks, resulting in a physiologic anemia. The resultant decrease in blood viscosity further decreases resistance to flow and in turn allows improved placental perfusion to support the growing fetus. In addition, plasma volume increases to 50% greater than nonpregnant values near term, allowing a reserve against blood loss during delivery. Heart rate peaks in the late third trimester, with a 20% to 25% increase relative to baseline.[7] During active labor, systolic and diastolic blood pressures can increase an additional 15% to 25% and 10% to 15% respectively. Cardiac output is increased by 15% in early labor and 25% during the active phase.

MEASURING BLOOD PRESSURE IN PREGNANCY

As previously described, each trimester of pregnancy involves marked hemodynamic changes, so the accurate measurement of blood pressure in pregnant women is essential for the diagnosis and treatment of hypertension. Although considered the gold standard for blood pressure measurement, the mercury sphygmomanometer is rarely available in the modern clinical setting where oscillometric devices are in widespread use. Note that all blood pressure monitor validation protocols recommend devices be specifically validated for accuracy in pregnant women in light of the previously mentioned alterations in the vasculature that occur and that may result in inaccuracies.[10] Best practices for blood pressure measurement include taking blood pressure using an appropriately sized cuff, in a patient with an empty bladder, preferably at least 30 minutes after ingestion of

caffeine or nicotine use, and after 5 minutes of quiet rest. The patient should be comfortably seated with uncrossed feet resting on the floor, in a chair with appropriate back and arm support, with the arm comfortably resting at the level of the heart (**Fig. 3**).[11,12]

DIAGNOSING AND CLASSIFYING HYPERTENSION IN PREGNANCY

In contrast with nonpregnant adults, the diagnosis of hypertension in pregnancy is based primarily on office blood pressure measurements, and concordant diagnostic thresholds between office and ambulatory or home blood pressure measurements have not been defined.[13] American College of Obstetricians and Gynecologists (ACOG) defines hypertension in pregnant women as clinic maternal systolic blood pressure greater than or equal to 140 mm Hg and/or diastolic blood pressure greater than or equal to 90 mm Hg on 2 or more occasions at least 4 hours apart. ACOG further categorizes severe-range hypertension as sustained systolic blood pressure greater than or equal to 160 mm Hg and/or diastolic blood pressure greater than or equal to 110 mm Hg; in this setting, verification should be performed in as few as 15 minutes to avoid delays in treatment[11] (**Table 1**).

Classification of Hypertensive Disorders During Pregnancy

Another distinction in the classification of pregnant women with hypertension compared with nonpregnant adults is that the category of HDP depends on how far along in pregnancy the woman is when first diagnosed. Twenty weeks' gestation is the cut point used, reflecting the return to an approximate baseline blood pressure after the first-trimester decline (**Fig. 4**).[11]

Chronic Hypertension

Chronic hypertension is defined as systolic blood pressure greater than or equal to 140 mm Hg and/or diastolic blood pressure greater than or equal to 90 mm Hg before pregnancy or before

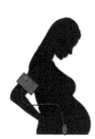

Causes	Effect on Blood Pressure Reading
Improper cuff size	Too large: decreases by 2–10 mm Hg Too small: increases by 2–10 mm Hg
Improper cuff placement	Increases by 5–50 mm Hg
Talking during measurement	Increases by up to 10 mm Hg
Patient positioning: • Unsupported back or improperly supported arm • Feet not resting flat on floor • Arm not supported	Increases by 10 mm Hg
Full bladder	Increases by 10 mm Hg

Fig. 3. Identifying inaccuracies resulting from improper blood pressure measurement.

20 weeks of gestation, the use of antihypertensives before pregnancy, or the persistence of hypertension more than 12 weeks after delivery.[11] Around 3% to 5% of pregnancies are estimated to be afflicted with chronic hypertension.

Gestational Hypertension

Gestational hypertension is defined as systolic blood pressure greater than or equal to 140 mm Hg and/or diastolic blood pressure greater than or equal to 90 mm Hg after 20 weeks of gestation in a woman who was at baseline normotensive.[12] If

a woman diagnosed with gestational hypertension has persistent postpartum increases in blood pressure, she should be reclassified as having chronic hypertension.

Preeclampsia with and Without Severe Features

Preeclampsia is an HDP that is typically associated with new-onset hypertension with proteinuria, which occurs most often after 20 weeks of gestation.[12] Proteinuria is defined by ACOG as (1) 300 mg or more per 24-hour urine collection; (2)

Table 1
Classification of hypertensive disorders of pregnancy

Chronic hypertension	• SBP ≥140 mm Hg and/or DBP ≥90 mm Hg before pregnancy or 20 wk of gestation Or • Use of antihypertensive medication before pregnancy Or • Persistence of hypertension >12 wk after delivery
Chronic hypertension with superimposed preeclampsia	• SBP ≥140 mm Hg and/or DBP ≥90 mm Hg before pregnancy or 20 wk of gestation Or • Use of antihypertensives before pregnancy Or • Persistence of hypertension >12 wk after delivery And • Target organ involvement (develops proteinuria or thrombocytopenia, increased transaminase levels, renal insufficiency, pulmonary edema, or new-onset headache)
Gestational hypertension	• SBP ≥140 mm Hg and/or DBP ≥90 mm Hg after 20 wk of gestation in a woman who was at baseline normotensive
Preeclampsia	• SBP ≥140 mm Hg and/or DBP ≥90 mm Hg after 20 wk of gestation in a woman who was at baseline normotensive and develops proteinuria or thrombocytopenia, increased transaminase levels, renal insufficiency, pulmonary edema, or new-onset headache (target organ involvement)

Abbreviations: DBP, diastolic blood pressure; SBP, systolic blood pressure.

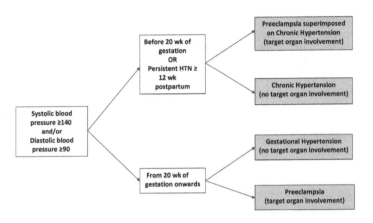

Fig. 4. Classification of hypertensive disorders in pregnancy. HTN, hypertension.

protein to creatinine ratio greater than or equal to 0.3 mg/dL; or (3) a dipstick reading of 2+ if quantitative methods are not available. However, preeclampsia can also manifest in the absence of proteinuria, and additional diagnostic criteria include (1) thrombocytopenia, defined as a platelet count less than 100,000 × 10⁹/L; (2) impaired hepatic function, defined as transaminase level greater than 2 times the upper limit of normal; (3) severe right upper right quadrant or epigastric pain that is not associated with other diagnoses; (4) renal insufficiency, defined as serum creatinine greater than 1.1 mg/dL or a doubling of serum creatinine level in the absence of other renal disease; (5) pulmonary edema; (6) new-onset headache unresponsive to acetaminophen and not associated with other diagnosis or visual symptoms.

Preeclampsia with severe features is defined as systolic blood pressure of 160 mm Hg or more and diastolic blood pressure of 110 mm Hg or more. The clinical presentation of hemolysis, increased liver enzyme levels, and low platelet count (HELLP syndrome) is a form of preeclampsia with severe features that generally occurs in the third trimester and has been associated with increased maternal morbidity and mortality. The diagnostic criteria for HELLP are (1) lactate dehydrogenase increased to 60 IU/L or more; (2) aspartate aminotransferase and alanine aminotransferase levels increased more than twice the upper limit of normal; (3) platelet count less than 100,000 × 10⁹/L.[12] However, right upper quadrant pain and generalized fatigue are the main presenting symptoms in 90% of cases.

Chronic Hypertension with Superimposed Preeclampsia

Chronic hypertension occurs in 1% to 5% of pregnant women, and 20% to 50% of these women go on to develop superimposed preeclampsia.[14] The

risk of superimposed preeclampsia in women with chronic hypertension is increased in women who are Black, obese, smoke, have a diastolic blood pressure greater than 100 mm Hg, have had chronic hypertension for more than 4 years, and have a history of preeclampsia during a prior pregnancy.[15] The incidence of superimposed preeclampsia is even higher in women with end-organ failure or secondary hypertension and approaches 75%.[16] However, in women with chronic hypertension and baseline proteinuria, superimposed preeclampsia can be difficult to distinguish from worsening chronic hypertension, and a high index of suspicion is required. The presence of new-onset thrombocytopenia or a sudden increase of liver enzyme levels is often the first sign of superimposed preeclampsia in this group.[11]

TREATMENT OF HYPERTENSIVE DISORDERS DURING PREGNANCY

The treatment of HDPs is mostly based on expert opinion and observational studies because there are few randomized controlled trials in this population, which was traditionally considered by institutional review boards to be a vulnerable population. Balancing the risks and benefits of the treatment of increased blood pressure in pregnant women on both the mother and fetus is an important consideration. In turn, the exact blood pressure at which pharmacologic treatment is initiated in pregnant women is the subject of ongoing research. Overall, based on the current evidence, ACOG recognizes that pregnant women with severe hypertension (blood pressure ≥160/110 mm Hg) should be treated with antihypertensives to prevent maternal vascular complications such as stroke and placental abruption.

Chronic Hypertension

There remains a controversy about treatment of pregnant women with chronic hypertension. This article presents the best evidence underscoring the major recommendations for antihypertensive use among pregnant women with nonsevere and severe chronic hypertension. First, a 2014 Cochrane Review of 49 trials noted that treatment of pregnant women with mild to moderate hypertension did not reduce the incidence of complications such as developing preeclampsia, preterm birth, or maternal and fetal mortality. However, treatment did reduce their risk of developing severe hypertension.[17] Second, the 2015 Control of Hypertension in Pregnancy Study (CHIPS) trial, which randomized 987 pregnant women to less tight control (target diastolic blood pressure of 100 mm Hg) versus tight control (target diastolic blood pressure <85 mm Hg) found that tight control of hypertension again reduced progression to severe hypertension.[18] There was no benefit or increased risk of harm to the fetus from tight diastolic blood pressure control, though a secondary analysis found severe hypertension was associated with an increased risk of adverse perinatal outcomes (birth weight <10th percentile, preeclampsia, preterm delivery, increased liver enzyme levels, low platelet count, and prolonged hospital stay) in both arms of the trial, and has been used to promote tighter diastolic blood pressure control in this population.[19] The third pivotal trial is currently ongoing. The Chronic Hypertension and Pregnancy (CHAP) project (clinicaltrials. gov NCT02299414) is a multicenter, pragmatic randomized trial with the primary aim to evaluate the benefits and harms of pharmacologic treatment of mild chronic hypertension in pregnancy treated to a goal blood pressure less than 140/90 mm Hg compared with current ACOG recommendation (no initiation of antihypertensive medication unless blood pressure ≥160/110 mm Hg). It is anticipated that the results of this trial will be available in 2021.

Because the current data show no direct benefit to the fetus with tight control of hypertension, according to ACOG, the initiation of antihypertensive medications is only recommended for persistent chronic hypertension when systolic pressure is greater than or equal to 160 mm Hg or diastolic is greater than or equal to 110 mm Hg. For pregnant women without a prior diagnosis of chronic hypertension with stage 1 hypertension (systolic blood pressure of 130–139 mm Hg or diastolic blood pressure of 80–89 mm Hg) before 20 weeks of gestation, antihypertensive initiation is not recommended.

The effects of continuing antihypertensive therapy for women with chronic hypertension diagnosed previous to pregnancy and with less than severe hypertension remain unclear. The current evidence base is conflicting and, at the current time, this decision is left to the treating physician's discretion. One prospective observational study noted that the discontinuation of antihypertensive treatment during pregnancy did not affect the incidence of preeclampsia or fetal complications such as growth restriction and perinatal death, but it was associated with a higher incidence of severe hypertension, placental abruption, and preterm delivery.[20] Another study found no increase in preeclampsia, placental abruption, and perinatal death with discontinuation of antihypertensive therapy during pregnancy.[21] High-quality, large, randomized controlled trials examining risks and benefits of antihypertensive treatment of both mothers and babies in nonsevere hypertension are sorely needed. The CHAP trial is working to respond to that demand.

Gestational Hypertension and Preeclampsia

The management of pregnant women with gestational hypertension, with no evidence of severe hypertension or progression to preeclampsia, can safely be performed as outpatients. Other than weekly in-office blood pressure monitoring and urine protein excretion, as well as twice-weekly home blood pressure measurements, nonpharmacologic interventions are deemed by ACOG to be appropriate for management. Nonpharmacologic interventions include monitoring activity and diet. However, up to 50% of women with gestational hypertension may develop preeclampsia. Women with gestational hypertension with severe-range blood pressures should start antihypertensive therapy and be managed as women with severe preeclampsia.[12]

PRIMARY AND SECONDARY PREVENTION OF PREECLAMPSIA

Numerous studies have been performed examining potential preventive therapies for preeclampsia. including supplementation with aspirin, calcium, vitamin C, vitamin E, fish oil, garlic, vitamin D, and folic acid. Low-dose aspirin is the 1 agent that has consistently been shown to provide a significant reduction in the risk of preeclampsia.[22] When administered before 16 weeks of gestation, low-dose aspirin (60–150 mg daily) has a modest impact on the risk of preeclampsia, severe preeclampsia, and fetal growth restriction.[23] Therefore, both ACOG and the United States Preventive Services Task Force (USPSTF) recommend the use of low-dose aspirin for women at increased risk of preeclampsia. ACOG recommends women at high risk, or with more than 1 moderate-risk factor, start aspirin

81 mg/d between 12 and 28 weeks of gestation, preferably before 16 weeks, to be continued through delivery.[24] The USPSTF recommends the use of low-dose aspirin (60–150 mg daily) between 12 and 28 weeks of gestation for women with 1 or more high-risk factors and consideration for use in women with more than 1 moderate-risk factor for preeclampsia.[25] High-risk factors for the development of preeclampsia according to both the USPSTF and ACOG include history of preeclampsia, multifetal gestation, chronic hypertension, type 1 or 2 diabetes, renal disease, and autoimmune disease. ACOG and the USPSTF both consider the following moderate-risk factors: first pregnancy, body mass index greater than 30 kg/m^2, family history of preeclampsia, and age greater than or equal to 35 years, whereas the USPSTF additionally recognizes low socioeconomic status, black race, history of low birthweight, and history of adverse pregnancy outcome to be moderate-risk factors. Current evidence does not support the universal use of low-dose aspirin for preeclampsia prevention.[24]

CHOICE OF ANTIHYPERTENSIVE MEDICATIONS IN PREGNANCY

There are no large randomized trials on which to base recommendations for the use of one antihypertensive medication rather than any other. All antihypertensive medications cross the placenta, but there is scant evidence on the impact of most antihypertensive medication classes on pregnancy outcomes and fetal risk. The exception to this is the known teratogenicity of angiotensin receptor blockers, angiotensin-converting enzyme (ACE) inhibitors, and direct renin inhibitors, which are always contraindicated in pregnancy. A large 2017 systemic review and meta-analysis of newborn outcomes after exposure to antihypertensive medications found there were inadequate data to recommend any specific therapy because of methodologic weakness of the available evidence.[26] A 2018 international cohort study with pooled data from 6 countries, the International Pregnancy Safety Study (InPreSS) consortium, found no relative or absolute risks for major congenital malformations, including cardiac malformations, with first-trimester β-blocker exposure.[27]

ACOG recommends the use of β-blockers and calcium channel blockers as first-line agents for the treatment of HDPs. Labetalol, a mixed alpha-adrenergic and beta-adrenergic blocker, is the most common beta-blocker used in pregnancy (**Table 2**).[28] In addition, pindolol and long-acting metoprolol are less studied in pregnancy but are considered acceptable alternatives, especially for women with concurrent heart failure who are chronically treated with metoprolol.[29] Atenolol should be avoided in pregnancy because of its association with a heightened risk of fetal growth restriction and low birth weight.[30]

Extended-release nifedipine, a dihydropyridine calcium channel blocker, is also recommended by ACOG to treat hypertension in pregnant women.[11] Extended-release nifedipine reduces blood pressure within an hour. A 2019 randomized control trial noted that nifedipine reduced blood pressure more rapidly and was easier to administer, although it was equal in efficacy and safety to labetalol.[31]

Alpha-methyldopa has been widely used in pregnant women around the globe because it has a long safety record and is available generically. A follow-up study on children of women treated with methyldopa during pregnancy noted its long-term safety.[32] However, it is less favored in the United States, where other options are readily available because of decreased efficacy compared with β-blockers and its association with adverse effects such as depression.[17]

Second-line agents for the treatment of HDPs include thiazide diuretics and hydralazine. The use of thiazide diuretics can be associated with significant volume depletion within the first 2 weeks, and close monitoring of volume status is recommended. Although this effect has not been noted within randomized control trials, the concern for potential fetal growth restriction or oligohydramnios is the reason thiazide diuretics are a second-line agent.[33] Care should be taken when using hydralazine in pregnancy because approximately half of women have associated side effects, including hypotension, headaches, flushing, tremors, and fluid retention. It is also associated with reflex tachycardia and therefore should never be used in isolation without a nodal blocking agent. A 2003 meta-analysis found hydralazine was more effective in reducing blood pressure than labetalol, but was also associated with more adverse maternal and fetal outcomes because of the unpredictable nature of resultant extreme hypotension in some patients.[34]

Other agents, such as clonidine, can be considered for recalcitrant hypertension but are considered third line. As previously mentioned, the use of ACE inhibitors, angiotensin II receptor blockers, direct renin inhibitors, and mineralocorticoid receptor antagonists are absolutely contraindicated in pregnancy because of their significant associations with fetal renal abnormalities and failure, growth restriction, congenital malformations, and death.

Table 2
Antihypertensive medications for pregnant women with nonsevere hypertension

	Agent	Dose	Side Effects
First line	Labetalol (PO)	100–200 mg BID (increase Q 2–3 d to max dosage 2400 mg/d)	Hypotension, increased liver enzyme Levels, persistent fetal bradycardia, and neonatal hypoglycemia Avoid in asthma because of risk of bronchospasm
	Extended-release nifedipine (PO)	30–60 mg Q day (increase Q 7–14 d to max dosage 120 mg/d)	Severe headache, peripheral edema
	Methyldopa (PO)	250 mg BID or TID (increase Q 2 d to max dose 3000 mg/d)	Sedative, peripheral edema, anxiety, nightmares, dry mouth, hypotension, Contraindicated in depression
Second or Third line	Hydrochlorothiazide	12.5 mg Q day (increase Q 7-14 d to max dosage 50 mg/d)	Volume depletion, fetal growth restriction, oligohydramnios
	Hydralazine	10 mg QID (increase Q 2–5 d to max dosage 200 mg/d)	Tachycardia, headache, flushing, fetal distress, hypotension, and inhibition of labor especially when combined with magnesium sulfate Should never be used in isolation because of reflex tachycardia

Abbreviations: BID, twice a day; PO, by mouth; max, maximum; Q, every; QID, 4 times a day; TID, 3 times a day.

Nonpharmacologic Interventions to Reduce Blood Pressure in Pregnant Women

Moderate exercise can be continued in pregnancy, and ACOG recommends that 30 minutes of moderate exercise several days of the week can offer benefits such as decreased risk of developing gestational diabetes, operative vaginal delivery, risk of cesarean birth, postpartum recovery time, and risk of postpartum depression.[35]

Weight loss and extremely low-sodium diets (<100 mEq/d) are not recommended for the management of HDPs. Overall, evidence is limited, but few studies of diet and lifestyle modification to reduce blood pressure have shown any effects on pregnancy outcomes. A 2020 observational study on the relationship between the DASH (Dietary Approaches to Stop Hypertension) diet and maternal blood pressure in pregnancy found that the DASH dietary pattern was associated with lower maternal blood pressure in women without HDPs.[36] However, in the 2013 executive summary, ACOG reports that there is no adequate evidence that salt restriction reduces preeclampsia risk.[37]

TREATMENT OF SEVERE-RANGE HYPERTENSION AND HYPERTENSIVE EMERGENCIES IN PREGNANCY

Severe-range hypertension is defined as blood pressure values exceeding 160 and/or 110 mm Hg. Hypertensive emergency of pregnancy is classified as (1) acute increase in blood pressures greater than or equal to 160/110 mm Hg, (2) development of symptoms consistent with severe preeclampsia, and (3) symptoms of end-organ damage. Severe hypertension is noted to cause central nervous system injury, and two-thirds of maternal deaths during 2003 to 2005 were caused by cerebral hemorrhage or infarction.[38] Therefore, any pregnant women with acute-onset severe hypertension that is persistent (15 minutes or more) should be initiated on antihypertensive treatment within 30 to 60 minutes to acutely reduce blood pressure. First-line agents include intravenous (IV) labetalol and hydralazine for management of acute-onset, severe hypertension in pregnant women and women in the postpartum period. IV hydralazine has been used for the acute treatment of severe hypertension for more than 65 years and is recommended by ACOG (**Table 3**).[39] In addition,

Table 3
Antihypertensive medications for pregnant women with severe hypertension

Agent	Dose	Side Effects
Labetalol (IV)	5–20 mg (increase every 10–15 min to max ag 220 mg/d)	Hypotension, increased liver enzyme levels, persistent fetal bradycardia, and neonatal hypoglycemia Avoid in asthma because of risk of bronchospasm and congestive heart failure
Hydralazine (IV)	5–10 mg (increase every 20 min to max dosage 30 mg/d)	Severe headache, peripheral edema, flushing, reflex bradycardia, hypotension. Avoid use in isolation because of reflex tachycardia
Immediate-release nifedipine (PO)	5–10 mg (increase every 30 min to max dosage 50 mg/d)	First-line alternative to labetalol only in the absence of IV access for treatment of acute, severe hypertension

Abbreviation: IV, intravenous.

immediate-release oral nifedipine may also be used. Current ACOG guidelines recommend the use of immediate-release oral nifedipine as a first-line alternative to labetalol in the absence of IV access for the treatment of acute, severe hypertension. IV nitroglycerin can also be used in the treatment of severe pregnancy-induced hypertension complicated by pulmonary edema.[40]

If blood pressure remains increased or initial blood pressure is greater than or equal to 180/120 mm Hg, then accelerated maternal and obstetric management should occur. In addition, if the blood pressure exceeds 240/150 mm Hg or there is any evidence of acute end-organ damage, accelerated management by a maternal fetal medicine or a critical care specialist is highly recommended.[39]

IV magnesium sulfate is not recommended as an antihypertensive agent, although it has blood pressure–reducing effects.[41] Magnesium remains the most common seizure prophylaxis in pregnant women with acute-onset severe hypertension, because it has been shown to be more effective than phenytoin, diazepam, and nimodipine in reducing the risk of eclampsia and is the drug of choice to prevent eclampsia in intrapartum and postpartum women.[42] The current preferred dosage is a loading dose of 4 to 6 g intravenously followed by a maintenance dosage of 1 to 2 g/h. The use of nifedipine with magnesium sulfate should be avoided or used cautiously because of the risk of synergistic hypotension.

For women with preeclampsia who have severely increased blood pressure that is unresponsive to treatment, the definitive treatment is delivery. Delivery is always beneficial for the mother but may be harmful to the fetus depending on its gestational age. Decisions weighing the risks of being born premature with the potential benefit of removing the fetus from the preeclamptic environment where it is at risk for intrauterine growth restriction and stillbirth must be made in collaboration with maternal fetal medicine specialists and neonatologists. For women with a preterm fetus who have gestational hypertension or preeclampsia without severe features, continued observation is often appropriate. However, the Hypertension and Preeclampsia Intervention Trial At Near Term (HYPITAT) trial found that women with gestational hypertension and preeclampsia without severe features after 36 weeks who had induction of labor had a significant reduction of adverse maternal outcomes, including HELLP syndrome, eclampsia, pulmonary edema, and placental abruption. In addition, induction of labor versus expectant management resulted in no significant differences in neonatal complications.[43]

THE FOURTH TRIMESTER

The postpartum period, defined as the 12 weeks after delivery, is now commonly referred to as the fourth trimester. Marked fluid shifts occur during the early postpartum period and they are associated with fluctuations in blood pressure.[7] There is an initial decrease in the first 48 hours and subsequent increase during postpartum days 3 to 6 as fluids mobilize. Contributing factors include IV fluid administration and loss of pregnancy-associated vasodilation. The use of nonsteroidal antiinflammatory drugs and ergot derivatives, which are used to treat postpartum hemorrhage, can also contribute to blood pressure variability.[44] Blood volume returns to nonpregnant values by 8 weeks postpartum because of diuresis. Pregnancy-related hypertension should resolve within 12 weeks; for increases in blood pressure beyond this period, clinicians should consider a secondary cause of hypertension because it is found in around 10% of patients.[45]

The weeks following birth are a critical period for a woman and her infant. There are scarce data regarding the evaluation and management of blood pressure in the fourth trimester, although ACOG recommends that women with severe hypertension should have a blood pressure evaluation within 72 hours after delivery, and no more than 7 to 10 days postpartum for women with HDPs.[46] The incidence of new-onset postpartum hypertension is uncertain, with an estimate ranging from 0.3% to 28%. In 1 study of 203 women with planned postpartum inpatient stays of 1 week or longer, 12% of previously normotensive women became hypertensive and more than 50% of women with a hypertensive disorder of pregnancy had a systolic/diastolic blood pressure greater than or equal to 150/100 mm Hg.[47] Since those studies were performed, the length of a hospital admission for delivery has shortened and most women are now discharged within 24 hours of delivery. In addition, many do not return for a blood pressure check until the standard 6-week postpartum visit, leading to missed blood pressure measurements and adjustment of treatment.

Hypertension is a leading cause of postpartum readmission in the United States.[48] More than one-half of pregnancy-related maternal deaths occur in the fourth trimester.[49] Postpartum maternal complications also include de novo postpartum preeclampsia; around one-third of eclampsia occurs postpartum. Women with postpartum preeclampsia most often present with new-onset headaches or visual changes in addition to increases in blood pressure. Early identification and management is pivotal, because these women are at an increased risk of stroke, seizures, pulmonary edema, renal failure, congestive heart failure, and death.[50] Half of all intracerebral hemorrhage caused by preeclampsia occurs in the postpartum period.[51]

As previously discussed, significant racial disparities exist in postpartum complication and readmission rates. Black women with cardiovascular risk factors are more likely to be readmitted postpartum, to have severe morbidity, and to have life-threatening complications, including pulmonary edema and acute heart failure, compared with white women.[52] Many of these complications are related to HDPs, and targeted interventions such as the use of self-measured blood pressure and telehealth may play an important role in prevention of postpartum hypertension and associated complications, such as postpartum stroke.[53] Future studies are needed to examine the impact and acceptability of these interventions.

In addition to the health burden imposed by pre-existing or new-onset hypertension, new mothers are often faced with other medical concerns, such as pain, depression, and anxiety. Despite the fourth trimester being a pivotal time of transition in the health of postpartum women and newborn infants, it is also frequently a time of health care transition and loss of coverage for many US women, which likely contributes to high rates of maternal mortality as well as disparities in care. Medicaid is the largest single payer of maternity care, covering 43% of all births in the United States in 2017. However, postpartum pregnancy-related coverage for mothers only lasts 60 days into the fourth trimester. Thirty-six states and Washington DC have expanded Medicaid under the Affordable Care Act (ACA), allowing pregnant women to remain covered beyond this period, but in the 14 non–Medicaid expansion states, many new mothers become uninsured because they no longer meet Medicaid income eligibility requirements (**Fig. 5**).[54,55] These women fall out of care and are at an even higher risk for adverse outcomes; uninsured women are more likely to have advanced-stage diseases such as HDPs and higher associated mortality.[56,57] At baseline, pregnant women with Medicaid have an increased risk for complications in pregnancy and poor fetal outcomes compared with women with private insurance, thus the most vulnerable women are exposed to even greater adversity when they lose coverage.[57] Although a 2019 observational study of births from 2011 to 2016 found state Medicaid expansion did not result in significant changes in rates of low birth weight or preterm births, it did result in the reduction of health disparities experienced by black infants.[58] Further work is needed to examine the effects of Medicaid expansion on maternal health in the fourth trimester.

If all states were to implement Medicaid expansion, the percentage of uninsured women aged 19 to 64 years could decrease from 20% to 8%.[59] ACOG fully supports the expansion of Medicaid as proposed in the ACA to help reduce health disparities and improve outcomes.[57] Many steps were taken in 2019 to ensure that mothers were able to have Medicaid coverage through 12 months postpartum, including the passage of the bipartisan legislation H.R. 4996, the Helping

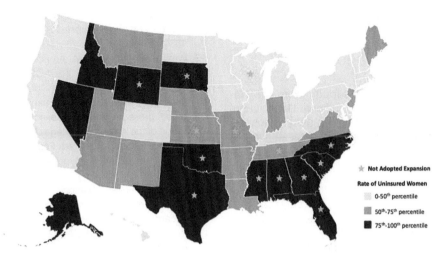

Fig. 5. Map of the United States showing the relationship between rate of uninsured women by state in 2019 and the Medicaid expansion status of the state as of March 2020. (*Data from* Status of State Medicaid Expansion Decisions: Interactive Map. Kaiser Family Foundation. Published 2020. Accessed 2020 and America's Health Rankings analysis of U.S. Census Bureau. United Health Foundation. Published 2019. Accessed2020.)

MOMs Act. Expanded fourth-trimester coverage is a pivotal part of care for pregnant women and new mothers, and further legislative steps need to be taken to ensure equitable outcomes for all women in the United States.

HYPERTENSIVE DISORDERS DURING PREGNANCY AND FUTURE CARDIOVASCULAR RISK

HDPs are associated with an increased risk of complications for both mother and baby during pregnancy and beyond.[60] Whether the HDP itself leads to increased risk or it is merely a marker of underlying increased risk remains an area of intense debate and ongoing research. Despite this debate, it is irrefutable that a history of HDP is associated with an increased risk of future maternal myocardial infarction, heart failure, chronic hypertension, and stroke.[61] In addition, the severity of preeclampsia has been shown to be positively correlated with severity of cardiovascular disease and earlier age of onset of disease.[62] These findings have led many professional societies, including the American Heart Association, American College of Cardiology, American Stroke Association, and ACOG, to include preeclampsia as a clinical risk factor that should be screened for as part of a comprehensive cardiovascular risk assessment.[12,63] The increased time between diagnosis of HDP and management is associated with an increased risk of maternal cardiovascular risk.[64] Therefore, early identification and treatment of women at risk for and with HDPs is important to prevent not only immediate but also future

mortality and morbidity. As such, the authors recommend the inclusion of a reproductive history as part of the comprehensive assessment of all women, to identify risk-modifying factors such as HDP, and appropriately risk stratify women for primary cardiovascular disease prevention.

SUMMARY

HDPs are a significant cause of maternal and fetal morbidity and mortality, and their prevalence is increasing. Moreover, the prevalence as well as the morbidity and mortality associated with HDP vary by race/ethnicity. Improvements in the prevention, diagnosis, and management of HDPs are needed to reduce maternal morbidity and mortality and reduce disparities in care for pregnant and postpartum women.

CLINICS CARE POINTS

- Good blood pressure measurement technique is essential for the accurate diagnosis of HDP as improper techniques are likely to falsely elevate blood pressure.
- Labetalol and nifedipine are the preferred first line agents for the treatment of hypertension in pregnancy.
- Postpartum hypertension is a leading cause of readmission in the United States. Headache or visual changes in a post-partum woman should raise concern for post-partum preeclampsia.
- An accurate reproductive history is an essential part of a woman's medical record and

should always be inquired about to appropriately risk stratify women for CVD.

DISCLOSURE

N.A. Bello reports grant support from the National Institutes of Health, National Heart, Lung, and Blood Institute (K23 HL136853), and the Katz Foundation. A.M. Khedagi has nothing to disclose.

REFERENCES

1. Hutcheon JA, Lisonkova S, Joseph KS. Epidemiology of pre-eclampsia and the other hypertensive disorders of pregnancy. Best Pract Res Clin Obstet Gynaecol 2011;25(4):391–403.

2. Data on Selected pregnancy complications in the United States. Center for Disease Control and Prevention: Center for Disease Control and Prevention; 2019.

3. Kuklina EV, Ayala C, Callaghan WM. Hypertensive disorders and severe obstetric morbidity in the United States. Obstet Gynecol 2009;113(6):1299–306.

4. Singh GK, Siahpush M, Liu L, et al. Racial/ethnic, nativity, and sociodemographic disparities in maternal hypertension in the United States, 2014-2015. Int J Hypertens 2018;2018:7897189.

5. Petersen EE, Davis NL, Goodman D, et al. Vital signs: pregnancy-related deaths, United States, 2011–2015, and strategies for prevention, 13 states, 2013–2017. MMWR Morb Mortal Wkly Rep 2019;68:423–9.

6. Miller EC, Espinoza MDZ, Huang Y, et al. Maternal race/ethnicity, hypertension, and risk for stroke during delivery admission. J Am Heart Assoc 2020;9(3):e014775.

7. Mustafa R, Ahmed S, Gupta A, et al. A comprehensive review of hypertension in pregnancy. J Pregnancy 2012;2012:105918.

8. Fisher C, MacLean M, Morecroft I, et al. Is the pregnancy hormone relaxin also a vasodilator peptide secreted by the heart? Circulation 2002;106(3):292–5.

9. Lumbers ER, Pringle KG. Roles of the circulating renin-angiotensin-aldosterone system in human pregnancy. Am J Physiol Regul Integr Comp Physiol 2014;306(2):R91–101.

10. Bello NA, Woolley JJ, Cleary KL, et al. Accuracy of blood pressure measurement devices in pregnancy: a systematic review of validation studies. Hypertension 2018;71(2):326–35.

11. ACOG practice Bulletin No. 203: chronic hypertension in pregnancy. Obstet Gynecol 2019;133(1):e26–50.

12. ACOG practice Bulletin No. 202: gestational hypertension and preeclampsia. Obstet Gynecol 2019;133(1):e1–25.

13. Whelton PK, Carey RM, Aronow WS, et al. 2017 ACC/AHA/AAPA/ABC/ACPM/AGS/APhA/ASH/ASPC/NMA/PCNA guideline for the prevention, Detection, evaluation, and management of high blood pressure in adults: executive summary: a report of the American College of Cardiology/American heart association Task Force on clinical practice guidelines. Hypertension 2018;71(6):1269–324.

14. Seely EW, Ecker J. Chronic hypertension in pregnancy. Circulation 2014;129(11):1254–61.

15. Lecarpentier E, Tsatsaris V, Goffinet F, et al. Risk factors of superimposed preeclampsia in women with essential chronic hypertension treated before pregnancy. PLoS One 2013;8(5):e62140.

16. Chappell LC, Enye S, Seed P, et al. Adverse perinatal outcomes and risk factors for preeclampsia in women with chronic hypertension: a prospective study. Hypertension 2008;51(4):1002–9.

17. Abalos E, Duley L, Steyn DW. Antihypertensive drug therapy for mild to moderate hypertension during pregnancy. Cochrane Database Syst Rev 2014;(2):Cd002252.

18. Magee LA, von Dadelszen P, Rey E, et al. Less-tight versus tight control of hypertension in pregnancy. N Engl J Med 2015;372(5):407–17.

19. Magee LA, von Dadelszen P, Singer J, et al. The CHIPS randomized controlled trial (control of hypertension in pregnancy study): is severe hypertension just an elevated blood pressure? Hypertension 2016;68(5):1153–9.

20. Rezk M, Ellakwa H, Gamal A, et al. Maternal and fetal morbidity following discontinuation of antihypertensive drugs in mild to moderate chronic hypertension: a 4-year observational study. Pregnancy Hypertens 2016;6(4):291–4.

21. Nakhai-Pour HR, Rey E, Berard A. Discontinuation of antihypertensive drug use during the first trimester of pregnancy and the risk of preeclampsia and eclampsia among women with chronic hypertension. Am J Obstet Gynecol 2009;201(2):180.e1-8.

22. Meher S, Duley L, Hunter K, et al. Antiplatelet therapy before or after 16 weeks' gestation for preventing preeclampsia: an individual participant data meta-analysis. Am J Obstet Gynecol 2017;216(2):121–8.e2.

23. Roberge S, Nicolaides K, Demers S, et al. The role of aspirin dose on the prevention of preeclampsia and fetal growth restriction: systematic review and meta-analysis. Am J Obstet Gynecol 2017;216(2):110–20.e6.

24. ACOG committee opinion No. 743: low-dose aspirin use during pregnancy. Obstet Gynecol 2018;132(1):e44–52.

25. LeFevre M. Low-dose aspirin use for the prevention of morbidity and mortality from preeclampsia: U.S. Preventive Services Task Force recommendation statement. Ann Intern Med 2014;161:819–26.

26. Boesen EI. Consequences of in-utero exposure to antihypertensive medication: the search for definitive answers continues. J Hypertens 2017;35(11):2161–4.

27. Bateman BT, Heide-Jorgensen U, Einarsdottir K, et al. Beta-blocker use in pregnancy and the risk for congenital malformations: an international cohort study. Ann Intern Med 2018;169(10):665–73.

28. Webster LM, Myers JE, Nelson-Piercy C, et al. Labetalol versus nifedipine as antihypertensive treatment for chronic hypertension in pregnancy: a randomized controlled trial. Hypertension 2017;70(5):915–22.

29. Ferrer RL, Sibai BM, Mulrow CD, et al. Management of mild chronic hypertension during pregnancy: a review. Obstet Gynecol 2000;96(5, Part 2):849–60.

30. Easterling TR, Carr DB, Brateng D, et al. Treatment of hypertension in pregnancy: effect of atenolol on maternal disease, preterm delivery, and fetal growth. Obstet Gynecol 2001;98(3):427–33.

31. Zulfeen M, Tatapudi R, Sowjanya R. IV labetalol and oral nifedipine in acute control of severe hypertension in pregnancy–A randomized controlled trial. Eur J Obstet Gynecol Reprod Biol 2019;236:46–52.

32. Cockburn J, Moar VA, Ounsted M, et al. Final report of study on hypertension during pregnancy: the effects of specific treatment on the growth and development of the children. Lancet 1982;1(8273):647–9.

33. Collins R, Yusuf S, Peto R. Overview of randomised trials of diuretics in pregnancy. Br Med J (Clin Res Ed 1985;290(6461):17–23.

34. Magee LA, Cham C, Waterman EJ, et al. Hydralazine for treatment of severe hypertension in pregnancy: meta-analysis. BMJ 2003;327(7421):955–60.

35. Physical activity and exercise during pregnancy and the postpartum period: ACOG committee opinion, number 804. Obstet Gynecol 2020;135(4):e178–88.

36. Courtney AU, O'Brien EC, Crowley RK, et al. DASH (Dietary Approaches to Stop Hypertension) dietary pattern and maternal blood pressure in pregnancy. J Hum Nutr Diet 2020;33(5):686–97.

37. Hypertension in pregnancy. Report of the American College of Obstetricians and Gynecologists' Task Force on hypertension in pregnancy. Obstet Gynecol 2013;122(5):1122–31.

38. Cantwell R, Clutton-Brock T, Cooper G, et al. Saving mothers' lives: reviewing maternal deaths to make motherhood safer: 2006-2008. the eighth report of the confidential enquiries into maternal deaths in the United Kingdom. BJOG 2011;118(Suppl 1):1–203.

39. ACOG committee opinion No. 767: Emergent therapy for acute-onset, severe hypertension during pregnancy and the postpartum period. Obstet Gynecol 2019;133(2):e174–80.

40. Cotton DB, Jones MM, Longmire S, et al. Role of intravenous nitroglycerin in the treatment of severe pregnancy-induced hypertension complicated by pulmonary edema. Am J Obstet Gynecol 1986;154(1):91–3.

41. Crowther CA, Brown J, McKinlay CJ, et al. Magnesium sulphate for preventing preterm birth in threatened preterm labour. Cochrane Database Syst Rev 2014;(8):Cd001060.

42. Euser AG, Cipolla MJ. Magnesium sulfate for the treatment of eclampsia: a brief review. Stroke 2009;40(4):1169–75.

43. Koopmans CM, Bijlenga D, Groen H, et al. Induction of labour versus expectant monitoring for gestational hypertension or mild pre-eclampsia after 36 weeks' gestation (HYPITAT): a multicentre, open-label randomised controlled trial. Lancet 2009;374(9694):979–88.

44. Bramham K, Nelson-Piercy C, Brown MJ, et al. Postpartum management of hypertension. BMJ 2013;346:f894.

45. Powles K, Gandhi S. Postpartum hypertension. CMAJ 2017;189(27):E913.

46. ACOG committee opinion No. 736: Optimizing postpartum care. Obstet Gynecol 2018;131(5):e140–50.

47. Walters BN, Walters T. Hypertension in the puerperium. Lancet 1987;2(8554):330.

48. Clapp MA, Little SE, Zheng J, et al. A multi-state analysis of postpartum readmissions in the United States. Am J Obstet Gynecol 2016;215(1):113.e1-10.

49. Creanga AA, Syverson C, Seed K, et al. Pregnancy-related mortality in the United States, 2011-2013. Obstet Gynecol 2017;130(2):366–73.

50. Sibai BM. Etiology and management of postpartum hypertension-preeclampsia. Am J Obstet Gynecol 2012;206(6):470–5.

51. Bateman BT, Schumacher HC, Bushnell CD, et al. Intracerebral hemorrhage in pregnancy: frequency, risk factors, and outcome. Neurology 2006;67(3):424–9.

52. Aziz A, Gyamfi-Bannerman C, Siddiq Z, et al. Maternal outcomes by race during postpartum readmissions. Am J Obstet Gynecol 2019;220(5):484.e1-10.

53. Bello NA, Miller E, Cleary K, et al. Out of office blood pressure measurement in pregnancy and the postpartum period. Curr Hypertens Rep 2018;20(12):101.

54. Status of state Medicaid expansion decisions: Interactive Map. Kaiser Family Foundation; 2020. Accessed, 2020.

55. America's health Rankings analysis of U.S. Census Bureau. United Health Foundation; 2019. Accessed, 2020.

56. Hadley J. Sicker and poorer–the consequences of being uninsured: a review of the research on the relationship between health insurance, medical care use, health, work, and income. Med Care Res Rev 2003;60(2 Suppl):3S–75S [discussion: 76S–112S].

57. ACOG Committee opinion no. 552: benefits to women of Medicaid expansion through the Affordable Care Act. Obstet Gynecol 2013;121(1):223–5.

58. Brown CC, Moore JE, Felix HC, et al. Association of state medicaid expansion status with low birth weight and preterm birth. JAMA 2019;321(16):1598–609.

59. Lyon SM, Douglas IS, Cooke CR. Medicaid expansion under the Affordable Care Act. Implications for insurance-related disparities in pulmonary, critical care, and sleep. Ann Am Thorac Soc 2014;11(4):661–7.

60. Thoulass JC, Robertson L, Denadai L, et al. Hypertensive disorders of pregnancy and adult offspring cardiometabolic outcomes: a systematic review of the literature and meta-analysis. J Epidemiol Community Health 2016;70(4):414–22.

61. Vahedi FA, Gholizadeh L, Heydari M. Hypertensive disorders of pregnancy and risk of future cardiovascular disease in women. Nurs Womens Health 2020;24(2):91–100.

62. Craici I, Wagner S, Garovic VD. Preeclampsia and future cardiovascular risk: formal risk factor or failed stress test? Ther Adv Cardiovasc Dis 2008;2(4):249–59.

63. Mosca L, Benjamin EJ, Berra K, et al. Effectiveness-based guidelines for the prevention of cardiovascular disease in women–2011 update: a guideline from the american heart association. Circulation 2011;123(11):1243–62.

64. Rosenbloom JI, Lewkowitz AK, Lindley KJ, et al. Expectant management of hypertensive disorders of pregnancy and future cardiovascular morbidity. Obstet Gynecol 2020;135(1):27–35.

Ischemic Heart Disease in Pregnancy

Charishma Nallapati, MD[a], Ki Park, MD[b],*

KEYWORDS

- Ischemic heart disease • Pregnancy • SCAD

KEY POINTS

- Ischemic heart disease during pregnancy or the early postpartum period, although rare, is associated with increased maternal morbidity and mortality.
- Most medications and considerations for procedural evaluation are largely similar in pregnant and nonpregnant patients, with a few important differences.
- Proper cardiac assessment, evaluation, and management, ideally in a multidisciplinary approach with cardiology and obstetric specialist, is essential.

INTRODUCTION

Ischemic heart disease (IHD) accounts for a third of all female deaths globally and affects nearly 48 million women in the United States.[1,2] Although IHD in women of childbearing age is low, current trends, including older age at time of childbirth as well as increases in prevalence of maternal diabetes, obesity, and hypertension, have all correlated with an increase in coronary artery disease in this population.[3–5] In addition, pregnancy itself has been shown to more than double the risk of acute myocardial infarction (AMI) compared with the risk in nonpregnant women of similar age.[4,6] At present, cardiac disease is the single leading cause of maternal death, with IHD accounting for more than one-fifth of cardiac causes.[7] Given the increasing rates of IHD in pregnancy, especially with the higher risk of mortality and morbidity,[3–5] further insight into evaluation and management with a multidisciplinary approach is needed.

PATHOPHYSIOLOGY

The underlying pathogenesis for the increased risk for AMI during pregnancy remains unclear. Although atherosclerotic disease is the single largest cause of myocardial infarction, accounting for nearly 40% of cases, alternative causes, including intracoronary thrombus without atherosclerosis, coronary spasm (normal coronary arteries), and spontaneous coronary artery dissection (SCAD), are seen more commonly in pregnancy than in nonpregnant women of the same age.[8,9]

Normal changes in cardiovascular hemodynamics and hormonal balance during pregnancy as well as the postpartum period create a spectrum of changes that may increase the risk for acute coronary syndromes. These changes include an increase in blood volume by approximately 50% to meet the demands of uteroplacental circulation, as well as an increase in cardiac output.[10,11] These changes create a physiologic anemia, and, when coupled with a decrease in diastolic blood pressure, reduce myocardial oxygen supply. This decrease in myocardial oxygen supply could potentially contribute to the development of myocardial ischemia, more profoundly when coronary blood supply is already compromised. In addition, during pregnancy there is an increase in stroke volume and heart rate, and both of these changes increase myocardial oxygen demand.[12]

[a] Department of Medicine, University of Florida College of Medicine, PO Box 100277, Gainesville, FL 32610, USA; [b] Division of Cardiovascular Medicine, University of Florida College of Medicine, 1329 Southwest Archer Road., P.O. Box 100288, Gainesville, FL 32610-0288, USA
* Corresponding author.
E-mail address: Ki.park@medicine.ufl.edu

Cardiol Clin 39 (2021) 91–108
https://doi.org/10.1016/j.ccl.2020.09.006
0733-8651/21/© 2020 Elsevier Inc. All rights reserved.

Furthermore, there are progressive progesterone-mediated and estrogen-mediated effects, specifically in the last months of pregnancy and the postpartum period, which possibly alter the integrity of coronary arteries, leading to increased rates of dissection.[9] These structural changes in the intima and media of the arterial wall include loss of normal corrugation in the elastic fibers, fragmentation of reticular fibers, and a decrease in the amount of acid mucopolysaccharide ground substance.[13-15] These hormonal changes are thought to be more profound in multiparous women, perhaps explaining the higher incidence of SCAD during pregnancy.[9,16]

PREVALENCE AND TYPE OF MYOCARDIAL INFARCTION IN PREGNANCY

The reported rate of myocardial infarction is 6.2 per 100,000 pregnancies.[4] Although atherosclerosis continues to be the single largest cause of AMI in pregnancy, other causes are more common than in the nonpregnant population. The prevalence of each cause within pregnant women with AMI are as follows: coronary atherosclerosis with or without intracoronary thrombus (27%–40%), SCAD (27%–43%), intracoronary thrombus without atherosclerosis (8%–17%), and coronary artery spasm (normal coronary arteries) (2%).[8,9,17,18] A review of the type and timing of AMI in 150 patients between 2006 and 2011 found that most patients presented with ST-segment elevation myocardial infarction (STEMI) (75%) and the rest with non–ST-elevation myocardial infarction (NSTEMI). Most events occurred during the third trimester of pregnancy (STEMI, 25%; NSTEMI, 32%) or postpartum period (STEMI, 45%; NSTEMI, 55%). The infarct involved the anterior wall of left ventricle in 69%, inferior wall in 27%, and lateral wall in 4%.[17]

PREEXISTING ISCHEMIC HEART DISEASE

Women with underlying IHD are classified as high risk; however, data regarding outcomes are limited. A recent review of 116 women with preexisting IHD noted a 32% chance of cardiovascular complications, including maternal mortality, and only a 21% chance of an uncomplicated pregnancy.[19] A true estimation of the incidence of AMI during pregnancy in women with known IHD is challenging because most studies only report the total incidence of AMI during pregnancy without distinguishing women with prior history of IHD.[3] Given the increased risk of morbidity and mortality, women with preexisting IHD should undergo thorough prepregnancy cardiac assessment and evaluation.

Risk Stratification

A comprehensive detailed history is important when assessing pregnant women with suspected IHD because most studies report AMI in those with at least 1 underlying risk factor.[19] Existing tools for assessing maternal cardiac risk in pregnancy are as listed in **Table 1**. Risk tools including Cardiac Disease in Pregnancy (CARPREG) I, CARPREG II, ZAHARA (Pregnancy and Congenital Heart Disease [translation from the Dutch]), and the modified World Health Organization (WHO) classification have traditionally been used to examine outcomes in women with congenital heart disease, valve disease, and cardiomyopathy.[20] There is limited assessment in women with IHD.

A few important risk factors are listed here:

(1) Advanced maternal age: the number of women becoming pregnant after the age of 35 years increased from 8% in 1985 to 19% in 2003.[21] Women more than 40 years of age were found to have a 30-fold higher AMI risk compared with less than 20 years of age.[21]

(2) Multiparity: multiparous women have been shown to have higher AMI risk, with some studies showing that ~66% of patients with AMI were multigravidas.[4,8] Even in direct comparison of pregnancy-associated SCAD (P-SCAD) and non–pregnancy-associated SCAD (NP-SCAD), P-SCAD occurred more often in multiparous women.[16] The aforementioned hormonal changes are more profound in women with multiple pregnancies.

(3) Hypertension/preeclampsia/eclampsia: hypertension is thought to exacerbate damage to blood vessels that have already undergone adverse remodeling because of the hemodynamic stress of pregnancy and endothelial activation.[9,22] Endothelial dysfunction is more pronounced in the preeclamptic and eclamptic states, with increased vascular reactivity in the presence of noradrenaline and angiotensin II.[23] Preeclampsia itself was noted in 16% of cases of AMI in pregnancy.[24]

(4) Use of fertility medications: there is no definitive evidence that fertility medications, including in vitro fertilization, intrauterine insemination, ovulation induction, and controlled ovarian stimulation, are associated with higher risk for cardiovascular disease.[25] Although it is plausible that the repeated cycles of hormonal hyperstimulation could cause endothelial dysfunction and renin-angiotensin system activation, thereby causing increased

Table 1

Risk models for assessing maternal cardiac outcomes in pregnant women with heart disease

Risk Model	Risk Factors	Interpretation	Additional Comments
CARPREG I[81]	• Poor functional class (NYHA functional class III or IV) or cyanosis • Systemic ventricular ejection fraction <40% • Left heart obstruction • Cardiac event before pregnancy	Each risk factor is worth 1 point. Women with risk scores of 0, 1, or >1 had event rates during pregnancy of 5%, 25%, or 75%, respectively	Outcomes in women with congenital and acquired heart disease based on general clinical and echocardiographic findings; does not incorporate lesion-specific risks
CARPREG II[82]	• Prior cardiac events or arrhythmias (3 points) • Baseline NYHA class (III–IV, 3 points) • Mechanical valve (3 points) • Ventricular dysfunction (2 points) • High-risk left-sided valve disease/left ventricular outflow tract obstruction (2 points) • Pulmonary hypertension (2 points) • Coronary artery disease (2 points) • High-risk aortopathy (2 points) • No prior cardiac intervention (1 point) • Late pregnancy assessment (1 point)	0–1 point (5%), 2 points (10%), 3 points (15%), 4 points (22%), >4 points (41%)	Compared with CARPREG I, CARPREG II has weighted risk scores and incorporates additional risk factors such as mechanical valves, coronary artery disease, and high-risk aortopathy. Increased predictive accuracy compared with CARPREG I[82]
ZAHARA[83]	• History of arrhythmias (weighted score 1.5) • Cardiac medications before pregnancy (weighted score 1.5) • NYHA functional class before pregnancy >II, left heart obstruction (weighted score 0.75) • Left heart obstruction (weighted score 2.5) • Systemic atrioventricular valve regurgitation (weighted score 0.75) • Pulmonary atrioventricular valve regurgitation (weighted score 0.75) • Mechanical valve prosthesis (weighted score 4.25) • Cyanotic heart disease (weighted score 1.0)	Weighted risk score. Women with risk scores of 0–0.50, 0.51–1.5, 1.51–2.5, 2.51–3.5, and >3.51 had event rates of 2.9%, 7.5%, 17.5%, 43.1%, and 70.0%, respectively	Pregnancy outcomes in women with congenital heart disease

(continued on next page)

Table 1
(continued)

Risk Model	Risk Factors	Interpretation	Additional Comments
Modified WHO classification[22]	WHO classification I • Uncomplicated small or mild pulmonary stenosis • Patent ductus arteriosus • Mitral valve prolapse • Successfully repaired simple lesions (atrial or ventricular septal defect, patent ductus arteriosus, anomalous pulmonary venous connection) WHO classification II (if otherwise well and uncomplicated) • Unrepaired atrial or ventricular septal defect • Unrepaired tetralogy of Fallot WHO classification II–III (depending on individual) • Mild left ventricular impairment • Native or tissue valvular heart disease not considered WHO I or IV • Marfan syndrome without aortic dilatation • Aorta<45 mm with bicuspid AV disease • Repaired coarctation WHO classification III • Mechanical valve • Systemic right ventricle • Fontan circulation • Unrepaired cyanotic heart disease • Other complex congenital heart disease • Aortic dilatation 40–45 mm in Marfan syndrome	WHO classification I: no detectable increased risk of maternal mortality and no/mild increase in morbidity WHO classification II: small increase in maternal risk of mortality or moderate increase in morbidity WHO classification III: significantly increased risk of maternal mortality or severe morbidity. Expert counseling required. If pregnancy is decided on, intensive specialist cardiac and obstetric monitoring needed throughout pregnancy, childbirth, and the puerperium WHO classification IV: extremely high risk of maternal mortality or severe morbidity; pregnancy contraindicated. If pregnancy occurs, termination should be discussed. If pregnancy continues, care as for WHO class III	Lesion-specific risk classification

- Aortic dilatation 45–50 mm in bicuspid AV disease

WHO classification IV (pregnancy contraindicated)

- Pulmonary arterial hypertension from any cause
- Severe systemic ventricular dysfunction (LVEF<30%, NYHA functional class III–IV)
- Severe mitral stenosis; severe symptomatic aortic stenosis
- Marfan syndrome with aorta dilated >45 mm
- Aortic dilatation >50 mm in aortic disease associated with bicuspid AV
- Native severe coarctation of the aorta

Abbreviations: AV, aortic valve; CARPREG, Cardiac Disease in Pregnancy; LVEF, left ventricular ejection fraction; NYHA, New York Heart Association; WHO, World Health Organization; ZAHARA, Pregnancy and Congenital Heart Disease (translation from the Dutch).
(*Data from* Refs.[22,81–83]).

risk, the current studies are limited because of small sample sizes as well as multiple confounding factors, including variability for the initial indication for fertility treatments.[25,26]

Medications for Coronary Artery Disease and Safety During Pregnancy

Most medications for IHD for treatment of AMI or for secondary prevention of cardiovascular disease can be continued in pregnancy and breastfeeding, with important exceptions. Cessation of certain medications is recommended because of teratogenicity or other unwanted effects for the fetus. In addition, dose adjustments may be needed because of hemodynamic changes during pregnancy that can influence the pharmacokinetics of the drug[9] (**Table 2**). As seen in **Table 2**, the use of statins is currently contraindicated (women are generally advised to stop taking statins in pregnancy); however, these women may be at higher risk for AMI in pregnancy and postpartum on discontinuation.[27,28]

Assessment of Suspected Ischemia

AMI in pregnancy presents with atypical features because many patients do not present with the typical central chest pain that radiates to the jaw or arms with associated autonomic features. These atypical features may be ascribed to symptoms of dyspepsia and gastroesophageal reflux disease. Given these atypical features and confounding presentations, there should be a low threshold to thoroughly investigate women with chest pain, especially those with the aforementioned cardiovascular risk factors.[9,29]

It is important to note variability in various cardiac tests during normal pregnancy as reference. For example, normal electrocardiogram (ECG) changes include 15° left-axis deviation as a result of diaphragmatic elevation, T-wave inversion in lead III and aVF, small nonpathologic Q waves, and presence of supraventricular and ventricular ectopic beats.[9,21,30] ST elevation on an ECG, as in cases outside of pregnancy, requires prompt treatment. Increased troponin level, even in patients with preeclampsia, should be taken seriously because preeclampsia alone does not cause increase in troponin levels above the diagnostic threshold for AMI.[31] However, levels of serum total creatinine phosphokinase and its MB isoenzyme are increased during normal labor and vaginal delivery and may not indicate myocardial infarction.[32] In addition, during induction of anesthesia for a cesarean delivery, ECG changes, including ST depression mimicking myocardial infarction, may be seen.[8,33] Therefore, it is

important to rely on clinical presentation as well as additional diagnostic and laboratory studies to guide assessment and management.

In patients with stable symptoms, noninvasive investigations are preferred. Exercise testing is considered safe in pregnancy provided there are no obstetric complications (vaginal bleeding, placenta previa); the disadvantage to exercise testing is a high false-positive rate, which is known from investigation in nonpregnant women.[21] Alternatively, dobutamine stress echo is an option because there are no reported adverse effects noted (pregnancy category B).[21]

Cardiac MRI offers superior imaging of cardiac structure and function and is particularly useful for the assessment of viability and myocardial scars.[34] However, because of limited data on MRI safety during organogenesis (first trimester), it is currently recommended to use MRI during the second and third trimester only when considering the risks/benefit ratio.[35] The use of gadolinium is more controversial because it is a category C drug; it should be avoided and used only when necessary.[36]

The use of computed tomography angiography (CTA) during pregnancy is also controversial. In experienced centers, the total radiation dose during a CTA scan is equivalent to or slightly lower than invasive coronary catherization.[34] The benefit of CTA is that it provides an alternative to defining coronary anatomy and reducing the procedural risk of iatrogenic coronary artery dissection associated with coronary angiography and stenting, which seems to be higher during the pregnancy and postpartum period.[17] Although CTA provides a noninvasive diagnostic approach, as in the nonpregnant population, the sensitivity of CTA for coronary dissection is unknown and there is a potential to miss nonproximal coronary dissection. In patients in whom CTA would need to be followed by an invasive procedure, there would have been a delay in treatment and an increase in maternal and fetal radiation exposure.[37] Therefore, the indication for CTA should be guided by clinical presentation and suspicion for severe proximal disease. In low-risk, stable pregnant women with likely pregnancy-associated NSTEMI where further risk stratification is indicated, CTA may be considered.[38]

Nuclear imaging studies, including myocardial perfusion imaging, during pregnancy should be avoided. The radiation dose is approximately 10 to 12 mSv, which is greater than a diagnostic coronary angiogram (5–7 mSv).[39]

Coronary Angiography

In acute plaque rupture leading STEMI, timely coronary reperfusion by percutaneous coronary

Table 2
Cardiac medications during pregnancy, delivery, and lactation

Drug	Use in Pregnancy	FDA Class	Use in Delivery	Breast Feeding	Dose Adjustment	Adverse Effects
Aspirin	First choice antiplatelet agent; also indicated for prevention of premature birth and preeclampsia	Nonclassified[27]	Discontinuation generally recommended before delivery because of risk of maternal bleeding. Controversial because no current evidence that low-dose aspirin increases maternal or fetal bleeding risks at time of neuraxial anesthesia during delivery.[84,85]	Appears in subclinical amounts in human milk; limited data; can be used with caution[27,86]	Up to 100 mg daily	In first trimester may cause 2-fold to 3 fold increased risk of gastroschisis[87]; also risk for premature closure of ductus arteriosus, fetal bleeding risk. Lower risk when dose is <100 mg[27]
Clopidogrel	May be used for shortest duration possible.[88] Animal studies do not note adverse effects; limited human data	B[27]	Discontinue 7 d before delivery because of risk of epidural hematoma[89]	Unknown in humans; caution advised[89]	None	Not expected to cause congenital anomalies based on animal studies[29]
Prasugrel Ticagrelor Eptifibatide	Little data; Ticagrelor does cross placenta. Not recommended	Prasugrel B Ticagrelor C[27] Eptifibatide C[90]	Not recommended	Prasugrel and ticagrelor placental transfer noted in rat studies; unknown risk[27]	None	No reported complications with prasugrel. Eptifibatide's short half-life may allow safe use proximal to delivery

(continued on next page)

Table 2
(continued)

Drug	Use in Pregnancy	FDA Class	Use in Delivery	Breast Feeding	Dose Adjustment	Adverse Effects
Ranexa	Unknown	C	—	Unknown	—	Maternal toxicity and misshapen sternebrae and reduced ossification in animal studies; no adequate well-controlled studies in pregnant women; current recommendation is used during pregnancy only when potential benefit to patient justifies potential risk to fetus[91]
Tirofiban	Unknown	C	Possible use in recently implanted DES and high-risk characteristics for stent thrombosis needing urgent surgery Discontinuation until 4 h before C-section and resumed at same schedule (including 30-min bolus)[92,93]	Unknown	—	No current guidelines; not well studied; there is case report stating that it could be safe, but not many studies[92]

Drug	Recommendations	Pregnancy category	Can be used if indicated	Transfers to breast milk	Comments
β-Blockers Labetalol Atenolol Metoprolol Carvedilol	Metoprolol succinate recommended (avoids interfering with B2-mediated uterine relaxation and peripheral vasodilation) Atenolol contraindicated	C; with exception of atenolol (D)	None	Labetalol and metoprolol safe; carvedilol is unknown risk[27,86]	Does not seem to increase risk of congenital malformations[94], possible fetal growth retardation.[95] Atenolol associated with birth defects; IUGR.[96] Hypoglycemia, bradycardia, respiratory depression, and hypotension in neonates[29,97-100]
CCBs Nifedipine Verapamil Diltiazem Amlodipine	Diltiazem not recommended Nifedipine is first line for hypertension and tocolysis (when used with magnesium) Verapamil considered fairly safe (second line after β-blockers for rate control and treatment of idiopathic sustained ventricular tachycardia). Amlodipine is probably safe for hypertension	C	—	Minimal transfer in breast milk; nifedipine safe; limited data on verapamil and diltiazem[27,101]	Prematurity, IUGR, fetal bradycardia in some CCBs; 1 study noted increased risk of neonatal seizures[102] Diltiazem noted as teratogenic in animals (few data in humans) Has tocolytic effect (delays contraction and suppresses labor); can cause maternal hypotension and placental hypoperfusion
Nitrates	Safe in pregnancy	C	—	Limited data; unknown[9,27]	None; Crosses placenta; potential hypotension[103]

(continued on next page)

Table 2
(continued)

Drug	Use in Pregnancy	FDA Class	Use in Delivery	Breast Feeding	Dose Adjustment	Adverse Effects
Statins	Contraindicated	X	—	Contraindicated[9,104]	—	Potential teratogenicity; limited human data. Use in first trimester correlated with premature birth[28]
Bile acid sequestrants (cholestyramine and colestipol)	Considered safer than other lipid level–lowering agents; treatment of choice for hyperlipidemia[105]	C	—	Limited data; considered safe[106]	—	May lower fat-soluble vitamin levels
Warfarin	Not recommended after 36 wk; recommended use <5 mg (primary indication is mechanical valves)	X	Contraindicated with vaginal delivery; switch to LMWH or unfractionated heparin at 36 wk of gestation (lower risk for fetal hemorrhage); If still taking during labor, C-section should be performed to prevent fetal intraventricular hemorrhage during passage through birth canal	Considered safe[27,86]	Based on INR levels; if taking >5 mg; recommend switch to LMWH or unfrac-tionated heparin by end of 6 wk of gestation[27]	Crosses placenta; embryopathy during first trimester; dose dependent fetal risks (>5 mg) Lowest risk for adverse maternal outcomes[107]
NOACs	Contraindicated	C	—	Unknown; contraindicated[108]	—	Unknown in humans. Animal studies note teratogenicity

Drug	Placental transfer	FDA category	Delivery timing	Lactation	Monitoring	Adverse effects
LMWH	Does not cross placenta; safe in pregnancy	B: enoxaparin	Contraindicated for regional anesthesia within 24 h of last dose; timed delivery recommended	Unlikely to transfer into breast milk; not absorbed into infant GI tract because of large molecular weight; considered safe[109]	Need monitoring for peak and trough anti-Xa levels	Maternal bleeding, including intrauterine hematoma[110] Lowest risk for adverse fetal outcomes[107]
Unfractionated heparin	Does not cross placenta; safe in pregnancy	C	Discontinue 4–6 h before delivery	Unlikely to transfer into milk; not absorbed into infant GI tract because of large molecular weight; considered safe[109]	None	Maternal bleeding, including intrauterine hematoma[110]
ACE inhibitors ARBs	Contraindicated	D	—	Limited data for ACE inhibitors; does transfer to breast milk; captopril, benazepril, and enalapril may be considered with close follow-up Conflicting data for ARBs; currently contraindicated[9,27,88,109]	—	Fetal renal and cardiac abnormalities[111,112]

The US Food and Drug Administration criteria for pregnancy categories for pharmaceuticals are as follows: A, controlled clinical studies in humans show safety; B, human data reassuring (animal positive), animal studies show no risk; C, human data lacking, animal studies positive or not done (67%); D, human data show risk, benefit may outweigh risk; and X, animal or human data positive for unacceptable risk.[113]

Abbreviations: ACE, angiotensin-converting enzyme; ARBs, angiotensin receptor blockers; CCB, calcium channel blockers; C-section, cesarean section; DES, drug-eluting stent; FDA, US Food and Drug Administration; GI, gastrointestinal; INR, International Normalized Ratio; IUGR, intrauterine growth restriction; LMWH, low-molecular-weight heparin; NOACs, novel oral anticoagulants.

(*Data from* Refs[9,27,84–97,100–113]).

intervention (PCI) with stent implantation is recommended.[40] The selection between a drug-eluting stent (DES) and bare metal stent (BMS) is based on time of event during pregnancy and bleeding risk. DESs have a lower risk of restenosis; however, historically they have required longer periods of antiplatelet medications compared with BMSs (12 months vs 1 month). Given the reduced duration of anticoagulation, it may be advantageous to consider BMS, especially during labor and delivery.[21]

Angiography is the gold standard for the diagnosis of IHD in pregnancy; however, despite this, only 60% of women diagnosed with AMI underwent coronary angiography,[41] which was in part because of the perceived fetal risk. The current accepted cumulative dose of ionizing radiation during pregnancy is 50 mGy (equal to 50 mSv or 5 rad).[42,43] However, an important determinant for radiation exposure is timing in which it occurs during pregnancy. During the first 2 weeks of gestation (before implantation), spontaneous abortion, regardless of radiation dose, may cause demise of the embryo.[44–46] From the third to eighth week of pregnancy, the risks for birth defects, pregnancy loss, or growth retardation are lower unless the exposure is more than 200 mSv.[47] From the eighth to fifteenth week of pregnancy, there is a higher risk for central nervous system (CNS) effects, including microcephaly and other CNS malformations (threshold 300 mSv). Aside from the risks of spontaneous abortion and teratogenesis (which seem to be higher before 20 weeks), the relative risk of childhood cancer is also higher during early gestation. The relative risk for childhood cancer from a diagnostic level of radiation is approximately 3.19 in the first trimester, 1.29 in the second, and 1.3 in the third.[36,48,49] However, given the increasing risk of fetal harm with increasing radiation exposure, precautions, including low acquisition times, should be implemented.[34]

Other recommendations to decrease radiation exposure during pregnancy include reduction in fluoroscopy frame rate, keeping the intensifier as close as possible to the patient, and avoiding steep angulated views.[34] The use of maternal lead shielding is controversial. It was recently found that, as long as the fetus is not directly within the x-ray beam, the exposure to the fetus occurs mainly through scatter (indirect) radiation. Although placing an external shield reduced exposure to staff, it is not effective in protecting the fetus.[50,51]

Other modifications that should be implemented include using a radial approach for arterial access (lower risk of bleeding complications) and use of a wedge (to prevent caval compression while the patient is lying supine and to maintain cardiac output).[21,52] The use of intra-aortic balloon pump to improve left ventricular output and coronary perfusion is also considered safe.[17,53]

Thrombolysis with Recombinant Tissue Plasminogen Activator

In situations where PCI is unavailable, tissue plasminogen activator (TPA) may be considered when required. It was previously thought that thrombolysis was contraindicated during pregnancy, but new data (from primary cases of stroke and thromboembolism) suggest that the risk of TPA is no greater than in the nonpregnant state.[54] Note that, in patients with myocardial infarction secondary to coronary dissection, thrombolytics may worsen hemorrhage and dissection.[8]

Coronary Artery Bypass Grafting

The indication for coronary artery bypass grafting (CABG) is usually left main artery disease and/or multivessel disease, not amenable to PCI. Note that the maternal risk of cardiac surgery is comparable with the nonpregnant state, unless emergent. The risks of fetal complications, including prematurity and death, were associated with urgent, high-risk surgery; maternal comorbidity; and early gestational age.[55] Although it is difficult to specifically estimate the maternal and fetal mortalities because only 5% of patients with acute coronary syndrome may require CABG, it should only be considered if it is lifesaving and no other treatment options are available. Based on multiple studies, the maternal mortality ranges from 3% to 13%, and the fetal mortality from 19% to 30%.[21,56]

Labor Management

Labor and delivery in a patient with known IHD should be managed by a team of cardiologists, maternal-fetal medicine specialists, and obstetric anesthesiologists in a referral hospital capable of managing high-risk obstetric patients.[57] For women with a recent myocardial infarction, it is best to defer delivery for several weeks if possible; this allows for myocardial healing and reduced risk of delivery complications associated with AMI. Although outcomes data for women with known IHD are limited, based on a study of women with general structural heart disease, there is no benefit to planned cesarean delivery.[58] In general, the plan for delivery should be driven by obstetric indications and not cardiovascular indications. The exceptions include dilated aorta and use of oral anticoagulation with spontaneous labor.[58] Cesarean deliveries are associated with greater rates of maternal hemorrhage, infection, and thromboembolism, all of which may further increase risk of myocardial ischemia.[9]

Vaginal delivery and labor itself are associated with increased cardiac stress. However, allowing for passive descent of fetal head at full dilatation or use of forceps/vacuum could be considered to avoid excessive maternal efforts and reduce the duration of maternal pushing.[8,59] In addition, active management during the third stage of labor with early cord clamping and administration of a uterotonic agent is recommended because it reduces the risk of postpartum hemorrhage by 40%.[60] Other considerations include placement of the patient in left lateral position to improve cardiac output, and use of β-blockers and epidural anesthesia to prevent tachycardia.[9]

Analysis of Complications in Women with Known Ischemic Heart Disease

As previously mentioned, pregnant women with IHD are considered to have high-risk pregnancies. In a systematic review consisting of 116 women with preexisting IHD with a total of 124 pregnancies, there was a 21% chance of having an uncomplicated pregnancy without cardiovascular, obstetric, or fetal/neonatal complications. The primary (ischemic) end point occurred in 9% of the patients; women with atherosclerosis as the underlying disorder for IHD were found to have more cardiovascular complications.[19] Prepregnancy revascularization (PCI, CABG, or thrombolysis) did not influence primary end point outcome. The recurrence rate of acute coronary syndrome in women with IHD was 1 in 11 pregnancies; the risk was highest in women with coronary dissection as the underlying disorder because there was a 1 in 5 risk of redissection.[19] Compared with women with new-onset IHD during pregnancy with complications primarily toward the end of pregnancy/postpartum, women with preexisting IHD may have complications throughout pregnancy. In a review of 11 cases of maternal fatality (mortality of 11%), maternal death occurred at the time of infarction with an incidence twice as high in women diagnosed with AMI during the peripartum period compared with antepartum or postpartum periods. The incidence of fetal mortality was 9% (6 of 68).[8]

ACQUIRED ISCHEMIC HEART DISEASE DURING PREGNANCY
Spontaneous Coronary Artery Dissection

Although an uncommon cause of AMI outside of pregnancy, SCAD accounts for 27% to 43% of AMI during pregnancy.[8,17,18] SCAD is defined as a nontraumatic, noniatrogenic cause of dissection, with formation of an intimal tear resulting in an intramural hematoma. The hematoma then causes compression of the true coronary artery lumen. Typical presentation of SCAD is similar to that of AMI, with chest pain, dyspnea, and diaphoresis. Diagnosis is typically difficult because a typical patient is often young with no other identifiable cardiovascular risk factors. However, a higher level of suspicion is warranted for patients with fibromuscular dysplasia (25%–86%), pregnancy (2%–8%), connective tissue disorders (1.2%–3%), systemic inflammation (<1%–8.9%), exogenous hormones (10.7%–12.6%), and precipitating stressful events, given the reported prevalence in cohort studies. Interestingly, more than 50% of patients recall a precipitating factor, including labor and delivery, intense Valsalva, exogenous hormones, recreational drugs, or intense exercise.[61,62] The underlying mechanism for SCAD is not fully understood and may be a consequence of increased hemodynamic stress in the setting of hormonal weakening of the arterial wall during pregnancy.[9,18]

As previously mentioned, the initial clinical presentation ranges from cardiogenic shock (2%–5%), to STEMI (26%–87%), to ventricular arrhythmia or sudden cardiac death (3%–11%).[63–65] In a cohort of 168 patients, all patients presented with an increased troponin I level.[61] In addition, although overall left ventricular ejection fraction was often preserved, left ventricular wall motion abnormalities were detected on echocardiography or early angiography.[66]

Although any artery can be affected, the left anterior descending artery is the most common, accounting for 32% to 46% of cases.[67] Similar to the management of nonpregnant women, conservative management with inpatient monitoring is recommended for most patients. In an observational study of 131 SCAD lesions, spontaneous healing occurred in 88.5%; after 35 days, angiographic healing was observed in all patients.[68] In cases in which angiography is indicated, note that radial forces generated by balloon inflation or stent expansion may propagate the dissection.[69] In addition, increased precautions before PCI for SCAD are needed because higher rates of technical failure and increased risk of extending the dissection requiring emergency surgery have been reported.[67,70]

In a comparison of P-SCAD versus NP-SCAD, P-SCAD was associated with more acute presentations, including STEMI (57% vs 36%), left main or multivessel SCAD (24% vs 5%), and left ventricular function less than or equal to 35% (26% vs 10%). P-SCAD was most likely to occur during the first postpartum month. In a meta-analysis that specifically identified more than 120 cases of pregnancy-associated SCAD between 2000 and 2015, more than 87 patients (72.5%) presented in the postpartum period between day 3 and day 210 after delivery.[71] This finding highlights possible hormonal or hemodynamic mechanisms that could be contributing to P-SCAD. Aside from the initial presentation of P-SCAD, risk factors such as multiparity, history of infertility therapies, and preeclampsia were more common. In contrast, patients with P-SCAD compared with NP-SCAD were less likely to have a diagnosis of fibromuscular dysplasia and extracoronary vascular abnormalities.[16]

Coronary Spasm

Coronary artery spasm accounts for approximately 2% of all pregnancy-related AMI.[8,17] As defined by Koneru and colleagues,[72] coronary artery spasm is a "dynamic, transient reduction in the luminal diameter of the epicardial coronary arteries due to increased vasomotor tone leading to myocardial ischemia."[73] Although the underlying pathophysiology is not well understood, it is thought to be a multifactorial process involving several mechanisms, including endothelial dysfunction, increased vascular reactivity to constrictor stimuli (catecholamines, acetylcholine, and histamine), and/or use of prostaglandin analogues.[9,74] The pathophysiologic mechanisms during pregnancy that may induce coronary vasospasm include use of ergot derivatives that are used to control postpartum or postabortion hemorrhage or to suppress lactation.[75–77] Other mechanisms may include increased renin release and angiotensin production from uterine hypoperfusion that may occur in the supine position.[78]

As in the nonpregnant population, early diagnosis and treatment is important. Spasm management depends on clinical picture and hemodynamic stability. Similar to the nonpregnancy population, treatment of an acute attack of coronary spasm includes sublingual nitroglycerin or oral isosorbide dinitrate. Prevention and long-term management include calcium channel blockers. However, patients with multivessel coronary spasm tend to be resistant to treatment and often require larger amounts of calcium channel blockers to suppress attacks.[79,80]

SUMMARY AND FUTURE DIRECTIONS

The incidence of AMI in pregnancy, although currently only reported at 2.8 to 6.2 per 100,000 pregnancies,[6] is expected to increase given the current trends of older age at childbirth and increasing numbers of women of childbearing age with preexisting coronary artery disease. Further risk stratification and closer monitoring are needed, especially in women with preexisting coronary artery disease. A multidisciplinary approach with a team of maternal-fetal medicine specialists and cardiologists is essential.

CARE: CLINICS POINTS

- Women with preexisting IHD should undergo thorough cardiac assessment and evaluation before pregnancy.
- Existing tools such as CARPREG I, CARPREG II, ZAHARA, and the modified WHO classification, although traditionally used for women with congenital heart disease, valve disease, and cardiomyopathy, are limited in risk assessment in women with IHD.
- Current trends of older maternal age, use of fertility treatments, and increasing prevalence of medical comorbidities may contribute to greater rates of IHD.
- It is important to recognize and treat SCAD and coronary vasospasm during pregnancy because they may have atypical presentations.
- Most medications used for IHD or for secondary prevention of cardiovascular disease can be continued during pregnancy, with important exceptions.
- Labor and delivery in a patient with known IHD should be managed by a team of cardiologists, maternal-fetal medicine specialists, and obstetric anesthesiologists in a referral hospital capable of managing high-risk obstetric patients.

DISCLOSURE

The authors have nothing to disclose.

REFERENCES

1. Bots SH, Peters SAE, Woodward M. Sex differences in coronary heart disease and stroke mortality: a global assessment of the effect of ageing between 1980 and 2010. BMJ Glob Health 2017. https://doi.org/10.1136/bmjgh-2017-000298.
2. Benjamin EJ, Muntner P, Alonso A, et al. Heart disease and stroke statistics-2019 update: a report from the American heart association. Circulation 2019. https://doi.org/10.1161/CIR.0000000000000659.
3. Burchill LJ, Lameijer H, Roos-Hesselink JW, et al. Pregnancy risks in women with pre-existing coronary artery disease, or following acute coronary syndrome. Heart 2015;101(7):525–9.
4. Ladner HE, Danielsen B, Gilbert WM. Acute myocardial infarction in pregnancy and the

puerperium: a population-based study. Obstet Gynecol 2005;105(3):480–4.

5. Gelson E, Gatzoulis MA, Steer P, et al. Heart disease - why is maternal mortality increasing? BJOG 2009;116(5):609–11.

6. James AH, Jamison MG, Biswas MS, et al. Acute myocardial infarction in pregnancy: a United States population-based study. Circulation 2006. https://doi.org/10.1161/CIRCULATIONAHA.105.576751.

7. Outcome IC, Programme R. Saving lives, improving mother's care report. Midwifery 2015; 31(2):262–3.

8. Roth A, Elkayam U. Acute myocardial infarction associated with pregnancy. J Am Coll Cardiol 2008;52(3):171–80.

9. Cauldwell M, Baris L, Roos-Hesselink JW, et al. Ischaemic heart disease and pregnancy. Heart 2019;105(3):189–95.

10. Hytten F. Blood volume changes in normal pregnancy. Clin Haematol 1985;14(3):601–12.

11. Silversides CK, Colman JM. Physiological changes in pregnancy. In: Oakley C, Warnes CA, editors. Heart disease in pregnancy. 2nd edition. Blackwell Publishing; 2007. https://doi.org/10.1002/9780470994955.ch2.

12. Melchiorre K, Sharma R, Khalil A, et al. Maternal cardiovascular function in normal pregnancy: evidence of maladaptation to chronic volume overload. Hypertension 2016;67(4):754–62.

13. Ueland K. Maternal cardiovascular dynamics. VII. Intrapartum blood volume changes. Am J Obstet Gynecol 1976. https://doi.org/10.1016/0002-9378(76)90517-2.

14. Caton WL, Roby CC, Reid DE, et al. Plasma volume and extravascular fluid volume during pregnancy and the puerperium. Am J Obstet Gynecol 1949. https://doi.org/10.1016/0002-9378(49)90232-X.

15. Adams JQ. Cardiovascular physiology in normal pregnancy: studies with the dye dilution technique. Am J Obstet Gynecol 1954. https://doi.org/10.1016/0002-9378(54)90100-3.

16. Tweet MS, Hayes SN, Codsi E, et al. Spontaneous coronary artery dissection associated with pregnancy. J Am Coll Cardiol 2017;70(4):426–35.

17. Elkayam U, Jalnapurkar S, Barakkat MN, et al. Pregnancy-associated acute myocardial infarction: a review of contemporary experience in 150 cases between 2006 and 2011. Circulation 2014;129(16): 1695–702.

18. Petitti DB, Sidney S, Quesenberry CP, et al. Incidence of stroke and myocardial infarction in women of reproductive age. Stroke 1997. https://doi.org/10.1161/01.STR.28.2.280.

19. Lameijer H, Burchill LJ, Baris L, et al. Pregnancy in women with pre-existent ischaemic heart disease: a systematic review with individualised patient data. Heart 2019;105(11):873–80.

20. Elkayam U, Goland S, Pieper PG, et al. High-risk cardiac disease in pregnancy: Part I. J Am Coll Cardiol 2016;68(4):396–410.

21. Fryearson J, Adamson DL. Heart disease in pregnancy: ischaemic heart disease. Best Pract Res Clin Obstet Gynaecol 2014. https://doi.org/10.1016/j.bpobgyn.2014.03.011.

22. Van Hagen IM, Boersma E, Johnson MR, et al. Global cardiac risk assessment in the registry of pregnancy and cardiac disease: results of a registry from the european society of cardiology. Eur J Heart Fail 2016. https://doi.org/10.1002/ejhf.501.

23. Roth A, Elkayam U. Acute myocardial infarction associated with pregnancy. Ann Intern Med 1996. https://doi.org/10.7326/0003-4819-125-9-199611010-00009.

24. Mulla ZD, Wilson B, Abedin Z, et al. Acute myocardial infarction in pregnancy: a statewide analysis. J Registry Manag 2015;42(1):12–7.

25. Dayan N, Filion KB, Okano M, et al. Cardiovascular risk following fertility therapy: systematic review and meta-analysis. J Am Coll Cardiol 2017. https://doi.org/10.1016/j.jacc.2017.07.753.

26. Pepine CJ, Park K. Fertility therapy and long-term cardiovascular risk: raising more questions than answers? J Am Coll Cardiol 2017;70(10):1214–5.

27. Halpern DG, Weinberg CR, Pinnelas R, et al. Use of medication for cardiovascular disease during pregnancy: JACC state-of-the-art review. J Am Coll Cardiol 2019;73(4):457–76.

28. Winterfeld U, Allignol A, Panchaud A, et al. Pregnancy outcome following maternal exposure to statins: a multicentre prospective study. BJOG 2013. https://doi.org/10.1111/1471-0528.12066.

29. Turitz AL, Friedman AM. Ischemic heart disease in pregnancy. Semin Perinatol 2014;38(5):304–8.

30. Soma-Pillay P, Nelson-Piercy C, Tolppanen H, et al. Physiological changes in pregnancy. Cardiovasc J Afr 2016. https://doi.org/10.5830/CVJA-2016-021.

31. Pergialiotis V, Prodromidou A, Frountzas M, et al. Maternal cardiac troponin levels in pre-eclampsia: a systematic review. J Matern Fetal Neonatal Med 2016. https://doi.org/10.3109/14767058.2015.1127347.

32. Abramov Y, Abramov D, Abrahamov A, et al. Elevation of serum creatine phosphokinase and its MB isoenzyme during normal labor and early puerperium. Acta Obstet Gynecol Scand 1996. https://doi.org/10.3109/00016349609047097.

33. Mathew JP, Fleisher LA, Rinehouse JA, et al. ST segment depression during labor and delivery. Anesthesiology 1992. https://doi.org/10.1097/00000542-199210000-00004.

34. Vidovich MI, Gilchrist IC. Minimizing radiological exposure to pregnant women from invasive procedures. Interv Cardiol 2013. https://doi.org/10.2217/ica.13.27.

35. Kanal E, Barkovich AJ, Bell C, et al. ACR guidance document for safe MR practices: 2007. Am J Roentgenol 2007. https://doi.org/10.2214/AJR.06.1616.

36. Chen MM, Coakley FV, Kaimal A, et al. Guidelines for computed tomography and magnetic resonance imaging use during pregnancy and lactation. Obstet Gynecol 2008. https://doi.org/10.1097/AOG.0b013e318180a505.

37. Joshi FR. CT rather than invasive angiography for pregnant patients with NSTEMI? J Am Coll Cardiol 2016. https://doi.org/10.1016/j.jacc.2016.08.075.

38. Elkayam U. Reply: CT rather than invasive angiography for pregnant patients with NSTEMI? more delay and more radiation. J Am Coll Cardiol 2016. https://doi.org/10.1016/j.jacc.2016.09.955.

39. Limacher MC, Douglas PS, Germano G, et al. Radiation safety in the practice of cardiology. J Am Coll Cardiol 1998. https://doi.org/10.1016/S0735-1097(98)00047-3.

40. O'Gara PT, Kushner FG, Ascheim DD, et al. 2013 ACCF/AHA guideline for the management of ST-elevation myocardial infarction. J Am Coll Cardiol 2013. https://doi.org/10.1016/j.jacc.2012.11.019.

41. Bush N, Nelson-Piercy C, Spark P, et al. Myocardial infarction in pregnancy and postpartum in the UK. Eur J Prev Cardiol 2013;20(1):12–20.

42. Brent RL. Utilization of developmental basic science principles in the evaluation of reproductive risks from pre- and postconception environmental radiation exposures. Teratology 1999. https://doi.org/10.1002/(SICI)1096-9926(199904)59:4<182::AID-TERA2>3.0.CO;2-H.

43. Ntusi NAB, Samuels P, Moosa S, et al. Diagnosing cardiac disease during pregnancy: imaging modalities. Cardiovasc J Afr 2016;27(2):95–103.

44. Zanotti-Fregonara P, Jan S, Taieb D, et al. Absorbed 18F-FDG dose to the fetus during early pregnancy. J Nucl Med 2010. https://doi.org/10.2967/jnumed.109.071878.

45. Patel SJ, Reede DL, Katz DS, et al. Imaging the pregnant patient for nonobstetric conditions: algorithms and radiation dose considerations. Radiographics 2007;27(6):1705-22.

46. International Commission on Radiological Protection. Pregnancy and medical radiation. Ann ICRP 2000. https://doi.org/10.1016/s0146-6453(00)00037-3.

47. Toppenberg KS, Hill DA, Miller DP. Safety of radiographic imaging during pregnancy. Am Fam Physician 1999;59(7):1813–8.

48. Tirada N, Dreizin D, Khati NJ, et al. Imaging pregnant and lactating patients. Radiographics 2015;35(6):1751–65.

49. Gilman EA, Kneale GW, Knox EG, et al. Pregnancy x-rays and childhood cancers: effects of exposure age and radiation dose. J Radiol Prot 1988. https://doi.org/10.1088/0952-4746/8/1/301.

50. Damilakis J, Theocharopoulos N, Perisinakis K, et al. Conceptus radiation dose and risk from cardiac catheter ablation procedures. Circulation 2001. https://doi.org/10.1161/hc5790.094909.

51. Goldberg-Stein SA, Liu B, Hahn PF, et al. Radiation dose management: Part 2, estimating fetal radiation risk from CT during pregnancy. Am J Roentgenol 2012. https://doi.org/10.2214/AJR.11.7458.

52. Sharma GL, Loubeyre C, Morice MC. Safety and feasibility of the radial approach for primary angioplasty in acute myocardial infarction during pregnancy. J Invasive Cardiol 2002;14(6):359–62.

53. Garry D, Leikin E, Fleisher AG, et al. Acute myocardial infarction in pregnancy with subsequent medical and surgical management. Obstet Gynecol 1996;87(5 Pt 2):802–4.

54. Sousa Gomes M, Guimarães M, Montenegro N. Thrombolysis in pregnancy: a literature review. J Matern Fetal Neonatal Med 2019. https://doi.org/10.1080/14767058.2018.1434141.

55. John AS, Gurley F, Schaff HV, et al. Cardiopulmonary bypass during pregnancy. Ann Thorac Surg 2011. https://doi.org/10.1016/j.athoracsur.2010.11.037.

56. Roos-Hesselink JW, Duvekot JJ, Thome SA. Pregnancy in high risk cardiac conditions. Heart 2009. https://doi.org/10.1136/hrt.2008.148932.

57. Regitz-Zagrosek V, Blomstrom Lundqvist C, Borghi C, et al. ESC Guidelines on the management of cardiovascular diseases during pregnancy. Eur Heart J 2011. https://doi.org/10.1093/eurheartj/ehr218.

58. Ruys TPE, Roos-Hesselink JW, Pijuan-Domènech A, et al. Is a planned caesarean section in women with cardiac disease beneficial? Heart 2015. https://doi.org/10.1136/heartjnl-2014-306497.

59. Brancato RM, Church S, Stone PW. A meta-analysis of passive descent versus immediate pushing in nulliparous women with epidural analgesia in the second stage of labor. J Obstet Gynecol Neonatal Nurs 2008. https://doi.org/10.1111/j.1552-6909.2007.00205.x.

60. Begley CM, Gyte GML, Devane D, et al. Active versus expectant management for women in the third stage of labour. Cochrane Database Syst Rev 2015. https://doi.org/10.1002/14651858.CD007412.pub4.

61. Saw J. Coronary angiogram classification of spontaneous coronary artery dissection. Catheter Cardiovasc Interv 2014. https://doi.org/10.1002/ccd.25293.

62. Rogowski S, Maeder MT, Weilenmann D, et al. Spontaneous coronary artery dissection: angiographic follow-up and long-term clinical outcome in a predominantly medically treated population.

Catheter Cardiovasc Interv 2017. https://doi.org/10.1002/ccd.26383.

63. Tweet MS, Hayes SN, Pitta SR, et al. Clinical features, management, and prognosis of spontaneous coronary artery dissection. Circulation 2012. https://doi.org/10.1161/CIRCULATIONAHA.112.105718.

64. Lettieri C, Zavalloni D, Rossini R, et al. Management and long-term prognosis of spontaneous coronary artery dissection. Am J Cardiol 2015. https://doi.org/10.1016/j.amjcard.2015.03.039.

65. Nakashima T, Noguchi T, Haruta S, et al. Prognostic impact of spontaneous coronary artery dissection in young female patients with acute myocardial infarction: a report from the Angina pectoris-myocardial infarction multicenter investigators in Japan. Int J Cardiol 2016. https://doi.org/10.1016/j.ijcard.2016.01.188.

66. Franco C, Starovoytov A, Heydari M, et al. Changes in left ventricular function after spontaneous coronary artery dissection. Clin Cardiol 2017. https://doi.org/10.1002/clc.22640.

67. Tweet MS, Eleid MF, Best PJM, et al. Spontaneous coronary artery dissection: revascularization versus conservative therapy. Circ Cardiovasc Interv 2014. https://doi.org/10.1161/CIRCINTERVENTIONS.114.001659.

68. Prakash R, Starovoytov A, Heydari M, et al. Catheter-induced iatrogenic coronary artery dissection in patients with spontaneous coronary artery dissection. JACC Cardiovasc Interv 2016. https://doi.org/10.1016/j.jcin.2016.06.026.

69. Saw J, Aymong E, Sedlak T, et al. Spontaneous coronary artery dissection association with predisposing arteriopathies and precipitating stressors and cardiovascular outcomes. Circ Cardiovasc Interv 2014. https://doi.org/10.1161/CIRCINTERVENTIONS.114.001760.

70. Vijayaraghavan R, Verma S, Gupta N, et al. Pregnancy-related spontaneous coronary artery dissection. Circulation 2014. https://doi.org/10.1161/CIRCULATIONAHA.114.011422.

71. Havakuk O, Goland S, Mehra A, et al. Pregnancy and the risk of spontaneous coronary artery dissection: an analysis of 120 contemporary cases. Circ Cardiovasc Interv 2017. https://doi.org/10.1161/CIRCINTERVENTIONS.117.004941.

72. Koneru J, Cholankeril M, Patel K, et al. Postpartum coronary vasospasm with literature review. Case Rep Cardiol 2014. https://doi.org/10.1155/2014/523023.

73. Yasue H, Kugiyama K. Coronary spasm: clinical features and pathogenesis. Intern Med 1997. https://doi.org/10.2169/internalmedicine.36.760.

74. Teragawa H, Nishioka K, Higashi Y, et al. Treatment of coronary spastic angina, particularly medically refractory coronary spasm. Clin Med Cardiol 2008. https://doi.org/10.4137/cmc.s681.

75. Taylor GJ, Cohen B. Ergonovine-induced coronary artery spasm and myocardial infarction after normal delivery. Obstet Gynecol 1985. https://doi.org/10.1097/00132582-198606000-00034.

76. Liao JK, Cockrill BA, Yurchak PM. Acute myocardial infarction after ergonovine administration for uterine bleeding. Am J Cardiol 1991. https://doi.org/10.1016/0002-9149(91)90669-C.

77. Ruch A, Duhring JL. Postpartum myocardial infarction in a patient receiving bromocriptine. Obstet Gynecol 1989;74(3 Pt 2):448–51.

78. Sasse L, Wagner R, Murray FE. Transmural myocardial infarction during pregnancy. Am J Cardiol 1975. https://doi.org/10.1016/0002-9149(75)90040-5.

79. Yasue H, Nakagawa H, Itoh T, et al. Coronary artery spasm - clinical features, diagnosis, pathogenesis, and treatment. J Cardiol 2008;51(1):2–17.

80. Askandar S, Flatt D, Rosu D, et al. Postpartum coronary arterial spasm. J La State Med Soc 2017;169(4):101–5.

81. Siu SC, Sermer M, Colman JM, et al. Prospective multicenter study of pregnancy outcomes in women with heart disease. Circulation 2001. https://doi.org/10.1161/hc3001.093437.

82. Silversides CK, Grewal J, Mason J, et al. Pregnancy outcomes in women with heart disease: the CARPREG II study. J Am Coll Cardiol 2018. https://doi.org/10.1016/j.jacc.2018.02.076.

83. Drenthen W, Boersma E, Balci A, et al. Predictors of pregnancy complications in women with congenital heart disease. Eur Heart J 2010;31(17):2124–32.

84. Askie LM, Duley L, Henderson-Smart DJ, et al. Antiplatelet agents for prevention of pre-eclampsia: a meta-analysis of individual patient data. Lancet 2007. https://doi.org/10.1016/S0140-6736(07)60712-0.

85. CLASP. A randomised trial of low-dose aspirin for the prevention and treatment of pre-eclampsia among 9364 pregnant women. Lancet 1994. https://doi.org/10.1016/S0140-6736(94)92633-6.

86. Pieper PG. Use of medication for cardiovascular disease during pregnancy. Nat Rev Cardiol 2015;12(12):718–29.

87. Kozer E, Nikfar S, Costei A, et al. Aspirin consumption during the first trimester of pregnancy and congenital anomalies: a meta-analysis. Am J Obstet Gynecol 2002. https://doi.org/10.1067/mob.2002.127376.

88. Regitz-Zagrosek V, Roos-Hesselink JW, Bauersachs J, et al. 2018 ESC Guidelines for the management of cardiovascular diseases during pregnancy. Eur Heart J 2018. https://doi.org/10.1093/eurheartj/ehy340.

89. de Santis M, de Luca C, Mappa I, et al. Clopidogrel treatment during pregnancy: a case report and a

review of literature. Intern Med 2011. https://doi.org/10.2169/internalmedicine.50.5294.

90. Nallamothu BK, Saint M, Saint S, et al. Double jeopardy. N Engl J Med 2005;353(1):75–80.

91. Reed M, Kerndt CC, Nicolas D. Ranolazine. StatPearls publishing 2020. Available at: http://www.ncbi.nlm.nih.gov/pubmed/29939605. Accessed June 6, 2020.

92. Argentiero D, Savonitto S, D'Andrea P, et al. Ticagrelor and tirofiban in pregnancy and delivery: beyond labels. J Thromb Thrombolysis 2020; 49(1):145–8.

93. Savonitto S, D'Urbano M, Caracciolo M, et al. Urgent surgery in patients with a recently implanted coronary drug-eluting stent: a phase II study of "bridging" antiplatelet therapy with tirofiban during temporary withdrawal of clopidogrel. Br J Anaesth 2010. https://doi.org/10.1093/bja/aep373.

94. Yakoob MY, Bateman BT, Ho E, et al. The risk of congenital malformations associated with exposure to β-blockers early in pregnancy: a meta-analysis. Hypertension 2013. https://doi.org/10.1161/HYPERTENSIONAHA.111.00833.

95. Gelson E, Curry R, Gatzoulis MA, et al. Effect of maternal heart disease on fetal growth. Obstet Gynecol 2011. https://doi.org/10.1097/AOG.0b013e31820cab69.

96. Duan L, Ng A, Chen W, et al. Beta-blocker subtypes and risk of low birth weight in newborns. J Clin Hypertens 2018. https://doi.org/10.1111/jch.13397.

97. Chow T, Galvin J, McGovern B. Antiarrhythmic drug therapy in pregnancy and lactation. Am J Cardiol 1998. https://doi.org/10.1016/S0002-9149(98)00473-1.

98. Crooks BNA, Deshpande SA, Hall C, et al. Adverse neonatal effects of maternal labetalol treatment. Arch Dis Child Fetal Neonatal Ed 1998. https://doi.org/10.1136/fn.79.2.F150.

99. Gladstone GR, Hordof A, Gersony WM. Propranolol administration during pregnancy: effects on the fetus. J Pediatr 1975. https://doi.org/10.1016/S0022-3476(75)80236-8.

100. Klarr J, Bhatt-Mehta V, Donn S. Neonatal adrenergic blockade following single dose maternal labetalol administration. Am J Perinatol 1994. https://doi.org/10.1055/s-2007-994563.

101. Mitani GM, Steinberg I, Lien EJ, et al. The pharmacokinetics of antiarrhythmic agents in pregnancy and lactation. Clin Pharm 1987. https://doi.org/10.2165/00003088-198712040-00002.

102. Davis RL, Eastman D, McPhillips H, et al. Risks of congenital malformations and perinatal events among infants exposed to calcium channel and beta-blockers during pregnancy. Pharmacoepidemiol Drug Saf 2011. https://doi.org/10.1002/pds.2068.

103. David M, Walka MM, Schmid B, et al. Nitroglycerin application during cesarean delivery: plasma levels, fetal/maternal ratio of nitroglycerin, and effects in newborns. Am J Obstet Gynecol 2000. https://doi.org/10.1016/S0002-9378(00)70353-X.

104. Morton S, Thangaratinam S. Statins in pregnancy. Curr Opin Obstet Gynecol 2013. https://doi.org/10.1097/GCO.0000000000000026.

105. Jacobson TA, Maki KC, Orringer CE, et al. National lipid association recommendations for patient-centered management of dyslipidemia: Part 2. J Clin Lipidol 2015. https://doi.org/10.1016/j.jacl.2015.09.002.

106. (US) B (MD): NL of M. drugs and lactation database (LactMed). Cholestyramine. Available at: https://www.ncbi.nlm.nih.gov/books/NBK501394/. Accessed June 10, 2020.

107. Steinberg ZL, Dominguez-Islas CP, Otto CM, et al. Maternal and fetal outcomes of anticoagulation in pregnant women with mechanical heart valves. J Am Coll Cardiol 2017. https://doi.org/10.1016/j.jacc.2017.03.605.

108. Lameijer H, JJJ Aalberts, van Veldhuisen DJ, et al. Efficacy and safety of direct oral anticoagulants during pregnancy; a systematic literature review. Thromb Res 2018. https://doi.org/10.1016/j.thromres.2018.07.022.

109. Safety in lactation: drugs for thromboembolic disorders. Available at: https://www.sps.nhs.uk/articles/safety-in-lactation-drugs-for-thromboembolic-disorders/. Accessed June 6, 2020.

110. Lu E, Shatzel JJ, Salati J, et al. The safety of low-molecular-weight heparin during and after pregnancy. Obstet Gynecol Surv 2017. https://doi.org/10.1097/OGX.0000000000000505.

111. Bowen ME, Ray WA, Arbogast PG, et al. Increasing exposure to angiotensin-converting enzyme inhibitors in pregnancy. Am J Obstet Gynecol 2008. https://doi.org/10.1016/j.ajog.2007.09.009.

112. Cooper WO, Hernandez-Diaz S, Arbogast PG, et al. Major congenital malformations after first-trimester exposure to ACE inhibitors. N Engl J Med 2006. https://doi.org/10.1056/NEJMoa055202.

113. Food and Drug Administration. HHS. Content and format of labeling for human prescription drug and biological products; requirements for pregnancy and lactation labeling. Final rule. Fed Regist 2014;79(233):72063–103.

Pulmonary Arterial Hypertension in Pregnancy

Wenners Ballard III, MD[a], Brittany Dixon, MD[b], Colleen A. McEvoy, MD[c], Amanda K. Verma, MD[b],*

KEYWORDS

- Pulmonary arterial hypertension • Pregnancy • Heart failure • Management • Outcomes

KEY POINTS

- Pulmonary arterial hypertension (PAH) is largely driven by changes in the pulmonary vasculature.
- With the female predominance of PAH, some studies have focused on identifying sex-specific differences in the cause and pathophysiology of PAH.
- Several hemodynamic changes occur throughout pregnancy that need to be considered with underlying PAH.

INTRODUCTION

Pulmonary arterial hypertension (PAH) is a rare disease that has significant implications with regard to morbidity and mortality in those affected. With a prevalence of 15 to 60 cases per million individuals and an incidence of 2 to 10 cases per million per year,[1] PAH is largely a sex-specific disease because 60% to 80% of those affected are women.[2,3] Given the female predominance, this article provides a current overview of the pathophysiology and management of PAH in women, specifically in the setting of pregnancy.

PAH is classified as group 1 pulmonary hypertension (PH) based on the classification schema from the sixth World Symposium on Pulmonary Hypertension.[4] Group 1 PAH includes PH that is idiopathic, heritable, drug/toxin induced, or associated with certain conditions such as connective tissue disease, human immunodeficiency virus (HIV) infection, portal hypertension, congenital heart disease, or schistosomiasis. Importantly, group 1 PAH excludes PH caused by intrinsic lung disease and left-sided heart disease.

Idiopathic PAH and congenital heart disease–associated PAH are the most common subtypes of PAH. The diagnosis of PAH is based on meeting defined criteria for PH: mean pulmonary arterial pressure (mPAP) greater than 20 mm Hg at rest assessed by right heart catheterization, in addition to hemodynamics of precapillary PH, defined as pulmonary artery wedge pressure less than or equal to 15 mm Hg and pulmonary vascular resistance (PVR) greater than 3 Wood units in the absence of other precapillary PH causes, such as lung disease or chronic thromboembolism.[1]

PATHOPHYSIOLOGY

PAH is largely driven by changes in the pulmonary vasculature. On a cellular level, structural changes are related to medial and intimal hypertrophy and adventitial fibrosis secondary to vascular smooth cell and endothelial cell proliferation and inflammatory cell recruitment. These changes are mediated by underlying signaling pathways that cause impairment of vasodilation and concurrent enhancement of vasoconstriction. Three of these

[a] Division of Hospital Medicine, Department of Medicine, Washington University School of Medicine, 4523 Clayton Avenue, CB 8058, St Louis, MO 63110, USA; [b] Division of Cardiovascular Medicine, Department of Medicine, Washington University School of Medicine, 660 South Euclid Avenue, CB 8086, St Louis, MO 63110, USA; [c] Division of Pulmonary and Critical Care Medicine, Department of Medicine, Washington University School of Medicine, 4523 Clayton Avenue, CB 8052, St Louis, MO 63110, USA
* Corresponding author.
E-mail address: amanda.verma@wustl.edu

Cardiol Clin 39 (2021) 109–118
https://doi.org/10.1016/j.ccl.2020.09.007

pathways have been heavily studied and are the basis for current treatment strategies: nitric oxide, prostacyclin, and endothelin pathways.

Nitric oxide is a vasodilator that also plays a role in leukocyte adhesion inhibition, platelet aggregation, and vascular proliferation.[5,6] PAH is associated with reduced bioavailability of nitric oxide as well as upregulation of phosphodiesterases (PDEs) that inactivate cyclic guanosine monophosphate (cGMP), a key mediator through which nitric oxide acts, further contributing to endothelial dysfunction. PDE-5 inhibitors are used in PAH to promote antiproliferation and also allow endogenous nitric oxide to activate pathways for vasodilatation. Soluble guanylate cyclase (sGC) stimulators are another PAH therapy that work on this pathway by directly binding to guanylate cyclase, which, in turn, increases cGMP production independent of and/or in an enhanced manner with nitric oxide.[7]

Prostacyclins and prostanoids bind cell surface receptors to increase intracellular cyclic adenosine monophosphate, which in turn causes vasodilatation as well as antiplatelet, antithrombotic, antiproliferative, and antiinflammatory effects. In PAH, prostacyclin levels are reduced in the lungs because of decreased metabolism of its precursor arachidonic acid as well as decreased expression of the enzyme responsible for synthesis of prostacyclins in pulmonary arteries of patients with PAH. Synthetic prostacyclin analogues and nonprostanoid activators of prostacyclin receptors have been used for treatment in PAH.[5,6,8,9]

Endothelin is a vasoconstrictor that stimulates pulmonary artery smooth muscle cell proliferation and is overexpressed in lung tissue and plasma of patients with PAH. Interestingly, there is crosstalk of endothelin with nitric oxide and prostacyclin pathways. Thus, nonselective endothelin receptor antagonists (ERAs) can be used for treatment of PAH by enhancing vasodilation and reducing vascular remodeling and right ventricular hypertrophy.[5,6,10] Together, the changes these major pathways and others cause to the pulmonary arterial circulation in PAH over time lead to increased pulmonary pressures, which exert an effect on the right ventricle (RV). With the high afterload the RV experiences, maladaptive remodeling can occur which leads to RV failure and ultimately death.

Genetics

With the female predominance of PAH, some studies have focused on identifying sex-specific differences in the causes and pathophysiology of PAH. PAH can be inherited with variable penetrance in an autosomal dominant fashion. In particular, mutation in the BMPR2 gene is the cause of most hereditary PAH. BMPR2 encodes a cell surface receptor for bone morphogenetic protein ligands of the transforming growth factor-β family. This pathway has a role in regulating proliferation, migration, and apoptosis of pulmonary artery endothelial and smooth muscle cells. The imbalance of these processes that occurs with BMPR2 mutation can lead to PAH physiology.[11] Interestingly, penetration for this mutation is higher in women (42%) compared with men (14%).[12] In studies of BMPR2 in patients without PAH, expression of BMPR2 levels in women are reduced compared with men in addition to downregulation of downstream signaling pathways.[13] Overall, this suggests a baseline sex-specific predisposition that is further compounded by the effects of the mutation.

Hormonal Influences

Sex hormone differences may also have a role in PAH. Estrogen and estrogen metabolites have been studied in detail; however, the data are conflicting and difficult to reconcile. The so-called estrogen paradox refers to the idea that PAH affects mostly women with an assumption that estrogen is pathologic, although most studies have shown a protective effect of estrogen, which includes antiproliferative and vasodilatory properties.[14]

In terms of its pathogenesis, estrogen has been shown to reduce expression of BMPR2 by directly binding to an estrogen response element of the BMPR2 promotor region.[15] Inhibition of estrogen synthesis with an aromatase inhibitor reverses PH and restores BMPR2 signaling in female rat models of PAH,[16] and aromatase inhibitors are currently being studied in human clinical trials with preliminary data showing improvement in functional capacity.[17] Higher levels of 17β-estradiol (a type of estrogen produced endogenously) are associated with PAH in men.[18] Although there is a paucity of literature, animal models suggest that, rather than estrogen and estrogen metabolites playing a direct role in PAH, estrogen and estrogen metabolites exert a pathologic role in PAH in certain conditions (ie, hypoxia, oxidative stress, inflammation, medication exposure) that alter estrogen metabolism homeostasis and thereby can cause maladaptive changes in the RV and pulmonary vasculature remodeling.[14]

Alternatively, in male animal models of PAH, exogenously administered estrogen improved RV function by stimulating contractility in addition to having vasodilatory and antiproliferative effects on the pulmonary vasculature.[19] A recent study also showed that female patients with PAH have higher RV contractility and better RV–pulmonary artery coupling than male patients, which may contribute to a survival benefit in women. The molecular mechanism of this is unknown but may be related to hormonal differences.[20] There are also studies suggesting that 17β-estradiol helps inhibit proliferation of smooth muscle cells in a dose-dependent fashion and mitigates maladaptive remodeling of pulmonary arterial vasculature.[21,22]

Progesterone has not been well studied in PAH, although it seems to be protective. In vitro studies suggest that progesterone inhibits endothelin synthesis and reduces inflammatory response. This suggestion is also supported by in vivo studies that show that lack of progesterone is related to increased vascular medial hypertrophy and smooth muscle cell proliferation.[23–25] Testosterone similarly has a conflicting relationship with PAH. It has been shown to have a vasodilatory effect on pulmonary arteries but promotes maladaptive RV remodeling in the setting of high afterload exposure.[26–28]

HEMODYNAMICS OF PREGNANCY AND PULMONARY ARTERIAL HYPERTENSION

Several hemodynamic changes occur throughout pregnancy that need to be considered with underlying PAH. In a normal pregnancy, blood volume increases by about 45%, starting at 6 weeks' gestation and peaking at 32 weeks. The increase in blood volume is also accompanied by increased production of red blood cells that leads to increase of 17% to 40% of blood cell mass. Heart rate increases throughout pregnancy but is gradual, peaking at the third trimester. With increase in stroke volume and heart rate, there is also increase in cardiac output by as much as 50% in pregnancy, also peaking at the beginning of the third trimester. Blood pressure and systemic vascular resistance typically decrease early in pregnancy and then begin to gradually increase in midpregnancy with restoration to normal or exceeding pre-pregnancy values closer to term.[29,30]

The heart typically tolerates these changes without significant changes in the intracardiac pressures given the compliance, dilatation, and eccentric hypertrophy that occur.[30,31] The pulmonary vasculature also dilates during pregnancy such that PVR is reduced. In addition, nonperfused pulmonary vessels are recruited to decrease PVR. At time of delivery, cardiac output, heart rate, and blood pressure increase secondary to increased sympathetic tone and catecholamine surge. Initially postpartum, there is surge in cardiac output. Then, within the first few days after delivery, there is a rapid decline to prepregnancy

output along with reduction in systemic vascular resistance. This process is associated with a high-output state caused by transfer of blood from uterus to systemic circulation, improvement in venous return caused by lack of vena cava compression, and mobilization of extracellular fluid.[29,30]

These hemodynamic changes of pregnancy are largely a result of hormonal fluctuations. As noted earlier, estrogen has a complicated relationship with regard to the pathophysiology of PAH and RV function. In general, because of the increased progesterone and estrogen levels, there is increased vasodilatation and decreased systemic vascular resistance such that systemic blood pressure is reduced. The underlying mechanism of vasodilatation is thought to be secondary to increase in endothelial nitric oxide synthase activity, increased prostacyclin synthase activity, and decreased endothelin-1 activity.[32] Prolactin, which increases toward the end of pregnancy and the postpartum period, also may have an impact because patients with PAH with increased prolactin levels have been found to have decreased functional capacity.[33,34] In addition, the fluctuations of these hormones during pregnancy may unmask PAH during pregnancy. For instance, increased levels of testosterone during pregnancy may impair RV function, and rapid decline in estrogen postpartum may induce RV failure after delivery. However, the implications of hormonal changes in pregnancy with relation to PAH are not well understood on the molecular and cellular levels.[32]

In the clinical setting, the hemodynamic changes of pregnancy compounded by PAH can cause significant problems throughout and/or at different times of pregnancy. Most patients with PAH tolerate the first trimester without significant symptoms. During the second and the beginning of the third trimester, when most hemodynamic changes are at their peak, patients often develop heart failure symptoms, such as shortness of breath and edema. In PAH during pregnancy, the pulmonary vasculature does not vasodilate and thus the increase in plasma volume and cardiac output leads to increased pulmonary pressures and RV afterload. Depending on the state of RV function before pregnancy, the RV may not adapt appropriately to the increase in pressure and volume and thus can precipitate acute RV heart failure. RV failure can further lead to hypotension and hypoxemia (especially in the setting of right-to-left shunting via patent foramen ovale). In the postpartum state, given the change in cardiac output and volume shifts that increase preload, RV failure may persist or worsen. Furthermore, with pregnancy being a hypercoagulable state, patients with PAH have higher risk of decompensation if they develop pulmonary embolism.[32,35]

MANAGEMENT

Pregnancy is contraindicated in patients with PAH, and termination of pregnancy is recommended per guidelines.[36] If a patient continues with pregnancy or PAH is detected during pregnancy past the point of termination, close monitoring and follow-up is essential because managing PAH in pregnancy can be a particularly complex and delicate process. Early referral to an experienced PH treatment center using a team approach is associated with improved outcomes.[37–40] Treatment strategies may include a combination of conservative, pharmacologic, surgical, and even transplant consideration in select patients. The chosen course depends on the disease severity, cause, individual patient characteristics, as well as clinical response during treatment.

Antepartum

Contraception and termination
Proactive counseling regarding maternal-fetal risks during pregnancy, teratogenic effects of PAH medications, and contraceptive strategies should be discussed with all women at the time of PAH diagnosis. However, this does not routinely happen in clinical practice. In a 2010 study of 536 peripartum women with congenital heart disease, only 48% of patients could recall ever being counseled on increased risk for PAH complications caused by pregnancy and only 43% reported receiving contraceptive counseling from a health care provider.[41]

Progestin-only or copper intrauterine devices (IUDs) are the safest and most effective method of nonpermanent contraception in patients with PAH.[32,42] Providers should be aware of vasovagal response that may occur with insertion of an IUD, especially in patients with severe PAH, although the response is typically transient and easily treatable.[43] Because of increased susceptibility to thrombosis within the pulmonary vasculature secondary to endothelial dysfunction in PAH,[44] both oral and nonoral formulations of estrogen-containing contraceptives are contraindicated because of increased risk of venous thromboembolism (VTE), although the risk is still lower than that of pregnancy itself.[45] Progestin-only methods are thought to be safe and can be considered in patients with PAH, although they are less efficacious than long-acting reversible methods such as IUD.[32,43,46] Special attention should be made to the drug-drug interactions of contraceptive therapies and PAH medical therapies because

certain drugs, such as the ERA bosentan, reduce the efficacy of combined oral contraceptive pills.[47]

Termination of pregnancy should also be discussed with patients given poor maternal outcomes.[1] This discussion should occur early in pregnancy given the changing political climate that may affect the timing of termination.

Genetic counseling
The identification of several germline mutations involved in the pathogenesis of PAH has underscored genetic counseling's growing role in PAH management. As previously described, mutation of the BMPR2 gene represents most hereditary cases, accounting for 75% of hereditary PAH cases and 20% of cases initially thought to be idiopathic.[48] Genetic counseling provides information to children and family members to facilitate early diagnosis, proactive management, and information about estimated risk of PAH in future children. For these reasons, the American College of Chest Physicians and global leaders in PAH genetics strongly recommend genetic counseling in both heritable PAH and idiopathic PAH subgroups.[48–50]

Peripartum

Initial steps in management include early referral to a center with experience in PAH treatment and tertiary care centers that may be able to offer transplant and extracorporeal membrane oxygenation (ECMO) services. A multidisciplinary approach with input from PAH specialists, cardiologists, cardiothoracic surgeons, maternal-fetal obstetrician-gynecologists, anesthesiologists, and neonatologists should be incorporated early in the patient's clinical course.[40] Management is tailored uniquely to the individual patient's cause of PAH, degree of severity, response to drug therapies, and hemodynamics.

Monitoring
With the physiologic changes that occur with pregnancy, patients with PAH require close monitoring to identify and treat factors that lead to severe right heart failure, such as volume overload, hypoxemia, and hypotension.[36] To help understand and anticipate how a patient may respond to the physiologic changes of pregnancy, patients should have serial echocardiograms performed during pregnancy with special attention to monitoring RV function as well as RV and pulmonary artery pressures. Most patients generally tolerate the first trimester without any significant issues. During the second trimester, patients may start to experience the effects of increased volume. At the beginning of the third trimester, patients reach peak hemodynamic load and are most likely to experience heart

failure symptoms. Studies have shown that the most likely cardiac indication for hospitalization is heart failure and that this takes place during the end of the second/beginning of the third trimester at a median of 27 weeks.[51]

Special considerations and safety of pharmacologic agents in pregnancy

PAH-specific medical therapies in pregnancy are described in case reports and in small case series; thus, recommendations are based on these limited data.[52] Similar to nonpregnant patients with PAH, continuation of calcium channel blockers in pregnant patients with PAH (who are responsive to vasoreactivity tests) is associated with improved survival and overall outcomes.[53] The safety of calcium channel blockers in pregnancy has been established (category B drug) and their use has also been shown to decrease preterm labor, a complication that affects a significant number of patients with PAH.[53–56] Prostacyclins, inhaled nitric oxide, and PDE inhibitors can also be used safely during pregnancy (category B drugs). However, standard practice of management for these targeted therapies in pregnancy has not yet been described.[57,58] ERAs and sGC stimulators have significant teratogenicity and are contraindicated in pregnancy (category X). ERAs and sGC stimulators should be immediately discontinued if termination is not being pursued.[32,58] Future studies that implement advanced therapies before or early during pregnancy and in patients with varying disease severity may be useful in delineating potential outcome benefits.

For volume overload, loop diuretics (category C) are preferred to thiazides because of neonatal hemorrhagic complications and hyponatremia observed in infants exposed to thiazides.[59] Volume status should be carefully monitored while patients are on diuretic therapy because intravascular volume depletion increases risk of placental hypoperfusion.

Inotropic support for RV failure may be required during pregnancy as well. Although inotropes such as dobutamine (category B) and milrinone (category C) have been described and shown to be effective in peripartum cardiomyopathy, the data for their use in PAH and pregnancy are lacking. Nonetheless, it is reasonable to use these agents in patients with moderate to severe RV dysfunction.

With increased risk of VTE in pregnancy and the underlying risk in patients with PAH, patients with PAH should be started on prophylactic anticoagulation during pregnancy, although standard guidelines have not been widely established.[32,49] Warfarin (category X) should be discontinued on confirmation of pregnancy because it freely crosses the placenta, is teratogenic, and is associated with increased risk of early miscarriage.[60] In contrast, low-molecular-weight heparin (category B) does not cross the placenta and has been used safely in pregnancy.[32,49,61] There are limited data regarding direct oral anticoagulants (ie, apixaban is category B; rivaroxaban, dabigatran, and edoxaban are category C) in pregnancy. In a meta-analysis that included a total of 236 patients taking direct oral anticoagulants, 31% of patients had miscarriages and 4% had bone and facial abnormalities in patients who did not terminate pregnancy. Interestingly, all patients had discontinued direct oral anticoagulant therapy within the first 2 months of pregnancy, suggesting that these may be underestimates of miscarriage and birth defect rates.[62]

Delivery and Postpartum Care

Monitoring

Close monitoring is imperative during the intrapartum period given the aforementioned hemodynamic changes of pregnancy coupled with the catecholamine surge associated with delivery. There are limited data on optimal monitoring strategies, delivery conditions, and timing, but some approaches are relatively consistent in centers experienced in PAH.[32,49] Many experts advise scheduled delivery between 34 and 36 weeks to avoid emergent delivery at facilities not equipped to handle PAH and to ensure optimal monitoring and treatment during delivery.[63] In general, patients should stop anticoagulation 24 to 48 hours before induction, have baseline laboratory tests checked (including comprehensive metabolic panel, troponin, and N-terminal brain natriuretic peptide) on admission, and be placed on continuous telemetry and pulse oximetry during hospitalization. For patients with moderate to severe PAH, it is reasonable to place an arterial line to continuously monitor blood pressure in addition to Swan-Ganz catheter to measure pulmonary pressures at the time of delivery. In patients with severe PAH with RV dysfunction, arterial and venous access can be placed to allow rapid ECMO cannulation in the event of cardiovascular collapse at the time of delivery. These patients should typically deliver in an operating room with cardiothoracic surgeons on standby to cannulate for ECMO, if needed. Postpartum patients should be closely monitored in an intensive care unit setting for at least 72 hours given the fluid shifts and hormonal changes that manifest typically within 72 hours after delivery. This time period presents the highest risk for maternal complications and death. Given hypercoagulability and risk for hemodynamic collapse in the postpartum period, it is imperative to start anticoagulation for VTE prophylaxis as soon as safely possible in patients with PAH and to resume PAH therapies.

Mode of delivery

Because of the physiologic demands of vaginal labor and delivery, including Valsalva maneuver, which quickly decreases RV preload leading to decompensation, as well as the catecholamine surge during labor increasing cardiac output and possibly PVR, most experts recommend cesarean delivery.[32,37] However, the evidence remains unclear on the ideal mode of delivery. In a 2017 case study that included 30 patients with PAH, 3 patients (10%) died who underwent cesarean delivery compared with 1 patient (3%) who died after delivering vaginally.[64] Although this suggests caution in pursuing cesarean delivery, it seems that patients who delivered in this way had more severe PAH at baseline, which may have contributed to poor outcomes rather than mode of delivery. Data from the Registry of Pregnancy and Cardiac Disease (ROPAC) included 39 patients with PAH and, of those that delivered, only 1 patient died who had vaginal delivery.[51] If patients pursue vaginal delivery, an assisted second stage (ie, forceps) is advised to reduce risk of increased vagal tone, which can lead to cardiovascular collapse from suprasystemic pulmonary pressures.[36] Overall, cesarean delivery should be strongly considered for patients with moderate and severe PAH, especially in preterm induction and/or primiparous patients.

Anesthesia

Anesthesia can be helpful to mitigate the consequent hemodynamic effects of labor and delivery, and an experienced cardiac anesthesiologist can be particularly helpful with delivery in patients with PAH. Regional neuraxial anesthesia is recommended for patients with PAH. Because single-bolus epidural anesthesia may cause profound hypotension, low-dose spinal epidural or slow titration of epidural anesthetic is advised and has been used safely in patients with Eisenmenger syndrome.[32,36,63,65] General anesthesia is typically avoided because of the potential for severe hypotension, negative inotropic effects of some agents, as well as the possible need for intubation or positive pressure ventilation, which decreases RV preload and potentiates hemodynamic decompensation.[66] Data indicate a signal of increased maternal mortality risk in women who receive general anesthesia compared with those receiving regional or neuraxial blockade.[53] General anesthesia has been used in some cases successfully without maternal or fetal negative outcomes and may be necessary if rapid decompensation occurs.[64]

Breastfeeding

Although there are few data on drug safety of medical therapies for PAH in breastfeeding (with the exception of calcium channel blockers), there are also no reported adverse events of PAH medications in the literature.[36,38,67] In general, patients with PAH are encouraged to breastfeed if they desire to do so, with rare exceptions. Case reports have suggested safety and minimal transmission of drug in breast milk with regard to calcium channel blockers, PDE inhibitors, and prostacyclins.[67] Risks and benefits of breastfeeding should be discussed with patients to allow an informed decision to be made with the available data.

OUTCOMES

According to the modified World Health Organization (mWHO) classification of maternal cardiovascular risk, PAH is classified as mWHO class IV. These patients are at extremely high risk of maternal mortality or severe morbidity, with an estimated maternal cardiac event rate of 40% to 100% during pregnancy.[36] This category of risk is considered a contraindication for pregnancy altogether given high maternal and fetal risks and poor outcomes. Of note, the highest risk for maternal complications and death occurs in the postpartum period rather than during pregnancy, and thus providers should be cautioned about a false sense of security following a noncomplicated delivery.

The ROPAC study was an international registry of pregnant women with cardiac disease from 2007 to 2018 that evaluated underlying cardiovascular disease and cardiac, obstetric, and fetal outcomes. An interim subgroup analysis of 151 patients with PH was performed, 26% of whom had PAH.[51] Among the patients with PAH, there were 4 deaths (10%), all of which occurred in the postpartum setting and were primarily caused by acute heart failure. The most common complication of patients with PAH was heart failure (36%), followed by arrhythmias (10%). Among all patients with PH in the study, those with severely increased RV systolic pressures (>70 mm Hg) had significantly higher mortality (25%) compared with low and moderate RV systolic pressures, which had 0% mortality at 6 months. There were 14 fetal or neonatal deaths (9.3%), 19.3% were considered small birth weight (<2500 g), and 13.8% were small for gestational age.[51] These results were similarly reproduced in a small prospective study of 26 patients performed by Jais and colleagues[53] that focused specifically on PAH. No maternal or fetal complications were found in 62% of pregnancies. Three patients (12%) died, again all in the postpartum period, and 1 patient required ECMO and urgent heart-lung transplant. The patients with poor outcomes had significantly worse hemodynamics (mPAP, 71 mm Hg; PVR, 20.8 Wood units; vs mPAP, 36 mm Hg; PVR, 6.25 Wood units) compared with patients who had a successful pregnancy. This latter group was also more likely to be on medical treatment of PAH.[53] Patients with severe PAH have also been shown to deliver earlier than those with mild PAH, usually because of heart failure symptoms.[68] In this same study, New York Heart Association (NYHA) class was tracked during pregnancy and remained stable at NYHA class I to II during pregnancy for patients with mild PAH, whereas almost all those with severe PAH had progression of NYHA class to at least class III at time of delivery.[68]

Although it seems that maternal mortalities have improved from initial investigations and in the setting of better understanding of PAH, advanced therapies, and preconception counseling/contraception, the morbidity and mortality of PAH in pregnancy are still high. Data suggest that outcomes may vary based on severity of disease and thus perhaps risk should not all be considered the same across the disease spectrum. Long-term fetal outcomes are also not well understood.

SUMMARY

PAH is a largely sex-specific disease affecting more women than men. Although the pathophysiology generally includes established pathways involving nitric oxide, prostacyclins, and endothelin, there are also genetic factors involved that predispose women to having PAH. The estrogen paradox is challenging to reconcile given that estrogen is thought to be more protective than harmful in PAH. Pregnancy is generally contraindicated in patients with PAH given the prohibitively high risk for maternal and fetal morbidity and mortality. Thus, preconception counseling and effective contraception are essential in patients with PAH. In patients who desire to proceed with pregnancy, PAH compounded by the physiologic changes of pregnancy can pose a significant hemodynamic burden that requires a multidisciplinary approach for care throughout pregnancy. The highest-risk period is the immediate postpartum period, when close monitoring and management are crucial. Although therapies have advanced, outcomes of patients with PAH and pregnancy are still poor, although they are improving.

Clinics care points

- PAH predominantly affects women. The estrogen paradox describes how, despite PAH being a sex-specific disease of women, estrogen seems to be protective rather than harmful in the pathophysiology of the disease.

- Pregnancy causes significant hemodynamic changes that may not be well tolerated in PAH. These effects typically manifest in patients at the end of the second/beginning of the third trimester.

- During pregnancy, a team approach including PH specialists, cardiologists, maternal-fetal medicine specialists, and anesthesiologists is crucial for managing patients with PAH. Most PAH medications (except endothelin antagonists and sGC stimulators) can be used safely during pregnancy. Anticoagulation should be considered in patients given the increased risk of VTE.

- Delivery should be scheduled before reaching full term. In general, cesarean delivery is recommended with combined spinal epidural anesthesia. The postpartum time period is the highest-risk time for women with regard to maternal complications and death. Patients should be closely monitored in the postpartum period because fluid shifts and hormonal changes can lead to heart failure and its sequelae.

DISCLOSURE

The authors have nothing to disclose.

REFERENCES

1. Galiè N, Humbert M, Vachiery JL, et al. [2015 ESC/ERS guidelines for the diagnosis and treatment of pulmonary hypertension]. Kardiol Pol 2015;73(12):1127–206.
2. Lau EMT, Giannoulatou E, Celermajer DS, et al. Epidemiology and treatment of pulmonary arterial hypertension. Nat Rev Cardiol 2017;14(10):603–14.
3. Badesch DB, Raskob GE, Elliott CG, et al. Pulmonary arterial hypertension: baseline characteristics from the REVEAL Registry. Chest 2010;137(2):376–87.
4. Simonneau G, Gatzoulis MA, Adatia I, et al. Updated clinical classification of pulmonary hypertension. J Am Coll Cardiol 2013;62(25 Suppl):D34–41.
5. Montani D, Chaumais MC, Guignabert C, et al. Targeted therapies in pulmonary arterial hypertension. Pharmacol Ther 2014;141(2):172–91.

6. Humbert M, Morrell NW, Archer SL, et al. Cellular and molecular pathobiology of pulmonary arterial hypertension. J Am Coll Cardiol 2004;43(12 Suppl S):13S–24S.

7. Chester AH, Yacoub MH, Moncada S. Nitric oxide and pulmonary arterial hypertension. Glob Cardiol Sci Pract 2017;2017(2):14.

8. Tuder RM, Cool CD, Geraci MW, et al. Prostacyclin synthase expression is decreased in lungs from patients with severe pulmonary hypertension. Am J Respir Crit Care Med 1999;159(6):1925–32.

9. Christman BW, McPherson CD, Newman JH, et al. An imbalance between the excretion of thromboxane and prostacyclin metabolites in pulmonary hypertension. N Engl J Med 1992;327(2):70–5.

10. Dupuis J, Hoeper MM. Endothelin receptor antagonists in pulmonary arterial hypertension. Eur Respir J 2008;31(2):407–15.

11. Loyd JE, Parker B, Lecture F. Genetics and gene expression in pulmonary hypertension. Chest Mar 2002;121(3 Suppl):46S–50S.

12. Larkin EK, Newman JH, Austin ED, et al. Longitudinal analysis casts doubt on the presence of genetic anticipation in heritable pulmonary arterial hypertension. Am J Respir Crit Care Med 2012;186(9):892–6.

13. Mair KM, Yang XD, Long L, et al. Sex affects bone morphogenetic protein type II receptor signaling in pulmonary artery smooth muscle cells. Am J Respir Crit Care Med 2015;191(6):693–703.

14. Tofovic SP. Estrogens and development of pulmonary hypertension: interaction of estradiol metabolism and pulmonary vascular disease. J Cardiovasc Pharmacol 2010;56(6):696–708.

15. Austin ED, Hamid R, Hemnes AR, et al. BMPR2 expression is suppressed by signaling through the estrogen receptor. Biol Sex Differ 2012;3(1):6.

16. Mair KM, Wright AF, Duggan N, et al. Sex-dependent influence of endogenous estrogen in pulmonary hypertension. Am J Respir Crit Care Med 2014;190(4):456–67.

17. Kawut SM, Archer-Chicko CL, DeMichele A, et al. Anastrozole in pulmonary arterial hypertension. A randomized, double-blind, placebo-controlled trial. Am J Respir Crit Care Med 2017;195(3):360–8.

18. Ventetuolo CE, Baird GL, Barr RG, et al. Higher estradiol and lower dehydroepiandrosterone-sulfate levels are associated with pulmonary arterial hypertension in men. Am J Respir Crit Care Med 2016; 193(10):1168–75.

19. Liu A, Schreier D, Tian L, et al. Direct and indirect protection of right ventricular function by estrogen in an experimental model of pulmonary arterial hypertension. Am J Physiol Heart Circ Physiol 2014; 307(3):H273–83.

20. Tello K, Richter MJ, Yogeswaran A, et al. Sex differences in right ventricular-pulmonary arterial coupling in pulmonary arterial hypertension. Am J

Respir Crit Care Med 2020. https://doi.org/10.1164/rccm.202003-0807LE.

21. Lahm T, Albrecht M, Fisher AJ, et al. 17β-Estradiol attenuates hypoxic pulmonary hypertension via estrogen receptor-mediated effects. Am J Respir Crit Care Med 2012;185(9):965–80.

22. Tofovic SP, Zhang X, Zhu H, et al. 2-Ethoxyestradiol is antimitogenic and attenuates monocrotaline-induced pulmonary hypertension and vascular remodeling. Vascul Pharmacol 2008;48(4–6):174–83.

23. Morey AK, Razandi M, Pedram A, et al. Oestrogen and progesterone inhibit the stimulated production of endothelin-1. Biochem J 1998;330(Pt 3): 1097–105.

24. Karas RH, van Eickels M, Lydon JP, et al. A complex role for the progesterone receptor in the response to vascular injury. J Clin Invest 2001;108(4):611–8.

25. Hester J, Ventetuolo C, Lahm T. Sex, gender, and sex hormones in pulmonary hypertension and right ventricular failure. Compr Physiol 2019;10(1): 125–70.

26. Smith AM, Bennett RT, Jones TH, et al. Characterization of the vasodilatory action of testosterone in the human pulmonary circulation. Vasc Health Risk Manag 2008;4(6):1459–66.

27. Hemnes AR, Maynard KB, Champion HC, et al. Testosterone negatively regulates right ventricular load stress responses in mice. Pulm Circ 2012; 2(3):352–8.

28. Docherty CK, Harvey KY, Mair KM, et al. The role of sex in the pathophysiology of pulmonary hypertension. Adv Exp Med Biol 2018;1065:511–28.

29. Ouzounian JG, Elkayam U. Physiologic changes during normal pregnancy and delivery. Cardiol Clin 2012;30(3):317–29.

30. Sanghavi M, Rutherford JD. Cardiovascular physiology of pregnancy. Circ Sep 2014;130(12): 1003–8.

31. Ducas RA, Elliott JE, Melnyk SF, et al. Cardiovascular magnetic resonance in pregnancy: insights from the cardiac hemodynamic imaging and remodeling in pregnancy (CHIRP) study. J Cardiovasc Magn Reson 2014;16:1.

32. Hemnes AR, Kiely DG, Cockrill BA, et al. Statement on pregnancy in pulmonary hypertension from the pulmonary vascular Research Institute. Pulm Circ 2015;5(3):435–65.

33. Hönicke U, Albrecht S, Schrötter H, et al. Prolactin and its 16-kDa N-terminal fragment: are higher in patients with precapillary pulmonary hypertension than in a healthy control group. Tex Heart Inst J 2012;39(1):44–50.

34. Sokolova J, Zimmermann R, Kreuder J, et al. Impaired release of bioactive parathyroid hormone-related peptide in patients with pulmonary hypertension and endothelial dysfunction. J Vasc Res 2007; 44(1):67–74.

35. Sugishita Y, Ito I, Kubo T. Pregnancy in cardiac patients: possible influence of volume overload by pregnancy on pulmonary circulation. Jpn Circ J 1986;50(4):376–83.

36. Regitz-Zagrosek V, Roos-Hesselink JW, Bauersachs J, et al. 2018 ESC Guidelines for the management of cardiovascular diseases during pregnancy. Eur Heart J 2018;39(34):3165–241.

37. Kiely DG, Condliffe R, Webster V, et al. Improved survival in pregnancy and pulmonary hypertension using a multiprofessional approach. BJOG 2010; 117(5):565–74.

38. Kiely DG, Condliffe R, Wilson VJ, et al. Pregnancy and pulmonary hypertension: a practical approach to management. Obstet Med 2013;6(4):144–54.

39. ten Klooster L, Theodorou C, Wilson V, et al. Managing pregnancy in pulmonary hypertension using a multi-professional approach: a 16-year experience in a specialist referral centre. Eur Respir J 2017; 50(suppl 61):PA2424.

40. Verma AK, Williams D, Nelson DM, et al. A cardio-obstetric approach to management of the complex pregnant cardiac patient. JACC: Case Rep 2020; 2(1):86–90.

41. Vigl M, Kaemmerer M, Seifert-Klauss V, et al. Contraception in women with congenital heart disease. Am J Cardiol 2010;106(9):1317–21.

42. Hill W, Holy R, Traiger G. EXPRESS: intimacy, contraception, and pregnancy prevention in patients with pulmonary arterial hypertension: are we counseling our patients? Pulm Circ 2018. https://doi.org/10. 1177/2045894018785259. 2045894018785259.

43. Thorne S, Nelson-Piercy C, MacGregor A, et al. Pregnancy and contraception in heart disease and pulmonary arterial hypertension. J Fam Plann Reprod Health Care 2006;32(2):75–81.

44. Chaouat A, Weitzenblum E, Higenbottam T. The role of thrombosis in severe pulmonary hypertension. Eur Respir J 1996;9(2):356–63.

45. Dragoman MV, Tepper NK, Fu R, et al. A systematic review and meta-analysis of venous thrombosis risk among users of combined oral contraception. Int J Gynaecol Obstet 2018;141(3):287–94.

46. Banerjee D, Ventetuolo CE. Pulmonary hypertension in pregnancy. Semin Respir Crit Care Med 2017; 38(2):148–59.

47. van Giersbergen PL, Halabi A, Dingemanse J. Pharmacokinetic interaction between bosentan and the oral contraceptives norethisterone and ethinyl estradiol. Int J Clin Pharmacol Ther 2006;44(3):113–8.

48. Chung WK, Austin ED, Best DH, et al. When to offer genetic testing for pulmonary arterial hypertension. Can J Cardiol 2015;31(4):544–7.

49. McLaughlin VV, Archer SL, Badesch DB, et al. ACCF/AHA 2009 expert consensus document on pulmonary hypertension a report of the American College of Cardiology Foundation Task Force on expert Consensus Documents and the American Heart Association developed in collaboration with the American College of Chest Physicians; American Thoracic Society, Inc.; and the Pulmonary Hypertension Association. J Am Coll Cardiol 2009; 53(17):1573–619.

50. Leter EM, Boonstra AB, Postma FB, et al. Genetic counselling for pulmonary arterial hypertension: a matter of variable variability. Neth Heart J 2011; 19(2):89–92.

51. Sliwa K, van Hagen IM, Budts W, et al. Pulmonary hypertension and pregnancy outcomes: data from the Registry Of Pregnancy and Cardiac Disease (ROPAC) of the European Society of Cardiology. Eur J Heart Fail 2016;18(9):1119–28.

52. Taichman DB, Ornelas J, Chung L, et al. Pharmacologic therapy for pulmonary arterial hypertension in adults: CHEST guideline and expert panel report. Chest 2014;146(2):449–75.

53. Jaïs X, Olsson KM, Barbera JA, et al. Pregnancy outcomes in pulmonary arterial hypertension in the modern management era. Eur Respir J 2012;40(4):881–5.

54. Magee LA, Schick B, Donnenfeld AE, et al. The safety of calcium channel blockers in human pregnancy: a prospective, multicenter cohort study. Am J Obstet Gynecol 1996;174(3):823–8.

55. Weber-Schoendorfer C, Hannemann D, Meister R, et al. The safety of calcium channel blockers during pregnancy: a prospective, multicenter, observational study. Reprod Toxicol 2008;26(1):24–30.

56. Flenady V, Wojcieszek AM, Papatsonis DN, et al. Calcium channel blockers for inhibiting preterm labour and birth. Cochrane Database Syst Rev 2014;(6):CD002255.

57. Bendayan D, Hod M, Oron G, et al. Pregnancy outcome in patients with pulmonary arterial hypertension receiving prostacyclin therapy. Obstet Gynecol 2005;106(5 Pt 2):1206–10.

58. Briggs GG, Freeman RK, Towers CV, et al. 11th edition. Drugs in pregnancy and lactation: a reference guide to fetal and neonatal risk, vol. xiii. Wolters Kluwer; 2017. p. 1646.

59. Lindheimer MD, Katz AI. Sodium and diuretics in pregnancy. N Engl J Med 1973;288(17):891–4.

60. Schaefer C, Hannemann D, Meister R, et al. Vitamin K antagonists and pregnancy outcome. A multicentre prospective study. Thromb Haemost 2006; 95(6):949–57.

61. Forestier F, Daffos F, Capella-Pavlovsky M. Low molecular weight heparin (PK 10169) does not cross the placenta during the second trimester of pregnancy study by direct fetal blood sampling under ultrasound. Thromb Res 1984;34(6):557–60.

62. Lameijer H, Aalberts JJJ, van Veldhuisen DJ, et al. Efficacy and safety of direct oral anticoagulants during pregnancy; a systematic literature review. Thromb Res 2018;169:123–7.

63. Konstantinides SV. Trends in pregnancy outcomes in patients with pulmonary hypertension: still a long way to go. Eur J Heart Fail 2016;18(9):1129–31.

64. Meng ML, Landau R, Viktorsdottir O, et al. Pulmonary hypertension in pregnancy: a report of 49 cases at Four tertiary North American Sites. Obstet Gynecol 2017;129(3):511–20.

65. Martin JT, Tautz TJ, Antognini JF. Safety of regional anesthesia in Eisenmenger's syndrome. Reg Anesth Pain Med 2002;27(5):509–13.

66. Blaise G, Langleben D, Hubert B. Pulmonary arterial hypertension: pathophysiology and anesthetic approach. Anesthesiology 2003;99(6):1415–32.

67. Drugs and lactation Database (LactMed). National Library of Medicine. Available at: https://www.ncbi.nlm.nih.gov/books/NBK501922/.

68. Katsuragi S, Yamanaka K, Neki R, et al. Maternal outcome in pregnancy complicated with pulmonary arterial hypertension. Circ J 2012;76(9):2249–54.

Peripartum Cardiomyopathy

Erika J. Douglass, MPH[a,b], Lori A. Blauwet, MD[c],*

KEYWORDS

- Peripartum cardiomyopathy • PPCM • Postpartum cardiomyopathy • Pregnancy • Heart failure

KEY POINTS

- Diagnosing peripartum cardiomyopathy (PPCM) requires a high degree of suspicion, because presenting signs and symptoms tend to mimic those of normal pregnancy and the early postpartum period.
- Guideline-directed medical therapy for heart failure, with special considerations for use during pregnancy and lactation, is recommended, although efficacy and optimal duration of therapy have not been established.
- Outcomes of both mother and child are generally good, although a subset of women experience chronic heart failure, transplant, and/or cardiac death.
- Subsequent pregnancy is not contraindicated in all women with history of PPCM, because risk of cardiac complications associated with future pregnancy varies according to degree of left ventricular recovery.

INTRODUCTION

Peripartum cardiomyopathy (PPCM) is a form of heart failure with no known cause that occurs toward the end of pregnancy or in the months following pregnancy and is marked by left ventricular (LV) systolic dysfunction. Outcomes vary, because most women experience complete LV recovery, but a significant minority experience persistent cardiac dysfunction, transplant, or death.

CASE DEFINITION

The National Heart, Lung, and Blood Institute (NHLBI) and the Heart Failure Association (HFA) of the European Society of Cardiology (ESC) Working Group (WG) on PPCM have both published definitions for PPCM[1,2] (**Box 1**). These 2 definitions differ in terms of timing of diagnosis and the cutoff for LV ejection fraction (LVEF). Further investigation is needed to determine

potential differences between women diagnosed with PPCM using the NHLBI criteria and (1) women who present with previously undiagnosed cardiomyopathy before 1 month before delivery or greater than 5 months postdelivery, and (2) women who present with an initial LVEF greater than 45%, to determine whether or not pathophysiology and outcomes are similar. Having a clear and accurate definition of PPCM is crucial for determining optimal management strategies and prognosis and facilitating collaborative research.

EPIDEMIOLOGY

Estimates of PPCM incidence vary widely around the world, with many of the estimates coming from retrospective single-center cohort studies. **Fig. 1** presents selected incidence estimates from several countries. The highest reported rates occur in Nigeria, with 995 cases per

---

[a] Department of Cardiovascular Medicine, Mayo Clinic, 4500 San Pablo Road, Jacksonville, FL 32224, USA;
[b] Department of Environmental Health and Engineering, Johns Hopkins Bloomberg School of Public Health, Baltimore, MD, USA; [c] Department of Cardiovascular Medicine, Mayo Clinic, 200 First Street Southwest, Rochester, MN 55905, USA
* Corresponding author.
E-mail address: blauwetlori@gmail.com

Cardiol Clin 39 (2021) 119–142
https://doi.org/10.1016/j.ccl.2020.09.008

Box 1
Current peripartum cardiomyopathy definitions.

NHLBI[1]

- Development of cardiac failure in the last month of pregnancy or within 5 months of delivery
- Absence of an identifiable cause for the cardiac failure
- Absence of recognizable heart disease before the last month of pregnancy
- LV systolic dysfunction identified by classic echocardiographic criteria, such as ejection fraction less than 45% or fractional shortening less than 30%, or both

European Society of Cardiology[2]

- Heart failure secondary to LV systolic dysfunction with an LV ejection fraction less than 45%
- Occurrence toward the end of pregnancy or in the months following delivery (mostly in the months following delivery)
- No other identifiable cause of heart failure

(*Data from* Pearson GD, Veille JC, Rahimtoola S, et al. Peripartum cardiomyopathy: National Heart, Lung, and Blood Institute and Office of Rare Diseases (National Institutes of Health) workshop recommendations and review. Jama. 2000;283(9):1183-1188 and Sliwa K, Hilfiker-Kleiner D, Petrie MC, et al. Current state of knowledge on aetiology, diagnosis, management, and therapy of peripartum cardiomyopathy: a position statement from the Heart Failure Association of the European Society of Cardiology Working Group on peripartum cardiomyopathy. European journal of heart failure. 2010;12(8):767-778).

100,000 deliveries, and Togo, with 781 cases per 100,000 deliveries.[3,4] In the United States, nationwide estimates vary from 18 to 103 per 100,000 live births or deliveries.[5-9] Risk factors associated with increased risk of developing PPCM include black African descent, hypertensive diseases of pregnancy (HDPs), multifetal pregnancies, and advanced maternal age.[6,7,10-13]

PATHOPHYSIOLOGY, GENETICS, AND RISK FACTORS

The cause of PPCM is not fully understood but is most likely multifactorial. Current research suggests that hormones of late pregnancy cause a vasculotoxic environment that, in susceptible women, leads to the development of PPCM.[14,15] High levels of prolactin are secreted from the pituitary gland and can be cleaved into the vasculotoxic, proinflammatory, and proapoptotic 16-kDa form.[16] At the same time, antiangiogenic soluble fms-like tyrosine kinase-1 (sFlt-1) is secreted from the placenta, inhibiting vascular endothelial growth factor and placental growth factor. Both the 16-kDa form of prolactin and sFlt-1 have been shown to cause PPCM in mouse models.[17,18] sFlt-1 levels are significantly increased in women with PPCM, and higher levels at diagnosis are associated with worse outcomes.[19] Women with preeclampsia also have significantly increased sFlt-1 levels, which may at least partially explain why HDP increases risk for PPCM.[20]

A small percentage of women with PPCM have a family history of dilated cardiomyopathy (DCM). Family clustering has also been observed.[21-26] Studies have also shown that a subset of women with PPCM have genetic mutations linked to DCM, predominantly in the TTN gene, which encodes the titin protein, which is critical to cardiac muscle structure.[27-29] The Investigations of Pregnancy Associated Cardiomyopathy (IPAC) study found that 1 TTN mutation genotype was associated with lower LVEF at 6 and 12 months, especially in black women, which may help explain why black women have worse outcomes compared with white women.[30] High frequencies of mutations in the TTN gene have also been found in women with preeclampsia, which may help to explain the increased risk of PPCM in women diagnosed with HDP.[31] However, only 15% to 20% of women with PPCM have TTN mutations, and greater than 90% of individuals in the general population that have TTN mutations never develop any form of cardiomyopathy,[27-29,32] so the significance of TTN mutations in women with PPCM remains unclear. Other factors that may increase susceptibility for PPCM include oxidative stress, inflammation, viral infection, and antiangiogenic molecules.[33]

DIAGNOSIS

Because the exact cause remains unknown and no single test currently exists to confirm the diagnosis, PPCM remains a diagnosis of exclusion. Women generally present with symptoms that are common to pregnancy (orthopnea, dyspnea on exertion, fatigue, edema, paroxysmal nocturnal exertion, and chest tightness), so the diagnosis of PPCM may be delayed or missed altogether. Late diagnosis has been linked to worse outcomes, including persistent cardiac dysfunction and increased mortality.[13,34-40]

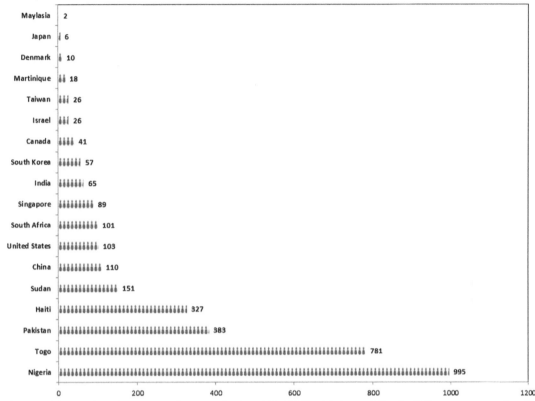

Fig. 1. Incidence of peripartum cardiomyopathy (per 100,000 live births or deliveries.) Measurements using live births: Haiti,[127] United States,[9] Singapore,[77] India,[128] Canada,[119] Martinique,[129] Japan,[130] Malaysia.[131] Measurements using deliveries: Nigeria,[3] Togo,[4] Pakistan,[132] Sudan,[133] China,[134] South Africa,[135] South Korea,[136] Israel,[118] Taiwan,[39] Denmark.[64] *Data from* Refs.[3,4,9,39,64,77,118,119,127–136]

Diagnostic Tests

Echocardiogram, electrocardiogram (ECG), chest radiograph, cardiac MRI, and laboratory testing may all be useful in the diagnosis of PPCM. Echocardiography is the most important imaging modality, because it is readily available in many health care centers and can easily and comprehensively assess cardiac structure and function. By the NHLBI definition, LVEF must be less than 45%.[1] The left ventricle is usually, but not always, dilated.[33–35,41] Assessment of right ventricular (RV) function is essential, because 3 recent articles have reported that many women with PPCM also have RV dysfunction and that these women are at higher risk for adverse outcomes.[42–44] Additional echocardiographic findings may include RV dilatation, mitral and/or tricuspid valve regurgitation, atrial enlargement, increased pulmonary pressures, and intracardiac thrombus.[33–35,41] Cardiac MRI may be useful for the evaluation of biventricular structure and function or when echocardiography is nondiagnostic, but gadolinium is not recommended for use during pregnancy.[43,45,46] Suggested diagnostic testing is outlined in **Table 1**.

BIOMARKERS

Many biomarker levels have been shown to be abnormal in women with PPCM and may thus be useful in diagnosing PPCM (**Table 2**). Markers of cardiac function such as N-terminal prohormone of brain natriuretic peptide (NT-proBNP), brain natriuretic peptide (BNP), and cardiac troponin are likely the most clinically useful. No biomarkers can be used in isolation to confirm PPCM, because none are specific to this disease.

TREATMENT
Initial Management

Initial management strategies vary depending on pregnancy status (**Table 3**). A multidisciplinary team approach to management is recommended,

Table 1
Suggested evaluation for women with peripartum cardiomyopathy

Time Period[a]	History and Clinical Examination	Laboratory Tests[b]	Urinalysis[c]	Chest Radiograph	Chest CTA[d]	ECG	ECHO	Cardiac MRI[e]
Diagnosis	♥♥♥	♥♥♥	♥♥	♥♥♥	♥♥	♥♥♥	♥♥♥	♥♥
3 mo	♥♥♥	♥♥♥				♥♥♥		
6 mo	♥♥♥	♥♥♥				♥♥♥	♥♥♥	
12 mo	♥♥♥	♥♥♥				♥♥♥	♥♥♥	
18 mo	♥♥♥	♥♥♥				♥♥♥	♥♥♥	
24 mo	♥♥♥	♥♥♥				♥♥♥	♥♥♥	
>24 mo[f]	♥♥♥	♥♥♥				♥♥♥	♥♥♥	

♥♥♥, highly recommended.
♥♥, recommended in certain circumstances.
♥, consider in certain circumstances.

Abbreviations: CTA, computed tomography angiography; ECG, electrocardiogram; ECHO, echocardiogram.

[a] Timing of follow-up may vary according to presentation and clinical course.
[b] Suggested laboratory tests include complete blood count, basic metabolic panel, and brain natriuretic peptide (BNP) or N-terminal prohormone of BNP (NT-proBNP) at all times points plus aspartate aminotransferase, alanine aminotransferase, cardiac troponin, and thyroid-stimulating hormone at baseline and during follow-up, if indicated.
[c] Urinalysis is especially important for women presenting with increased blood pressure during pregnancy or the first 6 weeks postpartum.
[d] Consider chest CTA to assess for pulmonary embolism in patients presenting during pregnancy or the first 6 weeks postpartum.
[e] Consider cardiac MRI if patient presents during the postpartum period and echocardiography results are inconclusive.
[f] Annual follow-up should occur indefinitely.

Table 2
Biomarkers in peripartum cardiomyopathy

Biomarkers of Cardiac Function		
NT-ProBNP	May be increased[29,138,154]	Failure to decrease levels by 6 mo is associated with persistent LV dysfunction[138]
BNP	May be increased[104]	Higher levels at diagnosis are associated with persistent LV dysfunction[104,138] Higher levels at 6 mo are associated with persistent LV dysfunction[104] Higher levels at 6 mo may predict mortality[89,138] Increased levels at 3 and 6 mo may predict persistent dysfunction[69] Lower levels at 3 and 6 mo are associated with faster recovery[69]
Cardiac troponin	May be increased[154]	Higher levels at diagnosis are associated with persistent LV dysfunction[156]
Biomarkers of Inflammation		
C-reactive protein	May be increased[95,138,154,157]	Higher levels at baseline may predict mortality[157] Higher levels at baseline are correlated with worse disease[95] Increased levels at 3 and 6 mo may predict persistent dysfunction[69]
IL-6	May be increased[138,157]	Higher levels at baseline may predict mortality[157]
Tumor necrosis factor alpha	May be increased[95,138,157]	Higher levels at baseline may predict mortality[157]
IL-1β	May be increased[138]	—
Interferon gamma	May be increased[138]	Failure to decrease levels by 6 mo is associated with persistent LV dysfunction[138]
Pregnancy and Nursing Hormones		
Relaxin-2	May be decreased[158,159]	Higher levels at diagnosis are associated with recovery at 2 mo[19]
Prolactin	May be increased[138]	Failure to decrease levels by 6 mo is associated with persistent LV dysfunction[138]
Vasculotoxic Cause–related Biomarkers		
Oxidized low-density lipoprotein	May be increased[16,138]	Failure to decrease levels by 6 mo is associated with persistent LV dysfunction[138]
Fas/apoptosis antigen 1	May be increased[95,138]	Higher levels at baseline may predict mortality[95]

sFlt-1	May be increased[18]	Higher levels at diagnosis are associated with more severe disease and major adverse events[19,60]
Asymmetric dimethyl arginine	May be increased[29]	—
PlGF	May be increased[159]	—
sFlt1/PlGF ratio	May be low[159]	—
Plasminogen activator inhibitor-1	May be increased[160]	—
MicroRNAs		
miR-146a	May be increased[29,161]	—
miR-1991	May be increased[162]	—
Biomarkers of Fibrosis and Remodeling		
Galectin-3	May be increased[102]	High baseline levels are associated with poor outcomes[102]
Soluble ST2	May be increased[102]	High baseline levels are associated with poor outcomes[102]
Cleaved osteopontin	May be increased[102]	High baseline levels are associated with poor outcomes[102]
Matrix-metallo-proteinase-2	May be increased[138]	—

Abbreviations: IL, interleukin; PlGF, placental growth factor.
    (*Data from* Refs[16,18,19,29,60,89,95,96,102,104,138,154,156–160,162])

particularly if the woman is pregnant or in the early postpartum period.

Medical Therapy

Women diagnosed with PPCM should be treated with guideline-directed medical therapy (GDMT) for heart failure with reduced ejection fraction (HFrEF), bearing in mind the safety of specific medications during pregnancy and breastfeeding. Recommended medications may include β-blockers, angiotensin-converting enzyme inhibitors (ACE-Is)/angiotensin receptor II blocker (ARBs), angiotensin receptor neprilysin inhibitor (ARNIs), hydralazine/nitrates, mineralocorticoid receptor antagonists (MRAs), and diuretics. Anticoagulation should be initiated if LV thrombus is present and may be considered in women with LVEF less than 35%.

Whether or not initiating GDMT for HFrEF is necessary in all women with PPCM remains unclear, because some women recover LV function quickly and completely while taking only minimal to low doses of heart failure medications. Note that there has never been a randomized clinical trial testing the efficacy and safety of any heart failure medications in women with PPCM. Information regarding specific medications and their compatibility with pregnancy and breast feeding is reviewed Karen L. Florio and colleagues' article, "Cardiovascular Medications in Pregnancy: A Primer," in this issue.

Bromocriptine

Bromocriptine, which inhibits the nursing hormone prolactin, has been proposed as a novel treatment of PPCM in response to the hypothesis that the development of PPCM is driven by the antiangiogenic and proapoptotic 16-kDa cleaved form of prolactin. A small proof-of-concept study with 20 women in South Africa found that the addition of bromocriptine led to greater recovery of LVEF and lower mortality at 6 months.[47] A second study in Burkina Faso showed that treatment with bromocriptine was associated with increased LVEF at 2 weeks and at 3, 6, and 12 months, as well as decreased mortality.[48] However, both studies had unusually high rates of mortality in the control groups, limiting the ability to generalize the results. A multicenter randomized study with no control group conducted in Germany compared 2 dosing regimens (1 week vs 8 weeks) of bromocriptine in addition to GDMT for heart failure.[49] Both study groups had similar outcomes, with no women undergoing heart transplant and

Table 3
Initial management of peripartum cardiomyopathy

	Hemodynamically Stable	Hemodynamically Unstable	Hemodynamically Stable	Hemodynamically Unstable
Consult Cardio-obstetrics specialist	✓	✓	✓	✓
Consult High-risk obstetrics (maternal fetal medicine) specialist	✓	✓	—	—
Form multidisciplinary team to prepare delivery plan	✓	✓	—	—
Consider early delivery	—	✓	—	—
Arrange for fetal monitoring during labor and delivery	✓	✓	—	—
Initiate selected oral heart failure medications (eg, diuretics, nitrates, hydralazine, digoxin)	✓	✓	—	—
Initiate oral GDMT for HFrEF (eg, β-blocker, ACE-I, ARB, ARNI, MRA, diuretics [modify if lactating])	—	—	✓	✓ (after stabilized)
Consider using inotropes	—	✓	—	✓
Initiate anticoagulation if LV thrombus	✓	✓	✓	✓

(continued on next page)

Table 3
(continued)

	Hemodynamically Stable (pregnant)	Hemodynamically Unstable (pregnant)	Hemodynamically Stable (postpartum)	Hemodynamically Unstable (postpartum)
Consider anticoagulation if LVEF <35%	—	—	✓	✓
Plan for vaginal delivery	✓	—	—	—
Plan for probable cesarean delivery	—	✓	—	—
Provide supplemental oxygen and/or noninvasive ventilation, if hypoxic	✓	—	✓	—
Intubate and ventilate if hypoxic despite noninvasive ventilation	—	✓	—	✓
Consider advanced heart failure therapies[a] if failure to respond to medical therapy (and delivery)	—	✓	—	✓
Discuss lactation preferences	—	—	✓	—
Discuss contraception	—	—	✓	✓

Abbreviations: ACE-I, angiotensin-converting enzyme inhibitor; ARB, angiotensin receptor blocker; ARNI, angiotensin receptor neprilysin inhibitor; GDMT, guideline-directed medical therapy; HFrEF, heart failure with reduced ejection fraction; MRA, mineralocorticoid receptor antagonist.

[a] Mechanical circulatory support/ventricular assist device/cardiac transplant.

no mortality in either group. The lack of a control group limits the applicability of these results in current clinical practice.

In addition to the lack of rigorous clinical research showing the efficacy of bromocriptine for treatment of acute PPCM, concern regarding potential serious adverse effects has limited routine administration of bromocriptine in clinical practice. Treatment with bromocriptine has been associated with stroke, myocardial infarction, and seizures and, as a result, it is no longer marketed for elective lactation suppression in the United States.[34] If bromocriptine is used, anticoagulation should be administered for the duration of therapy because women are already in a hypercoagulable state during the peripartum period and bromocriptine may further increase hypercoagulability.

Of particular importance, women treated with bromocriptine cannot breastfeed their infants. The World Health Organization recommends exclusive breastfeeding for 6 months and continued breastfeeding for at least 1 to 2 years because of the importance of breastfeeding to the health of both mother and infant. Not breastfeeding is associated with increased risk of diabetes, ovarian and breast cancer, and postpartum depression for mothers, and higher rates of mortality, infections, eczema, asthma, childhood obesity, type 2 diabetes, leukemia, and lower intelligence in children.[50,51] Results of the IPAC study and 2 retrospective cohort studies suggest that breastfeeding has no detrimental effect on outcomes for women with PPCM.[52–54]

The most recent statement on PPCM by the HFA ESC WG PPCM lists treatment with bromocriptine as a class IIb recommendation.[41] In contrast, the American Heart Association (AHA) and the Canadian Cardiovascular Society (CCS) both recommend that bromocriptine should not routinely be used in the treatment of PPCM until more rigorous data that support the safety and effectiveness of its use are available.[35,55]

Chronic Management

Most experts agree that GDMT for HFrEF should be continued indefinitely in women with PPCM who have persistent cardiac dysfunction. The optimal duration of treatment of women who recover normal LV function is unknown. A 2016 AHA scientific statement on the diagnosis and treatment of dilated cardiomyopathies recommended indefinite continuation of treatment in women with PPCM, including those with recovered cardiac function, as well as yearly clinical follow-up and assessment of LV function even after

recovery.[35] More recent articles suggest that treatment duration should be considered on a case-by-case basis, with changes to or discontinuation of any cardiac medications to be completed slowly using a stepwise approach with frequent clinical and echocardiographic monitoring and follow-up.[34,41] The HFA ESC WG PPCM has published recommendations for women diagnosed with PPCM who have recovered LV function (LVEF>55%) and are New York Heart Association (NYHA) functional class I as follows: continuation of all cardiac drugs for at least 12 to 24 months after full recovery and then discontinue them in a stepwise fashion (first MRA, second ACE-I/ARB/ ARNI, and then β-blocker) with frequent monitoring of symptoms and LV function.[41] Thus, although both the AHA and HFA ESC WG PPCM guidelines agree that diuretics can be tapered and discontinued if there are no signs of fluid overload, there is no consensus regarding duration of other cardiac medications in individual women.

Several studies and case reports have shown that some women with PPCM who have recovered LV function can safely be tapered off medical therapy.[36,56–58] In 1 study, 5 women were tapered off all cardiac medications and none experienced deterioration of LV function over an average follow-up duration of 29 months (range, 5–63 months.)[58] Another report found that 2 women who had fully recovered LV function had deterioration of LVEF after discontinuation of all cardiac medications, with deterioration occurring at 24 and 34 months after diagnosis.[57] Two more recent studies found that women with LV recovery may have high rates of LV diastolic dysfunction and reduced exercise capacity[59] as well as ongoing angiogenic imbalance and residual myocardial injury,[60] suggesting that women who recover may benefit from long-term GDMT for HFrEF.

Long-term cardiology follow-up of women with history of PPCM who have recovered LV function is recommended regardless of whether or not LV recovery occurs and/or cardiac medications are discontinued (see **Table 1**).

Advanced Heart Failure Therapies

Women with PPCM who have severe myocardial disease may benefit from a wearable or implantable cardiac defibrillator, left ventricular assist device (LVAD), mechanical circulatory support (MCS), and/or transplant. Multiple factors affect the rates of each of these types of advanced heart failure therapy, including time to diagnosis, race, and availability. Rates of use of each of these advanced therapies in women with PPCM are difficult to discern, because studies often do not list these therapies separately and have combined these outcomes differently for reporting. A nationwide study conducted in the United States reported that, between 2004 and 2011, 1.5% of patients with PPCM required MCS and 0.5% of patients underwent transplant.[9] Study specific rates in the United States vary between 0% and 7.8% for defibrillator implantation, 0% to 17.2% for MCS (intra-aortic balloon pump, LVAD, and extracorporeal membrane oxygenation), and 0% to 8.8% for transplant.[11,36,40,61–63] Rates in other countries vary widely, often depending on the availability of these advanced treatment options.[39,56,63–71]

OUTCOMES
Mortality

Women with PPCM tend to have lower mortalities than women with other forms of DCM.[72,73] Reported mortalities related to PPCM vary widely both within and between countries and within similar follow-up durations (**Table 4**). A recent systematic review and meta-analysis by Kerpen and colleagues[74] found the overall PPCM mortality to be 9%, with higher rates in developing countries (14%) compared with more advanced countries (4%). **Fig. 2**, which includes 9 countries in addition to the 13 included in the meta-analysis by Kerpen and colleagues,[74] shows a similar trend of higher mortalities in developing countries. The higher PPCM mortalities in developing countries are most likely related to the impact of social determinants of health, including reduced access to care in general and access to advanced heart failure therapies in particular.

Mortalities in Taiwan and the United States seem to be exceptions among advanced countries, whereas rates in The Philippines, China, and Singapore do not follow the trend among developing countries. Small sample sizes[75–77] and differences in methodologies and populations, particularly among the US reports,[7–9,11–13,36,38,40,43,58,61,62,72,73,78–87] may account for these variations.

Left Ventricular Recovery

Similar to mortality, women with PPCM tend to have higher rates of LV recovery than women with other forms of DCM.[72,73] Recovery rates differ between countries, from 28% in Haiti[88] to 43% in Israel,[71] 48% in Turkey,[89] 47% in Germany,[29] 55% in South Africa,[90] 63% in Japan,[67] and 67% in Denmark.[64] There is a wide variation in recovery rates within the United States as well, with reported rates ranging between 23% and 72%.[38,40,58,61,78,84,86,91,92] Lack of consensus in

the definition of LV recovery (LVEF>45% vs 50%, vs 55%, or any recovery vs a specific percentage increase in LVEF) and follow-up time (6 months vs 12 months vs longer) contributes to the large range in reported LV recovery rates among studies across the globe.

Timing of LV recovery varies, with some women recovering in days to weeks, whereas other women require months to years. An article from Israel reported that 22% of women with PPCM achieved full recovery (LVEF $\geq$ 50%) within 2 weeks, a further 30.1% recovered by 1 year, and an additional 13.8% recovered between 1 and 10 years.[71] The mean time to recovery in a study of 44 women in the United States was 54 months.[86] In Haiti, reported recovery time ranged from 3 to 38 months and in Turkey from 3 to 42 months (mean, 19.3 months).[69,93] One study completed in the United States found that 83% of women who recovered did so after more than 6 months of follow-up, whereas another study reported that 25% of women who recovered did so between 2 and 8 years after diagnosis.[84,94] The wide range of time to LV recovery underlines the importance of long-term cardiac follow-up of women with PPCM.

Predictors of Outcome

Many factors have been evaluated for their potential to predict outcomes in PPCM, particularly the risks for persistent myocardial dysfunction and death. The most reliable predictor has been found to be LVEF at diagnosis, with studies consistently reporting that women with lower LVEF (particularly <30%) at diagnosis are less likely to recover and more likely to experience adverse outcomes, including death.[29,36,38,40,57,58,61,78,80,83,86,91,92,95,96] Studies have also reported that the degree of LV dilatation may be a useful predictor, with larger LV end-diastolic diameter (LVEDD) being associated with lack of LV recovery and death.[29,40,57,58,78,92,96,97] LV dilatation and LVEF were combined as predictors in the IPAC study, which found that 91% of women with LVEF greater than or equal to 30% and LVEDD less than 60 mm recovered.[40] The IPAC study also reported that LV global longitudinal strain at presentation was associated with clinical outcomes and may be useful for risk stratification in addition to LVEF.[98] RV fractional area change at diagnosis was shown to be a strong predictor of outcomes in the IPAC study,[44] whereas another study in the United States found that moderate to severe RV dysfunction was associated with more severe disease and higher risk of adverse outcomes.[43] T-wave abnormalities on

Table 4
Studies with greater than or equal to 50 subjects reporting mortality among women with peripartum cardiomyopathy

First Author	Follow-up Duration	Actual, Mean, Median	Country	Data Source	Study Years	Sample (n)	Mortality (%)
In Hospital							
Kolte et al,[9] 2014	NA	NA	United States	Nationwide Inpatient Sample database	2004–2011	34,219	0.0
Krisnamoorthy et al,[80] 2016	NA	NA	United States	Nationwide Inpatient Sample database	2009–2010	4871	0.0
Lee et al,[136] 2018	NA	NA	South Korea	Korean National Health Insurance Database	2010–2012	795	1.0
Masoomi et al,[8] 2018	NA	NA	United States	Nationwide Readmissions Database	2013	568	1.2
Kao et al,[11] 2013	NA	NA	United States	Inpatient administrative databases for 6 states	2003–2007	535	1.3
Mielniczuk et al,[7] 2006	NA	NA	United States	National Hospital Discharge Survey	1990–2002	16,269	1.9
1–6 mo							
Azibani et al,[102] 2020	6 mo	Actual	Germany	1 hospital	Missing	73	0.0
Dhesi et al,[119] 2017	6 mo	Actual	Canada	Multiple databases linked together covering all of Alberta	2005–2014	194	1.5

(continued on next page)

Table 4
(continued)

First Author	Follow-up Duration	Actual, Mean, Median	Country	Data Source	Study Years	Sample (n)	Mortality (%)
Huang et al,[154] 2012	21.6 d	Mean	China	1 hospital	2007–2009	52	1.9
Tibazarwa et al,[90] 2012	6 mo	Actual	South Africa	1 hospital	2003–2008	78	3.8
Libhaber et al,[97] 2015	6 mo	Actual	South Africa	2 hospitals	Missing	206	12.6
Blauwet et al,[106] 2013	6 mo	Actual	South Africa	1 hospital	Missing	162	13.0
Azibani et al,[102] 2020	6 mo	Actual	South Africa	1 hospital	Missing	56	14.3
Sliwa 2006 et al,[95] 2006	6 mo	Actual	South Africa	1 hospital	Missing	100	15.0
7–12 mo							
Kamiya et al,[67] 2011	9.6 mo	Mean	Japan	Nationwide survey of medical locations	2007–2008	102	3.9
Isezuo et al,[3] 2007	9.7 mo	Mean	Nigeria	1 hospital	2003–2005	65	12.3
1–2 y							
Phan et al,[79] 2020	1 y	Actual	United States	Southern California Kaiser Healthcare System	2003–2014	333	0.3
Erbsøll et al,[64] 2017	10–14 mo	Actual	Denmark	Danish National Patient Register, Medical Birth Registry, Causes of Death Registry	2005–2014	61	1.6

Study	Follow-up	Type	Country	Setting	Years	N	%
McNamara et al,[40] 2015	1 y	Actual	United States	IPAC: nationwide cohort of 100 women	2009–2012	100	4.0
Goland et al,[12] 2013	1.6 y	Mean	United States	2 hospitals	1993–2000	156	7.1
Wu et al,[39] 2017	1 y	Actual	Taiwan	National health insurance database	1997–2011	742	7.3
Elkayam et al,[38] 2015	1.9 y	Mean	United States	Survey mailed to doctors nationwide and data from 1 hospital	Missing	100	9.0
Sliwa et al,[140] 2011	2 y	Actual	South Africa	1 hospital	Missing	60	36.7
>2 y							
Amos et al,[58] 2006	3.6 y	Mean	United States	1 hospital	1990–2003	55	0.0
Habli et al,[78] 2018	3.4 y	Mean	United States	2 hospitals	2000–2006	70	0.0
Li et al,[104] 2016	3.6 y	Mean	China	1 hospital	2004–2011	71	0.0
Moulig et al,[152] 2019	5 y	Actual	Germany	1 hospital	2006–2013	66	1.5
Gunderson et al,[13] 2011	3 y	Actual	United States	Northern California Kaiser delivery hospitals	1995–2004	110	1.8
Peters et al,[43] 2018	3.6 y	Median	United States	1 hospital	1992–2016	53	1.9
Brar et al,[81] 2007	4.7 y	Mean	United States	Southern California Kaiser Healthcare System	1996–2005	60	3.3
Ekizler et al,[163] 2019	5.6 y	Median	Turkey	1 hospital	2009–2017	82	7.3

(continued on next page)

Table 4
(continued)

First Author	Follow-up Duration	Actual, Mean, Median	Country	Data Source	Study Years	Sample (n)	Mortality (%)
Pillarisetti et al,[84] 2014	2.9 y	Mean	United States	2 hospitals	1999–2012	100	11.0
Fett et al,[150] 2005	2.2 y	Mean	Haiti	1 hospital	2000–2005	98	15.3
Akil et al,[66] 2016	2.7 y	Mean	Turkey	3 hospitals	2002–2012	58	15.5
Harper et al,[62] 2012	7 y	Actual	United States	1 hospital	2002–20,030	85	16.5
Biteker et al,[69] 2020	3.4 y	Mean	Turkey	1 hospital	2005–2016	52	19.2
Mahowald et al,[61] 2019	6.3 y	Mean	United States	1 hospital	2000–2011	59	20.3
Mishra et al,[145] 2006	6.1 y	Mean	India	1 hospital	1995–2005	56	23.2

Abbreviation: NA, not available.
(*Data from* Refs. 3,7–9,11–13,38–40,43,58,61,62,64,66,69,78,79,81,84,90,95,97,102,104,106,119,136,140,145,150,152,154)

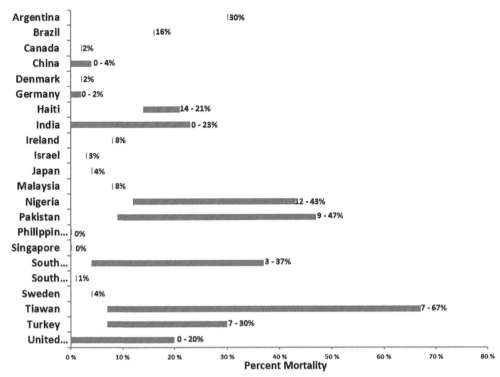

Fig. 2. Percentage mortality estimates for peripartum cardiomyopathy. Twenty-four countries are represented, 12 of which only had 1 estimate available, whereas each of the other 10 countries had between 2 and 25 estimates available. For countries with only 1 estimate available, that value is indicated. For the countries with multiple estimates available, ranges are presented showing the highest and lowest estimates for each country. *Data from* Refs.[7–9,11–13,36,38–40,42,43,47,56–58,61,62,64–70,73,75–87,95,97,99,102,106,119,131,136–155]

ECG have been suggested as a useful tool for predicting adverse outcome in PPCM, which could be advantageous in resource-poor settings in which echocardiographic evaluation may not be readily available.[90,99]

Other factors that also seem to affect outcomes include race, HDP, and body mass index (BMI). Studies in the United States show that, compared with nonblack women, black women have worse outcomes, including slower and less complete recovery of LV function and higher rates of defibrillator use, transplant, and mortality.[36,40,61,91,100–103] A recent meta-analysis found that studies with higher rates of African women tend to have higher mortalities.[74] History of HDP during index pregnancy may also be important, with multiple studies finding an association between HDP and improved rates of recovery and reduced mortality.[29,40,52,64,67,94,97,104] The IPAC study found that higher BMI is associated with less cardiac recovery at 6 and 12 months,[105] whereas a study including predominantly black African women in South Africa found that lower BMI was associated with a worse combined end point of death, LVEF less than 35%, or

remaining in NYHA functional class III/IV at 6 months.[106] Women with multiple predictors of poor outcome may be at increased risk of persistent cardiac dysfunction and death, but this remains speculative because of limited data. Multiple biomarkers have been investigated for their potential usefulness in predicting which women are more likely to experience adverse outcomes, but none have been validated for clinical use (see **Table 2**).

SUBSEQUENT PREGNANCY

Many women with history of PPCM desire to become pregnant again. One recent study found that 74% of women diagnosed with PPCM desire to have more children and 1 in 4 women with PPCM who are sexually active were not using birth control.[107] All women with PPCM are at risk of declining LV function during subsequent pregnancy, but the risk is not necessarily prohibitive. Although some women experience worsening LV function or even death with subsequent pregnancy, others are able to complete a subsequent pregnancy without cardiac complications. Having

1 subsequent pregnancy without heart failure relapse does not ensure that a woman will not experience worsening heart function during a future subsequent pregnancy and vice versa.[83,108–110] At present, there is no clear method to identify with certainty which women will experience adverse cardiac events with subsequent pregnancies. The risk of heart failure relapse is highest in women who have persistent LV dysfunction at the onset of a subsequent pregnancy, with up to 50% having further decline in LV function during subsequent pregnancies.[111–114] Women with recovered LV function have an approximately 20% chance of heart failure relapse as defined in various studies by either experiencing heart failure symptoms and/or decrease in LVEF.[108,111–114]

The AHA, the CCS, and the HFA ESC WG PPCM stratify recommendations regarding subsequent pregnancy based on LV function, recommending that women with partial or fully recovered LV function be advised that they may consider subsequent pregnancy, whereas women with lack of LV recovery should be advised against subsequent pregnancy.[35,55,113] Despite these recommendations, studies show that only 59% to 75% of women diagnosed with PPCM report receiving counseling on the risk of subsequent pregnancy.[107,115] Importantly, qualitative studies have shown that women report feeling that the counseling provided tends to be limited, with women simply being told that they should not get pregnant again rather than engaging in an informed discussion with a health care provider.[116,117] These findings indicate that discussions regarding contraception and potential risks of subsequent pregnancy should occur with informed health care providers who can provide accurate information and are willing to participate in a shared decision-making process.

All women considering or undergoing subsequent pregnancy, regardless of cardiac function before conception, should be closely monitored by a multidisciplinary team from before conception through to several months postpartum in order to identify potential cardiac compromise as early as possible so as to optimize management and improve outcomes.[35,111,113] Recommended cardiac monitoring includes clinical evaluation, BNP or NT-proBNP, and echocardiogram either just before conception or within the first trimester, at 6 months' gestation, 9 months' gestation, before hospital discharge after delivery, and 1 month after delivery, with the timeline and type of follow-up adjusted according to the patient's clinical status.

ADDITIONAL CLINICAL CONCERNS
Infant Outcomes

The few studies of PPCM that include infant outcomes suggest that PPCM diagnosis in mothers is related to increased adverse outcomes in the infants, including higher rates of preterm and premature birth,[13,87,118,119] increased risk of being born small for gestational age,[13,118] increased rates of low birth weight,[13,87,118,119] and lower Apgar scores at both 1 and 5 minutes.[13,87,118] In women with PPCM, rates of premature birth (<37 weeks' gestation) vary between 25% and 60%[13,38,87,104,119] and are significantly increased compared with controls (25.4% vs 8.6% $P<.01$[119] and 27.9% vs 7.3%; $P<.001$[13]). Mean birthweight for infants born to mothers with PPCM ranged between 2378 and 3178 g,[38,56,64,71,76,78,84,87,118,119] and 2 studies with controls found that birth weights were significantly lower in infants born to mothers with PPCM (2697 vs 3165 g, $P<.002$[118]; and 3188 vs 3331 g, $P<.01$[119]).[13,38,56,64,71,78,84,87,118,119] Two studies that examined Apgar scores at 1 and 5 minutes found both to be significantly lower in infants born to mothers with PPCM compared with those born to mothers without PPCM.[13,118]

Premature birth, low birth weight, and lower Apgar scores are all known to be associated with greater risk of infant mortality and a variety of early and late developmental and other medical issues.[120] However, information regarding these outcomes in children of women with PPCM remains limited because infant outcomes in PPCM have only rarely been assessed in research studies.

Mental Health

Depression is a well-known risk factor for heart disease, and depression and anxiety are linked to worse outcomes in heart failure.[121,122] Women diagnosed with PPCM tend to be young mothers who were previously in the prime of their lives and now must juggle a diagnosis of heart failure while caring for a newborn, a household, and possibly other children. These stresses increase the risk for mood disorders. High levels of generalized anxiety, cardiac anxiety, and quality-of-life concerns are present in more than 50% of women with PPCM, and 56% of women with PPCM never return to their baseline emotional states after PPCM diagnosis.[115] Although only 3% to 7% of women with PPCM have a history of depression before PPCM diagnosis,[9,64,80] the rate of depression in women after diagnosis with PPCM has been reported to be 32.3%,[123] which is higher than the reported rate of 11.5% among

---

Box 2
Knowledge gaps in peripartum cardiomyopathy requiring further evidence-based investigation

Research questions

Diagnosis

- How can women who are susceptible to developing PPCM be identified before pregnancy?

Pathophysiology and genetics

- What is the exact pathophysiology/pathophysiologies of PPCM?
- To what extent to do genetic variations contribute to the development of PPCM and influence outcomes?

Diagnosis

- Is there a PPCM-specific biomarker, or set of biomarkers, that can be used to diagnose PPCM with a high degree of certainty?

Treatment

- Which, if any, typical heart failure medications are beneficial for treating all women with PPCM?
- How long should GDMT for HFrEF be continued in women with PPCM who have completely recovered LV function?
- Is bromocriptine safe and effective for treatment of acute PPCM?
- When is the use of wearable defibrillators indicated?
- When should an implantable cardioverter defibrillator be recommended?
- What is the most appropriate type and timing of follow-up in women who have recovered LV function versus those who have not?

Outcomes

- What are the best clinical predictors of outcome for women with PPCM that could be available in various health care resource settings?
- What are the very-long-term (ie, decades after diagnosis) outcomes for women with history of PPCM?
- Do women with history of PPCM have higher risk of developing other types of cardiac disease as they age?

Subsequent pregnancy

- What are the risks of cardiac deterioration and death with subsequent pregnancy with women with history of PPCM and those who have recovered LV function versus those who have not?
- Are there management strategies that are useful to reduce the risk of adverse outcomes in women during a subsequent pregnancy?

Infant outcomes

- What are the short-term and long-term health risks for infants born of mothers with PPCM?
- Are there strategies than can mitigate these risks?

Mental and emotional health

- Are there safe and effective strategies that can be used to decrease the burden of mental and emotional health issues affecting women with PPCM and their families?

Issues to be addressed in order for future research to adequately address knowledge gaps

- Global agreement on the definition of PPCM
- Global agreement on the definition of LV recovery
- Global agreement on the definition of relapse during subsequent pregnancy
- Funding for large, multicenter, well-designed, and well-adjudicated prospective registries and clinical trials

postpartum women in the United States.[124] Notably, there has been an association reported between depression and lower adherence to appointments for PPCM.[123] Qualitative studies suggest that an underlying issue for ongoing emotional and mental distress is lack of inclusion of the women and their partners in discussions and decisions related to the women's care and prognosis, with 35% of women in 1 study thinking that they had not been adequately counseled and another 33% thinking they were left with unaddressed questions.[115–117,123,125,126]

The HFA ESC WG PPCM and AHA both advise that each woman with PPCM be assessed and followed during subsequent pregnancy by a multidisciplinary team including cardiology, obstetrics, maternal-fetal medicine, neonatology, anesthesiology, and possibly other specialties.[35,113] Given the high incidence of mood disorders in women with history of PPCM, including mental health specialists or social workers on the multidisciplinary team to help address the long lasting emotional and psychological impact of PPCM would be beneficial, not only during subsequent pregnancy but after initial diagnosis as well.

SUMMARY

Although rare, PPCM can have a profound effect on previously healthy young women. Numerous advances have been made in understanding the cause, pathophysiology, and natural history of this disease, but many knowledge gaps remain (**Box 2**). Large prospective studies and randomized clinical trials are needed to address these knowledge gaps and to facilitate development of evidence-based guidelines regarding the diagnosis and management of PPCM. In addition, it is of utmost importance that management decisions regarding women with PPCM be formulated among a multidisciplinary team using a shared decision-making approach with the patients and their families in order to optimize diagnosis, treatment, and outcomes for all concerned.

CLINICS CARE POINTS

- Women diagnosed with PPCM benefit from evaluation and treatment by a multidisciplinary team including members from cardiology, maternal fetal medicine, obstetrics, social work, mental health and other specialties as indicated.
- Obtaining a complete patient and family cardiac history is important in order to establish the diagnosis of PPCM, as PPCM is a diagnosis of exclusion.
- Clinicians should have a low threshold for obtaining cardiac testing, including an ECG, echocardiogram, and B-type natriuretic peptide (BNP) or N-terminal proBNP, in pregnant/postpartum women who present with signs/symptoms suggestive of heart failure, even though the signs/symptoms may seem typical for women who are pregnant or postpartum.
- No biomarkers, including troponin T, troponin I, B-type natriuretic peptide (BNP) or N-terminal proBNP, are specific for the diagnosis or PPCM.
- Bromocriptine may be helpful for treatment of acute PPCM, particularly in postpartum women with severely depressed LVEF, but the safety and efficacy of this medication for treatment of PPCM has not yet been established.
- Clinicians must be cognizant of which of the guideline directed mediations for heart failure are safe to use during pregnancy and which are safe to use during lactation.
- Contraceptive counseling during the postpartum period and on a regular basis thereafter is imperative in order to prevent unplanned pregnancy.
- Women with history of PPCM should be counseled about the risk of subsequent pregnancy, bearing in mind that women who have recovered normal LV function are generally able to complete a subsequent pregnancy without significant complications.
- Screening women with PPCM for anxiety and depression in both in the acute and chronic care setting is essential for optimizing management of their mental and physical health.

DISCLOSURE

The authors have nothing to disclose.

REFERENCES

1. Pearson GD, Veille JC, Rahimtoola S, et al. Peripartum cardiomyopathy: national heart, lung, and blood institute and office of rare diseases (National Institutes of Health) workshop recommendations and review. JAMA 2000;283(9):1183–8.
2. Sliwa K, Hilfiker-Kleiner D, Petrie MC, et al. Current state of knowledge on aetiology, diagnosis, management, and therapy of peripartum cardiomyopathy: a position statement from the heart failure association of the european society of cardiology working group on peripartum

cardiomyopathy. Eur J Heart Fail 2010;12(8): 767–78.

3. Isezuo SA, Abubakar SA. Epidemiologic profile of peripartum cardiomyopathy in a tertiary care hospital. Ethn Dis 2007;17(2):228–33.

4. Goeh Akue KE, Assou K, Kossidze K, et al. Peripartum myocardiopathy in lome (Togo). Int J Cardiol 2012;157(1):e12–3.

5. Kuklina EV, Callaghan WM. Cardiomyopathy and other myocardial disorders among hospitalizations for pregnancy in the United States: 2004-2006. Obstet Gynecol 2010;115(1):93–100.

6. Afana M, Brinjikji W, Kao D, et al. Characteristics and In-hospital outcomes of peripartum cardiomyopathy diagnosed during delivery in the United States from the nationwide inpatient sample (NIS) database. J Card Fail 2016;22(7):512–9.

7. Mielniczuk LM, Williams K, Davis DR, et al. Frequency of peripartum cardiomyopathy. Am J Cardiol 2006;97(12):1765–8.

8. Masoomi R, Shah Z, Arany Z, et al. Peripartum cardiomyopathy: an epidemiologic study of early and late presentations. Pregnancy Hypertens 2018;13: 273–8.

9. Kolte D, Khera S, Aronow WS, et al. Temporal trends in incidence and outcomes of peripartum cardiomyopathy in the United States: a nationwide population-based study. J Am Heart Assoc 2014; 3(3):e001056.

10. Elkayam U. Clinical characteristics of peripartum cardiomyopathy in the United States: diagnosis, prognosis, and management. J Am Coll Cardiol 2011;58(7):659–70.

11. Kao DP, Hsich E, Lindenfeld J. Characteristics, adverse events, and racial differences among delivering mothers with peripartum cardiomyopathy. JACC Heart Fail 2013;1(5):409–16.

12. Goland S, Modi K, Hatamizadeh P, et al. Differences in clinical profile of African-American women with peripartum cardiomyopathy in the United States. J Card Fail 2013;19(4):214–8.

13. Gunderson EP, Croen LA, Chiang V, et al. Epidemiology of peripartum cardiomyopathy: incidence, predictors, and outcomes. Obstet Gynecol 2011; 118(3):583–91.

14. Damp JA, Arany Z, Fett JD, et al. Imbalanced angiogenesis in peripartum cardiomyopathy (PPCM). Circ J 2018;82(10):2689.

15. Bello NA, Arany Z. Molecular mechanisms of peripartum cardiomyopathy: a vascular/hormonal hypothesis. Trends Cardiovasc Med 2015;25(6): 499–504.

16. Hilfiker-Kleiner D, Kaminski K, Podewski E, et al. A cathepsin D-cleaved 16 kDa form of prolactin mediates postpartum cardiomyopathy. Cell 2007; 128(3):589–600.

17. Hilfiker-Kleiner D, Struman I, Hoch M, et al. 16-kDa prolactin and bromocriptine in postpartum cardiomyopathy. Curr Heart Fail Rep 2012;9(3): 174–82.

18. Patten IS, Rana S, Shahul S, et al. Cardiac angiogenic imbalance leads to peripartum cardiomyopathy. Nature 2012;485(7398):333–8.

19. Damp J, Givertz MM, Semigran M, et al. Relaxin-2 and Soluble Flt1 levels in peripartum cardiomyopathy: results of the multicenter IPAC study. JACC Heart Fail 2016;4(5):380–8.

20. Bello N, Rendon IS, Arany Z. The relationship between pre-eclampsia and peripartum cardiomyopathy: a systematic review and meta-analysis. J Am Coll Cardiol 2013;62(18):1715–23.

21. Ntusi NB, Wonkam A, Shaboodien G, et al. Frequency and clinical genetics of familial dilated cardiomyopathy in Cape Town: implications for the evaluation of patients with unexplained cardiomyopathy. S Afr Med J 2011;101(6):394–8.

22. Massad LS, Reiss CK, Mutch DG, et al. Familial peripartum cardiomyopathy after molar pregnancy. Obstet Gynecol 1993;81:886–8, 5 (Pt 2).

23. Pearl W. Familial occurrence of peripartum cardiomyopathy. Am Heart J 1995;129(2):421–2.

24. Baruteau AE, Leurent G, Schleich JM, et al. Can Peripartum cardiomyopathy be familial? Int J Cardiol 2009;137(2):183–5.

25. Fett JD, Sundstrom BJ, Etta King M, et al. Mother-daughter peripartum cardiomyopathy. Int J Cardiol 2002;86(2–3):331–2.

26. van Spaendonck-Zwarts KY, van Tintelen JP, van Veldhuisen DJ, et al. Peripartum cardiomyopathy as a part of familial dilated cardiomyopathy. Circulation 2010;121(20):2169–75.

27. van Spaendonck-Zwarts KY, Posafalvi A, van den Berg MP, et al. Titin gene mutations are common in families with both peripartum cardiomyopathy and dilated cardiomyopathy. Eur Heart J 2014; 35(32):2165–73.

28. Ware JS, Li J, Mazaika E, et al. Shared genetic predisposition in Peripartum and dilated cardiomyopathies. N Engl J Med 2016;374(3):233–41.

29. Haghikia A, Podewski E, Libhaber E, et al. Phenotyping and outcome on contemporary management in a German cohort of patients with peripartum cardiomyopathy. Basic Res Cardiol 2013;108(4):366.

30. Sheppard R, Hsich E, Damp J, et al. GNB3 C825T Polymorphism and myocardial recovery in peripartum cardiomyopathy: results of the multicenter investigations of pregnancy-associated cardiomyopathy study. Circ Heart Fail 2016;9(3):e002683.

31. Gammill HS, Chettier R, Brewer A, et al. Cardiomyopathy and preeclampsia. Circulation 2018; 138(21):2359–66.

32. Haggerty CM, Damrauer SM, Levin MG, et al. Genomics-first evaluation of heart disease associated with titin-truncating variants. Circulation 2019; 140(1):42–54.

33. Ricke-Hoch M, Pfeffer TJ, Hilfiker-Kleiner D. Peripartum cardiomyopathy: basic mechanisms and hope for new therapies. Cardiovasc Res 2020; 116(3):520–31.

34. Davis MB, Arany Z, McNamara DM, et al. Peripartum cardiomyopathy: JACC state-of-the-art review. J Am Coll Cardiol 2020;75(2):207–21.

35. Bozkurt B, Colvin M, Cook J, et al. Current diagnostic and treatment strategies for specific dilated cardiomyopathies: a scientific statement from the american heart association. Circulation 2016; 134(23):e579–646.

36. Goland S, Modi K, Bitar F, et al. Clinical profile and predictors of complications in peripartum cardiomyopathy. J Card Fail 2009;15(8):645–50.

37. Fett JD. Earlier detection can help avoid many serious complications of peripartum cardiomyopathy. Future Cardiol 2013;9(6):809–16.

38. Elkayam U, Akhter MW, Singh H, et al. Pregnancy-associated cardiomyopathy: clinical characteristics and a comparison between early and late presentation. Circulation 2005;111(16):2050–5.

39. Wu VC, Chen TH, Yeh JK, et al. Clinical outcomes of peripartum cardiomyopathy: a 15-year nationwide population-based study in Asia. Medicine (Baltimore) 2017;96(43):e8374.

40. McNamara DM, Elkayam U, Alharethi R, et al. Clinical outcomes for peripartum cardiomyopathy in North America: results of the IPAC Study (Investigations of pregnancy-associated cardiomyopathy). J Am Coll Cardiol 2015;66(8):905–14.

41. Bauersachs J, Konig T, van der Meer P, et al. Pathophysiology, diagnosis and management of peripartum cardiomyopathy: a position statement from the Heart Failure Association of the European Society of Cardiology Study Group on peripartum cardiomyopathy. Eur J Heart Fail 2019;21(7): 827–43.

42. Karaye KM, Lindmark K, Henein M. Right ventricular systolic dysfunction and remodelling in Nigerians with peripartum cardiomyopathy: a longitudinal study. BMC Cardiovasc Disord 2016; 16:27.

43. Peters A, Caroline M, Zhao H, et al. Initial right ventricular dysfunction severity identifies severe peripartum cardiomyopathy phenotype with worse early and overall outcomes: a 24-year cohort study. J Am Heart Assoc 2018;7(9):e008378.

44. Blauwet LA, Delgado-Montero A, Ryo K, et al. Right ventricular function in peripartum cardiomyopathy at presentation is associated with subsequent left ventricular recovery and clinical outcomes. Circ Heart Fail 2016;9(5):e002756.

45. Haghikia A, Rontgen P, Vogel-Claussen J, et al. Prognostic implication of right ventricular involvement in peripartum cardiomyopathy: a cardiovascular magnetic resonance study. ESC Heart Fail 2015;2(4):139–49.

46. American College of Obstetricians and Gynecologists' Presidential Task Force on Pregnancy and Heart Disease and Committee on Practice Bulletins—Obstetrics. ACOG practice bulletin no. 212: pregnancy and heart disease. Obstet Gynecol 2019;133(5):E320–56.

47. Sliwa K, Blauwet L, Tibazarwa K, et al. Evaluation of bromocriptine in the treatment of acute severe peripartum cardiomyopathy: a proof-of-concept pilot study. Circulation 2010;121(13): 1465–73.

48. Yameogo NVK LJ, Seghda A, Owona A, et al. Bromocriptine in management of peripartum cardiomyopathy: a randomized study on 96 women in Burkina Faso. J Cardiol Clin Res 2017;5(2):1098.

49. Hilfiker-Kleiner D, Haghikia A, Berliner D, et al. Bromocriptine for the treatment of peripartum cardiomyopathy: a multicentre randomized study. Eur Heart J 2017;38(35):2671–9.

50. Victora CG, Bahl R, Barros AJ, et al. Breastfeeding in the 21st century: epidemiology, mechanisms, and lifelong effect. Lancet 2016;387(10017): 475–90.

51. Office of the Surgeon General (US). The Surgeon general's call to action to support breastfeeding. Rockville (MD): Center for Disease Control; Office of Women's Health; 2011.

52. Safirstein JG, Ro AS, Grandhi S, et al. Predictors of left ventricular recovery in a cohort of peripartum cardiomyopathy patients recruited via the internet. Int J Cardiol 2012;154(1):27–31.

53. Koczo A, Marino A, Jeyabalan A, et al. Breastfeeding, cellular immune activation, and myocardial recovery in peripartum cardiomyopathy. JACC Basic Transl Sci 2019;4(3):291–300.

54. Davis M, Kawamoto K, Langen E, et al. Breastfeeding is not associated with worse outcomes in peripartum cardiomyopathy. J Am Coll Cardiol 2017; 69(11 Supplement):842.

55. Ezekowitz JA, O'Meara E, McDonald MA, et al. 2017 Comprehensive update of the canadian cardiovascular society guidelines for the management of heart failure. Can J Cardiol 2017;33(11): 1342–433.

56. Barasa A, Goloskokova V, Ladfors L, et al. Symptomatic recovery and pharmacological management in a clinical cohort with peripartum cardiomyopathy. J Matern Fetal Neonatal Med 2018;31(10):1342–9.

57. Biteker M. Peripartum cardiomyopathy in Turkey. Int J Cardiol 2012;158(3):e60–1.

58. Amos AM, Jaber WA, Russell SD. Improved outcomes in Peripartum cardiomyopathy with contemporary. Am Heart J 2006;152(3):509–13.

59. Ersboll AS, Bojer AS, Hauge MG, et al. Long-term cardiac function after Peripartum cardiomyopathy and preeclampsia: a Danish nationwide, clinical follow-up study using maximal exercise testing and cardiac magnetic resonance imaging. J Am Heart Assoc 2018;7(20): e008991.

60. Goland S, Weinstein JM, Zalik A, et al. Angiogenic imbalance and residual myocardial injury in recovered peripartum cardiomyopathy patients. Circ Heart Fail 2016;9(11):e003349.

61. Mahowald MK, Basu N, Subramaniam L, et al. Long-term outcomes in Peripartum cardiomyopathy. Open Cardiovasc Med J 2019;13(1):13–23.

62. Harper MA, Meyer RE, Berg CJ. Peripartum cardiomyopathy: population-based birth prevalence and 7-year mortality. Obstet Gynecol 2012;120(5): 1013–9.

63. Dayoub EJ, Datwani H, Lewey J, et al. One-year cardiovascular outcomes in patients with Peripartum cardiomyopathy. J Card Fail 2018;24(10):711–5.

64. Ersboll AS, Johansen M, Damm P, et al. Peripartum cardiomyopathy in Denmark: a retrospective, population-based study of incidence, management and outcome. Eur J Heart Fail 2017;19(12): 1712–20.

65. Ntusi NB, Badri M, Gumedze F, et al. Pregnancy-associated heart failure: a comparison of clinical presentation and outcome between hypertensive heart failure of pregnancy and idiopathic Peripartum cardiomyopathy. PloS one 2015;10(8): e0133466.

66. Akil MA, Bilik MZ, Yildiz A, et al. Peripartum cardiomyopathy in Turkey: experience of three tertiary centres. J Obstet Gynaecol 2016;36(5):574–80.

67. Kamiya CA, Kitakaze M, Ishibashi-Ueda H, et al. Different characteristics of peripartum cardiomyopathy between patients complicated with and without hypertensive disorders. -Results from the Japanese Nationwide survey of peripartum cardiomyopathy. Circ J 2011;75(8):1975–81.

68. Horgan SJ, Margey R, Brennan DJ, et al. Natural history, management, and outcomes of peripartum cardiomyopathy: an Irish single-center cohort study. J Matern Fetal Neonatal Med 2013;26(2):161–5.

69. Biteker M, Ozlek B, Ozlek E, et al. Predictors of early and delayed recovery in peripartum cardiomyopathy: a prospective study of 52 Patients. J Matern Fetal Neonatal Med 2020;33(3):390–7.

70. Peradejordi MA, Favaloro LE, Bertolotti A, et al. Predictors of mortality or heart transplantation in peripartum cardiomyopathy. Revista Argentina de Cardiologia 2013;81(1):41–8.

71. Shani H, Kuperstein R, Berlin A, et al. Peripartum cardiomyopathy - risk factors, characteristics and long-term follow-up. J Perinat Med 2015;43(1): 95–101.

72. Cooper LT, Mather PJ, Alexis JD, et al. Myocardial recovery in peripartum cardiomyopathy: prospective comparison with recent onset cardiomyopathy in men and nonperipartum women. J Card Fail 2012;18(1):28–33.

73. Felker GM, Jaeger CJ, Klodas E, et al. Myocarditis and long-term survival in peripartum cardiomyopathy. Am Heart J 2000;140(5):785–91.

74. Kerpen K, Koutrolou-Sotiropoulou P, Zhu C, et al. Disparities in death rates in women with peripartum cardiomyopathy between advanced and developing countries: a systematic review and meta-analysis. Arch Cardiovasc Dis 2018;112(3): 187–98.

75. Hsieh CC, Chiang CW, Hsieh TT, et al. Peripartum cardiomyopathy. Jpn Heart J 1992;33(3):343–9.

76. Samonte VI, Ngalob QG, Mata GD, et al. Clinical and echocardiographic profile and outcomes of peripartum cardiomyopathy: the Philippine general hospital experience. Heart Asia 2013;5(1):245–9.

77. Lim CP, Sim DK. Peripartum cardiomyopathy: experience in an Asian tertiary centre. Singapore Med J 2013;54(1):24–7.

78. Habli M, O'Brien T, Nowack E, et al. Peripartum cardiomyopathy: prognostic factors for long-term maternal outcome. Am J Obstet Gynecol 2008; 199(4):415 e411–415.

79. Phan D, Duan L, Ng A, et al. Characteristics and outcomes of pregnant women with cardiomyopathy stratified by etiologies: a population-based study. Int J Cardiol 2020;305:87–91.

80. Krishnamoorthy P, Garg J, Palaniswamy C, et al. Epidemiology and outcomes of peripartum cardiomyopathy in the United States: findings from the Nationwide inpatient sample. J Cardiovasc Med (Hagerstown,) 2016;17(10):756–61.

81. Brar SS, Khan SS, Sandhu GK, et al. Incidence, mortality, and racial differences in peripartum cardiomyopathy. Am J Cardiol 2007;100(2): 302–4.

82. Ford RF, Barton JR, O'Brien JM, et al. Demographics, management, and outcome of peripartum cardiomyopathy in a community hospital. Am J Obstet Gynecol 2000;182(5):1036–8.

83. Chapa JB, Heiberger HB, Weinert L, et al. Prognostic value of echocardiography in peripartum cardiomyopathy. Obstet Gynecol 2005;105(6): 1303–8.

84. Pillarisetti J, Kondur A, Alani A, et al. Peripartum cardiomyopathy: predictors of recovery and current state of implantable cardioverter-defibrillator use. J Am Coll Cardiol 2014;63(25 Pt A):2831–9.

85. Bernstein PS, Magriples U. Cardiomyopathy in pregnancy: a retrospective study. Am J perinatol 2001;18(3):163–8.

86. Modi KA, Illum S, Jariatul K, et al. Poor outcome of indigent patients with peripartum cardiomyopathy in the United States. Am J Obstet Gynecol 2009; 201(2):171 e171–175.

87. Witlin AG, Mabie WC, Sibai BM. Peripartum cardiomyopathy: an ominous diagnosis. Am J Obstet Gynecol 1997;176(1 Pt 1):182–8.

88. Fett JD, Sannon H, Thelisma E, et al. Recovery from severe heart failure following peripartum cardiomyopathy. Int J Gynaecol Obstet 2009;104(2):125–7.

89. Biteker M, Ilhan E, Biteker G, et al. Delayed recovery in peripartum cardiomyopathy: an indication for long-term follow-up and sustained therapy. Eur J Heart Fail 2012;14(8):895–901.

90. Tibazarwa K, Lee G, Mayosi B, et al. The 12-lead ECG in peripartum cardiomyopathy. Cardiovasc J Afr 2012;23(6):322–9.

91. Lewey J, Levine LD, Elovitz MA, et al. Importance of early diagnosis in peripartum cardiomyopathy. Hypertension 2020;75(1):91–7.

92. Goland S, Bitar F, Modi K, et al. Evaluation of the clinical relevance of baseline left ventricular ejection fraction as a predictor of recovery or persistence of severe dysfunction in women in the United States with peripartum cardiomyopathy. J Card Fail 2011;17(5):426–30.

93. Fett JD. Long-term maternal outcomes in patients with peripartum cardiomyopathy (PPCM). Am J Obstet Gynecol 2009;201(6):e9. author reply e9-10.

94. Poppas A, French K, Tsiaras S, et al. Peripartum cardiomyopathy: longitudinal follow-up and continued recovery of ventricular function. J Am Coll Cardiol 2013;61(10):E585.

95. Sliwa K, Forster O, Libhaber E, et al. Peripartum cardiomyopathy: inflammatory markers as predictors of outcome in 100 prospectively studied patients. Eur Heart J 2006;27(4):441–6.

96. Duran N, Gunes H, Duran I, et al. Predictors of prognosis in patients with peripartum cardiomyopathy. Int J Gynaecol Obstet 2008;101(2):137–40.

97. Libhaber E, Sliwa K, Bachelier K, et al. Low systolic blood pressure and high resting heart rate as predictors of outcome in patients with peripartum cardiomyopathy. Int J Cardiol 2015;190: 376–82.

98. Sugahara M, Kagiyama N, Hasselberg NE, et al. Global left ventricular strain at presentation is associated with subsequent recovery in patients with peripartum cardiomyopathy. J Am Soc Echocardiogr 2019;32(12):1565–73.

99. Ekizler FA, Cay S. A novel marker of persistent left ventricular systolic dysfunction in patients with peripartum cardiomyopathy: monocyte count- to-

HDL cholesterol ratio. BMC Cardiovasc Disord 2019;19(1):114.

100. Elkayam U, Habakuk O. The search for a crystal ball to predict early recovery from peripartum cardiomyopathy? JACC Heart Fail 2016;4(5):389–91.

101. Irizarry OC, Levine LD, Lewey J, et al. Comparison of clinical characteristics and outcomes of peripartum cardiomyopathy between African American and Non-African American Women. JAMA Cardiol 2017;2(11):1256–60.

102. Azibani F, Pfeffer TJ, Ricke-Hoch M, et al. Outcome in German and South African peripartum cardiomyopathy cohorts associates with medical therapy and fibrosis markers. ESC Heart Fail 2020;7(2): 512–22.

103. Gentry MB, Dias JK, Luis A, et al. African-American women have a higher risk for developing peripartum cardiomyopathy. J Am Coll Cardiol 2010; 55(7):654–9.

104. Li W, Li H, Long Y. Clinical characteristics and long-term predictors of persistent left ventricular systolic dysfunction in peripartum cardiomyopathy. Can J Cardiol 2016;32(3):362–8.

105. Davis EM, Ewald G, Givertz MM, et al. Maternal obesity affects cardiac remodeling and recovery in women with peripartum cardiomyopathy. Am J perinatol 2019;36(5):476–83.

106. Blauwet LA, Libhaber E, Forster O, et al. Predictors of outcome in 176 South African patients with peripartum cardiomyopathy. Heart 2013;99(5):308–13.

107. Rosman L, Salmoirago-Blotcher E, Wuensch KL, et al. Contraception and reproductive counseling in women with peripartum cardiomyopathy. Contraception 2017;96(1):36–40.

108. Codsi E, Rose CH, Blauwet LA. Subsequent pregnancy outcomes in patients with peripartum cardiomyopathy. Obstet Gynecol 2018;131(2):322–7.

109. Elkayam U, Tummala PP, Rao K, et al. Maternal and fetal outcomes of subsequent pregnancies in women with peripartum cardiomyopathy. N Engl J Med 2001;344(21):1567–71.

110. Fett JD, Fristoe KL, Welsh SN. Risk of heart failure relapse in subsequent pregnancy among peripartum cardiomyopathy mothers. Int J Gynaecol Obstet 2010;109(1):34–6.

111. Elkayam U. Risk of subsequent pregnancy in women with a history of peripartum cardiomyopathy. J Am Coll Cardiol 2014;64(15):1629–36.

112. Elkayam U. Can I get pregnant again? Eur J Heart Fail 2017;19(12):1729–31.

113. Sliwa K, Petrie MC, Hilfiker-Kleiner D, et al. Long-term prognosis, subsequent pregnancy, contraception and overall management of peripartum cardiomyopathy: practical guidance paper from the heart failure association of the European society of cardiology study group on peripartum cardiomyopathy. Eur J Heart Fail 2018;20(6):951–62.

114. Fett JD, Shah TP, McNamara DM. Why do some recovered peripartum cardiomyopathy mothers experience heart failure with a subsequent pregnancy? Curr Treat Options Cardiovasc Med 2015; 17(1):354.

115. Koutrolou-Sotiropoulou P, Lima FV, Stergiopoulos K. Quality of life in survivors of peripartum cardiomyopathy. Am J Cardiol 2016; 118(2):258–63.

116. de Wolff M, Ersboll AS, Hegaard H, et al. Psychological adaptation after peripartum cardiomyopathy: a qualitative study. Midwifery 2018;62: 52–60.

117. Dekker RL, Morton CH, Singleton P, et al. Women's experiences being diagnosed with peripartum cardiomyopathy: a qualitative study. J Midwifery womens Health 2016;61(4):467–73.

118. Sagy I, Salman AA, Kezerle L, et al. Peripartum cardiomyopathy is associated with increased uric acid concentrations: a population based study. Heart Lung 2017;46(5):369–74.

119. Dhesi S, Savu A, Ezekowitz JA, et al. Association between diabetes during pregnancy and peripartum cardiomyopathy: a population-level analysis of 309,825 women. Can J Cardiol 2017;33(7):911–7.

120. Axelrad DA K, Chowdhury F, D'Amico L, et al. America's children and the environment. 3rd edition. Washington, DC: Agency UEP; 2013.

121. Nicholson L, Lecour S, Wedegartner S, et al. Assessing perinatal depression as an indicator of risk for pregnancy-associated cardiovascular disease. Cardiovasc J Afr 2016;27(2):119–22.

122. Celano CM, Villegas AC, Albanese AM, et al. Depression and anxiety in heart failure: a review. Harv Rev Psychiatry 2018;26(4):175–84.

123. Rosman L, Salmoirago-Blotcher E, Cahill J, et al. Depression and health behaviors in women with Peripartum cardiomyopathy. Heart Lung 2017; 46(5):363–8.

124. Ko JY, Rockhill KM, Tong VT, et al. Trends in postpartum depressive symptoms - 27 States, 2004, 2008, and 2012. MMWR Morb Mortal Wkly Rep 2017;66(6):153–8.

125. Hess RF, Weinland JA. The life-changing impact of peripartum cardiomyopathy: an analysis of online postings. MCN Am J Matern Child Nurs 2012; 37(4):241–6.

126. Patel H, Schaufelberger M, Begley C, et al. Experiences of health care in women with Peripartum Cardiomyopathy in Sweden: a qualitative interview study. BMC Pregnancy Childbirth 2016;16(1):386.

127. Fett JD. Unrecognized peripartum cardiomyopathy. Crit Care Med 2005;33(8):1892–3. author reply 1893.

128. Binu AJ, Rajan SJ, Rathore S, et al. Peripartum cardiomyopathy: an analysis of clinical profiles and outcomes from a tertiary care centre in southern India. Obstet Med 2019. https://doi.org/10.1177/1753495X19851397.

129. Sebillotte CG, Deligny C, Hanf M, et al. Is African descent an independent risk factor of peripartum cardiomyopathy? Int J Cardiol 2010; 145(1):93–4.

130. Isogai T, Kamiya CA. Worldwide incidence of peripartum cardiomyopathy and overall maternal mortality. Int Heart J 2019;60(3):503–11.

131. Chee KH. Favourable outcome after peripartum cardiomyopathy: a ten-year study on peripartum cardiomyopathy in a university hospital. Singapore Med J 2013;54(1):28–31.

132. Perveen S, Ainuddin J, Jabbar S, et al. Peripartum cardiomyopathy: frequency and predictors and indicators of clinical outcome. J Pak Med Assoc 2016;66(12):1517–21.

133. Suliman A. The state of heart disease in Sudan. Cardiovasc J Afr 2011;22(4):191–6.

134. Liu H, Xu JW, Zhao XD, et al. Pregnancy outcomes in women with heart disease. Chin Med J (Engl) 2010;123(17):2324–30.

135. Desai D, Moodley J, Naidoo D. Peripartum cardiomyopathy: experiences at king edward VIII hospital, durban, South Africa and a review of the literature. Trop doct 1995;25(3):118–23.

136. Lee S, Cho GJ, Park GU, et al. Incidence, risk factors, and clinical characteristics of peripartum cardiomyopathy in South Korea. Circ Heart Fail 2018; 11(4):e004134.

137. Sharieff S, Zaman KS. Prognostic factors at initial presentation in patients with peripartum cardiomyopathy. J Pak Med Assoc 2003;53(7):297–300.

138. Forster O, Hilfiker-Kleiner D, Ansari AA, et al. Reversal of IFN-gamma, oxLDL and prolactin serum levels correlate with clinical improvement in patients with peripartum cardiomyopathy. Eur J Heart Fail 2008;10(9):861–8.

139. Tibazarwa K, Sliwa K. Peripartum cardiomyopathy in Africa: challenges in diagnosis, prognosis, and therapy. Prog Cardiovasc Dis 2010;52(4):317–25.

140. Sliwa K, Forster O, Tibazarwa K, et al. Long-term outcome of peripartum cardiomyopathy in a population with high seropositivity for human immunodeficiency virus. Int J Cardiol 2011;147(2):202–8.

141. Sliwa K, Skudicky D, Bergemann A, et al. Peripartum cardiomyopathy: analysis of clinical outcome, left ventricular function, plasma levels of cytokines and Fas/APO-1. J Am Coll Cardiol 2000;35(3):701–5.

142. Hasan JA, Qureshi A, Ramejo BB, et al. Peripartum cardiomyopathy characteristics and outcome in a tertiary care hospital. J Pak Med Assoc 2010; 60(5):377–80.

143. Shah I, Shahzeb A, Shah ST, et al. Peripartum cardiomyopathy: risk factors, hospital course and prognosis; experiences at lady reading hospital Peshawar. Pakistan Heart J 2012;45(2):108–15.

144. Karaye KM, Yahaya IA, Lindmark K, et al. Serum selenium and ceruloplasmin in nigerians with peripartum cardiomyopathy. Int J Mol Sci 2015;16(4):7644–54.

145. Mishra TK, Swain S, Routray SN. Peripartum cardiomyopathy. Int J Gynaecol Obstet 2006;95(2):104–9.

146. Suri V, Aggarwal N, Kalpdev A, et al. Pregnancy with dilated and peripartum cardiomyopathy: maternal and fetal outcome. Arch Gynecol Obstet 2013;287(2):195–9.

147. Prasad GS, Bhupali A, Prasad S, et al. Peripartum cardiomyopathy - case series. Indian Heart J 2014; 66(2):223–6.

148. Pandit V, Shetty S, Kumar A, et al. Incidence and outcome of peripartum cardiomyopathy from a tertiary hospital in South India. Trop doct 2009;39(3):168–9.

149. Fett JD, Carraway RD, Dowell DL, et al. Peripartum cardiomyopathy in the hospital albert schweitzer district of Haiti. Am J Obstet Gynecol 2002; 186(5):1005–10.

150. Fett JD, Christie LG, Carraway RD, et al. Five-year prospective study of the incidence and prognosis of peripartum cardiomyopathy at a single institution. Mayo Clin Proc 2005;80(12):1602–6.

151. Fett JD, Christie LG, Murphy JG. Brief communication: outcomes of subsequent pregnancy after peripartum cardiomyopathy: a case series from Haiti. Ann Intern Med 2006;145(1):30–4.

152. Moulig V, Pfeffer TJ, Ricke-Hoch M, et al. Long-term follow-up in peripartum cardiomyopathy patients with contemporary treatment: low mortality, high cardiac recovery, but significant cardiovascular co-morbidities. Eur J Heart Fail 2019;21(12):1534–42.

153. Liu Y, Zeng Y. Clinical characteristics and prognosis of peripartum cardiomyopathy in 28 Patients. Zhongguo Yi Xue Ke Xue Yuan Xue Bao 2016; 38(1):78–82.

154. Huang GY, Zhang LY, Long-Le MA, et al. Clinical characteristics and risk factors for peripartum cardiomyopathy. Afr Health Sci 2012;12(1):26–31.

155. Carvalho A, Brandao A, Martinez EE, et al. Prognosis in peripartum cardiomyopathy. Am J Cardiol 1989;64(8):540–2.

156. Hu CL, Li YB, Zou YG, et al. Troponin T measurement can predict persistent left ventricular dysfunction in peripartum cardiomyopathy. Heart 2007;93(4):488–90.

157. Sarojini A, Sai Ravi Shanker A, Anitha M. Inflammatory markers-serum level of C-reactive protein, tumor necrotic factor-alpha, and interleukin-6 as predictors of outcome for peripartum cardiomyopathy. J Obstet Gynaecol India 2013;63(4):234–9.

158. Nonhoff J, Ricke-Hoch M, Mueller M, et al. Serelaxin treatment promotes adaptive hypertrophy but does not prevent heart failure in experimental peripartum cardiomyopathy. Cardiovasc Res 2017;113(6):598–608.

159. Mebazaa A, Seronde MF, Gayat E, et al. Imbalanced angiogenesis in peripartum cardiomyopathy- diagnostic value of placenta growth factor. Circ J 2017;81(11):1654–61.

160. Ricke-Hoch M, Hoes MF, Pfeffer TJ, et al. In peripartum cardiomyopathy Plasminogen Activator Inhibitor-1 is a potential new biomarker with controversial roles. Cardiovasc Res 2019;116(11):1875–86.

161. Halkein J, Tabruyn SP, Ricke-Hoch M, et al. MicroRNA-146a is a therapeutic target and biomarker for peripartum cardiomyopathy. J Clin Invest 2013; 123(5):2143–54.

162. Stapel B, Kohlhaas M, Ricke-Hoch M, et al. Low STAT3 expression sensitizes to toxic effects of beta-adrenergic receptor stimulation in peripartum cardiomyopathy. Eur Heart J 2016;38(5):349–61.

163. Ekizler FA, Cay S, Kafes H, et al. The prognostic value of positive T wave in lead aVR: a novel marker of adverse cardiac outcomes in peripartum cardiomyopathy. Ann Noninvasive Electrocardiol 2019; 24(3):e12631.

Hypertrophic Cardiomyopathy in Pregnancy

Sara Saberi, MD, MS

KEYWORDS

- Hypertrophic cardiomyopathy • Pregnancy • Pre-pregnancy counseling

KEY POINTS

- Prepregnancy risk assessment and counseling as well as genetic counseling are indicated in all women with hypertrophic cardiomyopathy.
- Advising against pregnancy is justified in only a small minority with left ventricular ejection fraction less than 30%, New York Heart Association classes III–IV with restrictive physiology, or severe symptomatic left ventricular outflow obstruction.
- β-Blockers (preferably metoprolol) should be continued in women who used them prior to pregnancy.
- Vaginal delivery is recommended as first choice in the vast majority of women with hypertrophic cardiomyopathy.

INTRODUCTION

Hypertrophic cardiomyopathy (HCM) is one of the most common inherited cardiovascular conditions, affecting 1:500 persons worldwide.[1,2] It often is genetic, caused by pathogenic variants in genes encoding the cardiac sarcomere, the contractile unit of the cardiomyocyte. HCM is an autosomal dominant condition, meaning first-degree relatives each have a 50% chance of inheriting the genetic variant that causes disease. Highly variable penetrance and pleiotropic effects play a large role in the final phenotype.

In an adult, HCM is defined by left ventricular (LV) hypertrophy, with a wall thickness greater than or equal to 15 mm in at least 1 myocardial segment that is not explained solely by loading conditions.[3] In most patients, hypertrophy is asymmetric and preferentially involves the interventricular septum in the basal and mid segments, but increased wall thickness can occur in any LV segment and also can involve the right ventricle (Fig. 1). Typically, LV hypertrophy does not appear in patients with pathogenic sarcomere variants until the second decade of life but can occur at any time.[4,5] Other core pathophysiologic features include a small hyperdynamic LV, reduced compliance, and, in 70% of patients, resting or dynamic LV outflow tract (LVOT) obstruction (LVOTO).[6–8] Patients often experience symptoms, including exercise intolerance in the form of dyspnea and fatigue, chest pain, lightheadedness, and palpitations. Although the disease course is highly variable, many experience heart failure and atrial fibrillation (AF), whereas relatively few experience potentially life-threatening ventricular arrhythmias resulting in sudden cardiac death (SCD).[6,9]

To date, no available pharmaceutical agents have been shown to modify disease development or outcomes in patients with HCM,[10] with the possible exception of diltiazem in preventing LV remodeling.[11] Current treatment focused on

Department of Internal Medicine, Division of Cardiovascular Medicine, University of Michigan School of Medicine, 1500 East Medical Center Drive, CVC Suite 2364, Ann Arbor, MI 48109-5853, USA
E-mail address: saberis@med.umich.edu
Twitter: @S2beri (S.S.)

Cardiol Clin 39 (2021) 143–150
https://doi.org/10.1016/j.ccl.2020.09.009
0733-8651/21/© 2020 Elsevier Inc. All rights reserved.

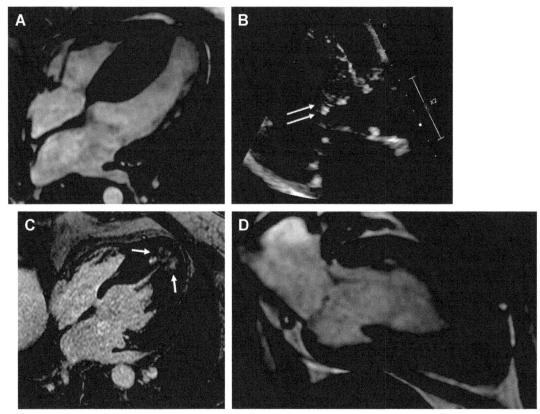

Fig. 1. HCM anatomic variants. (*A*) Asymmetric septal hypertrophy with reverse curve morphology. (*B*) Systolic anterior motion of the mitral valve leaflets (*arrows*), causing LV outflow obstruction. (*C*) Apical hypertrophy with delayed enhancement (*arrows*). (*D*) Midcavity hypertrophy with apical aneurysm.

relieving symptoms related to resting or dynamic LVOTO relies on β-blockers, nondihydropyridine calcium channel blockers, and disopyramide.[3] Marked symptomatic LVOTO with gradients greater than or equal to 50 mm Hg either at rest or with provocation despite medication and lifestyle modification is a threshold for surgical or percutaneous intervention. Clinical heart failure in HCM ranges from heart failure with preserved ejection fraction (EF), to severe restrictive cardiomyopathy, and to LV systolic dysfunction.[12] Patients with nonobstructive HCM and LV systolic dysfunction (EF <50%) should be treated with guideline-directed medical therapy for heart failure with reduced EF.[3] Symptoms related to diastolic dysfunction or microvascular ischemia in those with preserved LV systolic function are managed primarily with β-blockers, although nondihydropyridine calcium channel blockers may be used as an alternative.

AF significantly increases the risk of thromboembolism in patients with HCM, and oral anticoagulation is recommended as primary stroke prophylaxis regardless of CHA2DS2-VASc (congestive heart failure, hypertension, age ≥ 75 years, diabetes mellitus, stroke or transient ischemic attack, vascular disease, age 65 to 74 years, sex category) score, which does not correlate well with clinical outcomes.[13] Direct oral anticoagulants are superior to warfarin in terms of both effectiveness and safety in the primary prevention of stroke in HCM.[14]

Most contemporary series of adult patients with HCM report an annual incidence for cardiovascular death of 1% to 2%, with heart failure, thromboembolism, and SCD the main causes.[9,15,16] The implantable cardioverter-defibrillator (ICD) is universally recommended in secondary prevention; however, indications for primary prevention are hotly debated and the American College of Cardiology/American Heart Association guidelines differ in terms of their recommendations as compared with the European Society of Cardiology guidelines.[3,17]

Widespread use of echocardiography and both genetic and clinical screening of families with

HCM have led to earlier detection of the disease over time and HCM increasingly is diagnosed in women of childbearing age. Although the prevalence of HCM in the general population is 1:500, the observed incidence of HCM among pregnant women is less than 1:1000, posing challenges to obstetricians, cardiologists, and anesthesiologists in terms of evidence-based practice.[18–20] This review focuses on the management considerations for pregnant women with HCM.

PRECONCEPTION GENETIC TESTING

Identifying the genetic basis of disease allows the unique opportunity to identify risk and prevent disease. The development of faster and less expensive DNA sequencing methodology has fostered the transition of genetic testing for HCM from highly specialized academic research laboratories to the clinic. Currently all laboratories employ a candidate-gene strategy, analyzing the sequence of sarcomere genes as well as several genes associated with metabolic/storage and mitochondrial diseases that may mimic HCM.[21] Accurate interpretation of genetic testing results are complex, given their probabilistic rather than quantitative nature. It may be difficult to predict accurately if an identified DNA variant is truly disease causing, disease modifying, or simply a benign polymorphism present in a small proportion of the general population. Failing to identify a mutation does not exclude the possibility of genetic disease. Result interpretation may evolve over time as more experience is gained in sequencing reference populations in different ethnic backgrounds and in sequencing more patients and families with HCM, further complicating the ability to guide families accurately.

Assisted reproduction using preimplantation genetic diagnosis (PGD) based on genetic testing is the only method currently available for disease prevention. With PGD, in vitro fertilization is performed and a single cell is removed from early-stage embryos for genetic testing to determine if a family's pathogenic variant is present or absent. Only embryos without evidence of the pathogenic variant are then implanted. The decision to pursue PGD is a highly personal one and may be an option for particular consideration for families in whom disease expression is associated with a high burden of malignancy. Discussions regarding the intricacies of genetic testing and PGD must involve genetic counselors with expertise in cardiovascular genetics. When PGD is being considered, the risk of in vitro fertilization should be taken into account, because it can be associated with fluid retention.

PATHOPHYSIOLOGY RELATED TO PREGNANCY

Pregnancy is associated with many physiologic changes, including a 40% to 50% increase in plasma volume and cardiac output, a reduction in systemic vascular resistance, and a hypercoagulable state. The hypertrophied small LV can, in most cases, accommodate the physiologic increase in blood volume without clinically significant elevations in filling pressures. The increased volume load of pregnancy causes enlargement of the LV cavity, which theoretically may reduce LVOTO; however, increased cardiac output and tachycardia tends to counteract this effect and LVOT gradients increase with advancing gestation. Volume loading also increases dilation of the left atrium, thereby increasing the risk of atrial tachyarrhythmias. In the context of decreased myocardial compliance, the volume changes and increased heart rate that occur later in pregnancy can aggravate symptoms of dyspnea and peripheral edema and lower the threshold for development of congestive heart failure.

PRECONCEPTION CLINICAL EVALUATION AND RISK ASSESSMENT

Although most women with HCM have uncomplicated pregnancies, the physiologic changes are associated with increased risk for both mother and fetus. A meta-analysis of 9 observational studies from 1968 to 2012 of 408 pregnancies in 237 women with HCM reported maternal mortality of 0.5%, and complications or worsening of symptoms occurred in 29% of cases. These complications included heart failure in up to 30% and arrhythmias in up to 48%. Fetal mortality by spontaneous abortion (15%), therapeutic abortion (5%), or stillbirth (2%) is comparable to the general population. The risk of premature birth, however, is 2 times to 3 times higher compared with the general population (26% vs 10%–12%, respectively).[22,23] Among a group of 60 women with HCM enrolled in the contemporary, international Registry of Pregnancy and Cardiac Disease from 2007 to 2014, there were no maternal deaths and 15% developed heart failure, 10% developed ventricular tachyarrhythmias, and 1.7% developed AF.[24] Heart failure occurred mainly during the third trimester, highlighting the need for close follow-up.

Risk assessment should be performed before conception using the modified World Health Organization (WHO) classification (**Table 1**). Most women with HCM are modified WHO classes II and III, implying a moderate risk of morbidity.[25] Risk is increased where women are symptomatic

Table 1
Modified World Health Organization classification of maternal risk applied to hypertrophic cardiomyopathy

	Modified World Health Organization Classes II–III	Modified World Health Organization Class III	Modified World Health Organization Class IV
Application to HCM	Mild to moderate LVOTO NYHA I Normal or mild LV systolic dysfunction (EF >45%) Well-controlled arrhythmia Bioprosthetic valve repair/replacement	Severe LVOTO NYHA II Moderate LV systolic dysfunction (EF 30%–45%) Arrhythmias despite medical optimization Mechanical valve replacement	Severe symptomatic LVOTO Severe systemic ventricular systolic dysfunction (EF <30% or NYHA classes III–IV)
Maternal risk	Intermediate increased risk of mortality or moderate–severe increase in morbidity	Significantly increased risk of mortality or severe morbidity	Extremely high risk of maternal mortality or severe morbidity; pregnancy contraindicated
Pregnancy care	High-risk obstetrics and cardiologist or specialized HCM center and pregnancy heart team	Specialized HCM center Pregnancy heart team	Specialized HCM center pregnancy heart team
Minimum follow-up during pregnancy	Each trimester	Monthly or bimonthly	Bimonthly
Mode of delivery	Vaginal	Vaginal Cesarean if severe symptomatic LVOTO	Cesarean

prepregnancy or exhibit a high-risk profile, including significant diastolic dysfunction, severe LVOTO (LVOT gradient ≥50 mm Hg), and arrhythmias.[22,24] Advising against pregnancy is justified only in a small minority with significant LV dysfunction (systolic dysfunction with LV EF less than 30%, or severe diastolic dysfunction with restrictive physiology) or severe symptomatic LVOTO. With relief of LVOTO, pregnancy can be expected to carry reduced risk.

To aid in preconception risk assessment, all women should be assessed clinically and undergo echocardiography and exercise tolerance testing. Important features to note include measures of LV systolic and diastolic function, hypertrophy burden, left atrial size, LVOT gradients at rest and with provocation, systolic anterior motion of the mitral leaflets, and degree of mitral regurgitation. Maximum workload and peak oxygen consumption on cardiopulmonary exercise testing also are informative.

It is important to address potentially teratogenic medications during the preconception evaluation. β-Blockers and nondihydropyridine calcium channel blockers should be continued. Disopyramide should be used only when the potential benefits outweigh the risks, because it can cause uterine contractions.[26] Women taking direct-acting oral anticoagulants or vitamin K antagonists prior to conception should have a clear plan to switch to low-molecular-weight (LMW) heparin during attempted conception or immediately upon becoming pregnant.

MANAGEMENT DURING PREGNANCY

Women in WHO classes II to III should be assessed by a cardiologist each trimester, including physical examination and echocardiography.[25] Echocardiography additionally should be performed to further investigate the development of new symptoms or a significant change from baseline. For women in WHO class III, more frequent follow-up, monthly or bimonthly, is warranted (see **Table 1**). These women should be managed in a specialized HCM center with a multidisciplinary team.[17,25] Follow-up during pregnancy should focus on the development or progression of dyspnea, arrhythmias, LVOTO, and diastolic and systolic dysfunction.

In HCM, plasma levels of B-type natriuretic peptide (BNP) and N-terminal pro-brain natriuretic peptide are independent predictors of morbidity and mortality.[27,28] In pregnancy, the level of natriuretic peptides are relatively stable throughout pregnancy and similar to that of the nonpregnant state.[29,30] During pregnancy, many women with heart disease have increased BNP levels, and higher BNP during pregnancy can be associated with adverse maternal cardiac events.[31] These cardiac biomarkers have not been evaluated systematically in pregnant women with HCM or correlated with maternal morbidity or mortality; thus, their clinical utility is unknown.

Cardiac magnetic resonance imaging (MRI) does not have ionizing radiation and can be safely used in pregnant women.[32] Contrast-enhanced cardiac MRI with late gadolinium enhancement (LGE) identifies fibrosis but is not necessary for evaluation of cardiac structure. The prevalence of LGE in HCM is approximately 50% to 80% and its extent correlates with the adverse LV remodeling associated with systolic dysfunction.[33–36] A meta-analysis of cross-sectional studies investigating the relationship between LGE and long-term outcomes demonstrated a relationship between LGE and cardiovascular mortality, heart failure, and all-cause death but shows only a trend toward an increased risk of SCD.[37] Theoretic concerns about the safety of gadolinium-based contrast enhancement during pregnancy center on the fact that it is water soluble and can cross the placenta into the fetal circulation and amniotic fluid. Given use of gadolinium in evaluation of HCM primarily relates to prognosis, its use in pregnant women should be avoided. In patients with good echocardiographic images, cardiac MRI provides similar information on ventricular function and morphology,[38,39] but it is helpful in establishing the diagnosis of HCM in patients with poor acoustic windows or when some LV regions are poorly visualized, such as the LV apex.[40,41] Echocardiographic contrast agents are useful in outlining the endocardium and their use is recommended in patients with HCM whose acoustic windows are suboptimal. There are no data, however, regarding their safety in pregnancy and, as such, their uses should be avoided.[42] In pregnant women with HCM in whom an LV apical aneurysm is suspected on echocardiography but cannot be confirmed due to poor acoustic windows, it is reasonable to pursue diagnosis with cardiac MRI given the high associated risk for arrhythmic sudden death and thromboembolic events.[43] As such, diagnosis of

an LV apical aneurysm should prompt consideration for ICD implantation or wearable cardioverter-defibrillator and recommendation for anticoagulation.

For women whose symptoms and disease are well controlled with β-blockers, they should be continued. Side effects, such as intrauterine growth retardation, neonatal bradycardia, and hypoglycemia, usually are not severe and can be managed easily during pregnancy. Metoprolol is the most widely used; atenolol is not advised because it has been associated with more significant growth retardation. β-Blockers do not need to be introduced routinely in all pregnant women with HCM; however, they should be initiated when new symptoms occur, for rate control in the development of AF, and to suppress new ventricular arrhythmias. They also should be considered in those with more than mild LVOTO (ie, LVOT peak gradient $\geq$30 mm Hg) to prevent sudden pulmonary congestion.[25] Verapamil and diltiazem are classified by the Food and Drug Administration as class C and should be reserved as a second choice when β-blockers are not tolerated (with fetal monitoring for atrioventricular block).[3,44]

Hypovolemia is poorly tolerated in those women with LVOTO who suffer hyperemesis gravidarum. Aggressive oral hydration with at least 2000 mL of fluids a day is recommended. If oral intake is not tolerated or sufficient, intravenous fluid replacement and antiemetic therapy may be necessary. Hypervolemia and symptoms of CHF that may develop during later stages of pregnancy can be managed with loop diuretics. Initiation or up-titration of β-blockers and nondihydropyridine calcium channel blockers may help mitigate symptomatic LVOTO. Alcohol septal ablation with appropriate radiation shielding and limited fluoroscopy time have been performed successfully in the case of failed medical therapy in highly symptomatic severe LVOTO.[45]

Cardioversion should be considered for poorly tolerated persistent AF.[25] Immediate electrical cardioversion is recommended whenever ongoing AF results in maternal hemodynamic instability or fetal distress. Because a few cases of fetal distress immediately after electrical cardioversion have been described, elective electrical cardioversions should be carried out in facilities with the capacity to perform fetal monitoring and emergency cesarean delivery.[46] Cardioversion generally should be preceded by anticoagulation.

AF significantly increases the risk of thromboembolism in patients with HCM and oral anticoagulation is recommended as primary stroke prophylaxis regardless of CHA_2DS_2-VASc score, which does not correlate well with clinical outcomes.[13] Therapeutic anticoagulation is recommended for any pregnant woman with HCM who develops paroxysmal or persistent AF. The choice of anticoagulant during pregnancy needs to take into account fetal safety and risk of maternal hemorrhagic complications.

LMW heparin is the preferred anticoagulant for prevention of thromboembolism related to AF in most pregnant women because it does not cross the placenta, thus is not teratogenic and does not result in fetal anticoagulation.[47,48] LMW heparin usually is replaced with unfractionated heparin at 36 weeks to 37 weeks of gestation in order to minimize the risk of delivery within 24 hours of the last dose of LMW heparin and to increase the chance of being able receive neuraxial anesthesia.[49]

Warfarin generally is avoided during pregnancy because it crosses the placenta and exposure during the first trimester can result in embryopathy, whereas exposure later in pregnancy can cause fetal bleeding, including intracranial hemorrhage. An exception is a woman with a mechanical mitral valve who is considered at particularly high risk for thrombosis or thromboembolism. Women taking warfarin prior to conception for prevention of stroke related to AF should be counseled to switch to another anticoagulant (eg, LMW heparin) during attempted conception or immediately on becoming pregnant, to avoid teratogenic effects of the drug during the first trimester.

Direct oral anticoagulants are not used in pregnancy because of absence of information on efficacy and fetal safety. Although they have not been shown to be teratogenic, women taking these anticoagulants should be switched to LMW heparin prior to conception or immediately upon becoming pregnant.[50]

When indicated, pacemaker or ICD implantation during pregnancy should be performed.[3] A wearable cardioverter-defibrillator may be considered as a bridge to ICD implantation. Garment and belt fitting is crucial for electrocardiographic signal analysis and appropriate shock delivery and, given the body habitus changes that occur throughout the second and third trimesters of pregnancy, serial evaluations for appropriate fitting may be necessary. Furthermore, for wearable cardioverter-defibrillators to be effective in prevention of SCD, full compliance would be necessary.

DELIVERY

The preferred mode of delivery is vaginal, with an individualized delivery plan addressing timing of delivery (spontaneous/induced), method of induction, analgesia/regional anesthesia, and level of monitoring required.[25] Women in modified WHO classes II–III may have spontaneous labor and vaginal delivery. There is no need to deactivate an ICD during vaginal delivery.

Cesarean delivery should be considered in patients with severe symptomatic LVOTO or severe heart failure (WHO class IV). In elective cesarean deliveries, an ICD is programmed to monitor only to avoid electrical interference from diathermy and reprogrammed to full therapy mode immediately postoperatively.[51] Epidural and spinal anesthesia cause systemic vasodilation and hypotension and, therefore, must be used with caution in patients with severe LVOTO and may require continuous hemodynamic assessment with arterial line monitoring. Single-shot spinal anesthesia should be avoided.[25,52] Oxytocin should be given as a slow infusion and intravenous fluids must be given judiciously in order to avoid poorly tolerated volume overload in the setting of significant diastolic dysfunction.

SUMMARY

HCM generally is well tolerated in pregnancy with favorable maternal and fetal outcomes and a relatively low likelihood of complications of pregnancy. Heart failure and arrhythmias are the primary complications women with HCM experience. Prepregnancy counseling and risk evaluation in women with HCM are paramount to favorable maternal and fetal outcomes. Symptoms often can be managed safely with β-blockers. A majority of women with HCM can deliver vaginally, with cesarean delivery reserved only for those with high-risk features, such as severe symptomatic LVOTO or severe heart failure. Management during pregnancy and around delivery should be conducted by a multidisciplinary team consisting of a cardiologist, obstetrician, genetic counselor, and anesthesiologist.

CLINICS CARE POINTS

- Prepregnancy risk assessment and counseling as well as genetic counseling are indicated in all women with HCM.
- Advising against pregnancy is justified only in a small minority with LV EF less than 30%, New York Heart Association (NYHA) classes III–IV with restrictive physiology, or severe symptomatic LV outflow obstruction.
- β-Blockers (preferably metoprolol) should be continued in women who used them prior to pregnancy.

- Vaginal delivery is recommended as first choice in the vast majority of women with hypertrophic cardiomyopathy.

DISCLOSURE

The author has received honorarium and travel expense reimbursement for serving on an Advisory Board for MyoKardia, Inc.

REFERENCES

1. Maron BJ. Hypertrophic cardiomyopathy: an important global disease. Am J Med 2004;116(1):63–5.
2. Maron BJ, Gardin JM, Flack JM, et al. Prevalence of hypertrophic cardiomyopathy in a general population of young adults. Echocardiographic analysis of 4111 subjects in the CARDIA Study. Coronary Artery Risk Development in (Young) Adults. Circulation 1995;92(4):785–9.
3. Authors/Task Force Members, Elliott PM, Anastasakis A, et al. 2014 ESC guidelines on diagnosis and management of hypertrophic cardiomyopathy: the Task Force for the diagnosis and management of hypertrophic cardiomyopathy of the European Society of Cardiology (ESC). Eur Heart J 2014;35(39):2733–79.
4. Ho CY. Hypertrophic cardiomyopathy: preclinical and early phenotype. J Cardiovasc Transl Res 2009;2(4):462–70.
5. Olivotto I, Girolami F, Nistri S, et al. The many faces of hypertrophic cardiomyopathy: from developmental biology to clinical practice. J Cardiovasc Transl Res 2009;2(4):349–67.
6. Maron BJ. Clinical course and management of hypertrophic cardiomyopathy. N Engl J Med 2018; 379(7):655–68.
7. Maron MS, Olivotto I, Zenovich AG, et al. Hypertrophic cardiomyopathy is predominantly a disease of left ventricular outflow tract obstruction. Circulation 2006;114(21):2232–9.
8. Seferovic PM, Polovina M, Bauersachs J, et al. Heart failure in cardiomyopathies: a position paper from the heart failure association of the European Society of Cardiology. Eur J Heart Fail 2019;21(5):553–76.
9. Ho CY, Day SM, Ashley EA, et al. Genotype and Lifetime burden of disease in hypertrophic cardiomyopathy: Insights from the sarcomeric Human cardiomyopathy Registry (SHaRe). Circulation 2018;138(14):1387–98.
10. Spoladore R, Maron MS, D'Amato R, et al. Pharmacological treatment options for hypertrophic cardiomyopathy: high time for evidence. Eur Heart J 2012;33(14):1724–33.
11. Ho CY, Lakdawala NK, Cirino AL, et al. Diltiazem treatment for pre-clinical hypertrophic cardiomyopathy sarcomere mutation carriers: a pilot randomized trial to modify disease expression. JACC Heart Fail 2015;3(2):180–8.
12. Maron BJ, Ommen SR, Semsarian C, et al. Hypertrophic cardiomyopathy: present and future, with translation into contemporary cardiovascular medicine. J Am Coll Cardiol 2014;64(1):83–99.
13. Guttmann OP, Pavlou M, O'Mahony C, et al. Prediction of thrombo-embolic risk in patients with hypertrophic cardiomyopathy (HCM Risk-CVA). Eur J Heart Fail 2015;17(8):837–45.
14. Lee HJ, Kim HK, Jung JH, et al. Novel oral anticoagulants for primary stroke prevention in hypertrophic cardiomyopathy patients with atrial fibrillation. Stroke 2019;50(9):2582–6.
15. Elliott PM, Gimeno JR, Thaman R, et al. Historical trends in reported survival rates in patients with hypertrophic cardiomyopathy. Heart 2006;92(6):785–91.
16. Maron BJ, Rowin EJ, Casey SA, et al. How hypertrophic cardiomyopathy became a contemporary treatable genetic disease with low mortality: shaped by 50 years of clinical research and practice. JAMA Cardiol 2016;1(1):98–105.
17. Gersh BJ, Maron BJ, Bonow RO, et al. 2011 ACCF/AHA guideline for the diagnosis and treatment of hypertrophic cardiomyopathy: executive summary: a report of the American College of Cardiology Foundation/American heart association Task Force on practice guidelines. Circulation 2011;124(24): 2761–96.
18. Avila WS, Rossi EG, Ramires JA, et al. Pregnancy in patients with heart disease: experience with 1,000 cases. Clin Cardiol 2003;26(3):135–42.
19. Lima FV, Parikh PB, Zhu J, et al. Association of cardiomyopathy with adverse cardiac events in pregnant women at the time of delivery. JACC Heart Fail 2015;3(3):257–66.
20. Sikka P, Suri V, Aggarwal N, et al. Are we missing hypertrophic cardiomyopathy in pregnancy? Experience of a tertiary care hospital. J Clin Diagn Res 2014;8(9):OC13–5.
21. Arad M, Maron BJ, Gorham JM, et al. Glycogen storage diseases presenting as hypertrophic cardiomyopathy. N Engl J Med 2005;352(4):362–72.
22. Schinkel AF. Pregnancy in women with hypertrophic cardiomyopathy. Cardiol Rev 2014;22(5):217–22.
23. Drenthen W, Pieper PG, Roos-Hesselink JW, et al. Outcome of pregnancy in women with congenital heart disease: a literature review. J Am Coll Cardiol 2007;49(24):2303–11.
24. Goland S, van Hagen IM, Elbaz-Greener G, et al. Pregnancy in women with hypertrophic cardiomyopathy: data from the European Society of Cardiology initiated Registry of Pregnancy and Cardiac disease (ROPAC). Eur Heart J 2017;38(35): 2683–90.
25. Regitz-Zagrosek V, Roos-Hesselink JW, Bauersachs J, et al. 2018 ESC Guidelines for the

management of cardiovascular diseases during pregnancy. Eur Heart J 2018;39(34):3165–241.

26. Tadmor OP, Keren A, Rosenak D, et al. The effect of disopyramide on uterine contractions during pregnancy. Am J Obstet Gynecol 1990;162(2):482–6.

27. D'Amato R, Tomberli B, Castelli G, et al. Prognostic value of N-terminal pro-brain natriuretic Peptide in outpatients with hypertrophic cardiomyopathy. Am J Cardiol 2013;112(8):1190–6.

28. Geske JB, McKie PM, Ommen SR, et al. B-type natriuretic peptide and survival in hypertrophic cardiomyopathy. J Am Coll Cardiol 2013;61(24):2456–60.

29. Hameed AB, Chan K, Ghamsary M, et al. Longitudinal changes in the B-type natriuretic peptide levels in normal pregnancy and postpartum. Clin Cardiol 2009;32(8):E60–2.

30. Yurteri-Kaplan L, Saber S, Zamudio S, et al. Brain natriuretic peptide in term pregnancy. Reprod Sci 2012;19(5):520–5.

31. Tanous D, Siu SC, Mason J, et al. B-type natriuretic peptide in pregnant women with heart disease. J Am Coll Cardiol 2010;56(15):1247–53.

32. Expert Panel on MRS, Kanal E, Barkovich AJ, et al. ACR guidance document on MR safe practices: 2013. J Magn Reson Imaging 2013;37(3):501–30.

33. Choudhury L, Mahrholdt H, Wagner A, et al. Myocardial scarring in asymptomatic or mildly symptomatic patients with hypertrophic cardiomyopathy. J Am Coll Cardiol 2002;40(12):2156–64.

34. Maron MS, Appelbaum E, Harrigan CJ, et al. Clinical profile and significance of delayed enhancement in hypertrophic cardiomyopathy. Circ Heart Fail 2008;1(3):184–91.

35. Moon JC, McKenna WJ, McCrohon JA, et al. Toward clinical risk assessment in hypertrophic cardiomyopathy with gadolinium cardiovascular magnetic resonance. J Am Coll Cardiol 2003;41(9):1561–7.

36. Rubinshtein R, Glockner JF, Ommen SR, et al. Characteristics and clinical significance of late gadolinium enhancement by contrast-enhanced magnetic resonance imaging in patients with hypertrophic cardiomyopathy. Circ Heart Fail 2010;3(1):51–8.

37. Green JJ, Berger JS, Kramer CM, et al. Prognostic value of late gadolinium enhancement in clinical outcomes for hypertrophic cardiomyopathy. JACC Cardiovasc Imaging 2012;5(4):370–7.

38. Olivotto I, Maron MS, Autore C, et al. Assessment and significance of left ventricular mass by cardiovascular magnetic resonance in hypertrophic cardiomyopathy. J Am Coll Cardiol 2008;52(7):559–66.

39. Puntmann VO, Gebker R, Duckett S, et al. Left ventricular chamber dimensions and wall thickness by cardiovascular magnetic resonance: comparison with transthoracic echocardiography. Eur Heart J Cardiovasc Imaging 2013;14(3):240–6.

40. Moon JC, Fisher NG, McKenna WJ, et al. Detection of apical hypertrophic cardiomyopathy by cardiovascular magnetic resonance in patients with non-diagnostic echocardiography. Heart 2004;90(6):645–9.

41. Rickers C, Wilke NM, Jerosch-Herold M, et al. Utility of cardiac magnetic resonance imaging in the diagnosis of hypertrophic cardiomyopathy. Circulation 2005;112(6):855–61.

42. Muskula PR, Main ML. Safety with echocardiographic contrast agents. Circ Cardiovasc Imaging 2017;10(4):e005459.

43. Rowin EJ, Maron BJ, Haas TS, et al. Hypertrophic cardiomyopathy with left ventricular apical aneurysm: implications for risk stratification and management. J Am Coll Cardiol 2017;69(7):761–73.

44. Pieper PG, Walker F. Pregnancy in women with hypertrophic cardiomyopathy. Neth Heart J 2013;21(1):14–8.

45. Shaikh A, Bajwa T, Bush M, et al. Successful alcohol septal ablation in a pregnant patient with symptomatic hypertrophic obstructive cardiomyopathy. J Cardiol Cases 2018;17(5):151–4.

46. Tromp CH, Nanne AC, Pernet PJ, et al. Electrical cardioversion during pregnancy: safe or not? Neth Heart J 2011;19(3):134–6.

47. Forestier F, Daffos F, Capella-Pavlovsky M. Low molecular weight heparin (PK 10169) does not cross the placenta during the second trimester of pregnancy study by direct fetal blood sampling under ultrasound. Thromb Res 1984;34(6):557–60.

48. Forestier F, Daffos F, Rainaut M, et al. Low molecular weight heparin (CY 216) does not cross the placenta during the third trimester of pregnancy. Thromb Haemost 1987;57(2):234.

49. American College of Obstetricians and Gynecologists' Committee on Practice Bulletins—Obstetrics. ACOG practice bulletin no. 196: thromboembolism in pregnancy. Obstet Gynecol 2018;132(1):e1–17.

50. Cohen H, Arachchillage DR, Middeldorp S, et al. Management of direct oral anticoagulants in women of childbearing potential: guidance from the SSC of the ISTH. J Thromb Haemost 2016;14(8):1673–6.

51. Donnelly P, Pal N, Herity NA. Perioperative management of patients with implantable cardioverter defibrillators. Ulster Med J 2007;76(2):66–7.

52. Walker D, Kaur N, Bell R, et al. Hyperthrophic obstructive cardiomyopathy and pregnancy: University College London hospital experience. Minerva Anestesiol 2007;73(9):485–6.

Valvular Heart Disease in Pregnancy

Jennifer Lewey, MD, MPH[a],*, Lauren Andrade, MD[b], Lisa D. Levine, MD, MSCE[c]

KEYWORDS

- Valvular heart disease • Pregnancy • Mitral stenosis • Aortic stenosis • Mechanical heart valve
- Anticoagulation

KEY POINTS

- Pregnancy is well tolerated in most women with valvular heart disease. Cardiac output increases up to 50% and can lead to clinical decompensation in high-risk women.
- Women with mechanical heart valves need careful management of anticoagulation during pregnancy to minimize maternal and fetal risks.
- Vaginal delivery with epidural anesthesia is recommended for most women with stable valvular heart disease.
- All women with valvular heart disease should be managed by a multidisciplinary Pregnancy Heart Team before and during pregnancy.

INTRODUCTION

Cardiovascular (CV) disease complicates an estimated 1% to 4% of all pregnancies and is the leading cause of death in pregnant and postpartum women in the United States.[1,2] Valvular heart disease is a common cause of CV disease that affects women of childbearing age.[3,4] Congenital heart disease is the leading cause of valvular heart disease in the United States; however, rheumatic heart disease is a prevalent condition especially among immigrant populations.[5,6] Most women with valvular heart disease will do well during pregnancy, but high-risk conditions such as severe mitral stenosis (MS) or aortic stenosis (AS), can be associated with significant maternal morbidity and mortality. Management of anticoagulation of pregnant women with mechanical heart valves presents unique challenges to reduce the risk of maternal and fetal complications. Women with valvular heart disease who are pregnant or considering pregnancy should be managed by a multidisciplinary Pregnancy Heart Team consisting of cardiologists and high-risk obstetricians.

Hemodynamic changes start early in pregnancy. Cardiac output increases 30% to 50% and peaks between the second and third trimesters.[7,8] Changes in cardiac output are driven by an increase in stroke volume in the first half of pregnancy followed by a gradual rise in heart rate. As a result of placental maturation, systemic vascular resistance and blood pressure decrease in the first and second trimesters and returns to prepregnancy levels in the third trimester. Women with valvular heart disease, especially left-sided obstructive lesions, may have limited cardiac reserve to accommodate these hemodynamic changes. As a result, close serial monitoring during pregnancy is necessary to assess for clinical decompensation. The changes in flow can lead

[a] Division of Cardiology, Department of Medicine, University of Pennsylvania Perelman School of Medicine, Perelman Center for Advanced Medicine, 3400 Civic Center Boulevard, 2-East Pavilion, Philadelphia, PA 19104, USA; [b] Philadelphia Adult Congenital Heart Center, University of Pennsylvania, Children's Hospital of Philadelphia, Perelman Center for Advanced Medicine, 3400 Civic Center Boulevard, 2- East Pavilion, Philadelphia, PA 19104, USA; [c] Department of Obstetrics and Gynecology, Maternal and Child Health Research Center, University of Pennsylvania Perelman School of Medicine, 3400 Spruce Street, 2 Silverstein, Philadelphia, PA 19104, USA
* Corresponding author.
E-mail address: jennifer.lewey@pennmedicine.upenn.edu

Cardiol Clin 39 (2021) 151–161
https://doi.org/10.1016/j.ccl.2020.09.010
0733-8651/21/© 2020 Elsevier Inc. All rights reserved.

cardiology.theclinics.com

to increases in mitral and aortic transvalvular gradients and an overestimation of lesion severity. Direct valve planimetry for patients with AS or MS may more accurately reflect the degree of valve stenosis, especially for patients newly diagnosed during pregnancy. The hypercoagulable state of pregnancy increases the risk of thromboembolic events during pregnancy and the first 6 to 12 weeks postpartum, further complicating the anticoagulation management of women with mechanical valves.[9]

Labor and delivery is associated with sudden hemodynamic changes and increases in oxygen consumption. After delivery, dramatic changes in hemodynamics occur as a result of autotransfusion of uterine blood volume, relief of caval pressure, and mobilization of dependent edema. The sudden increase in preload can lead to clinical decompensation and women with high-risk lesions will need to be followed closely immediately after delivery and in the subsequent days post-delivery.

PRECONCEPTION COUNSELING

Reproductive age women with valvular heart disease should undergo counseling before conception by a collaborative Pregnancy Heart Team consisting of a maternal fetal medicine (MFM) specialist and cardiologist with experience in caring for pregnant women with heart disease.[10] The goal of preconception counseling is to review and individualize the maternal and fetal risk of pregnancy. Baseline cardiac function should be assessed with an electrocardiogram and echocardiogram to start. Exercise stress testing can be an important tool to assess exercise capacity, development of arrhythmias and symptomatic response, which may guide risk stratification and treatment before conception. Additional imaging modalities such as cardiac MRI or computed tomography may be used to further assess valvular function, anatomy of structures not well seen by echocardiogram, and associated aortopathies.

For women planning pregnancy, medications should be reviewed for safety during pregnancy. Angiotensin-converting enzyme inhibitors and angiotensin receptor blockers are teratogenic and can be changed to medications with a better safety profile during pregnancy. Bosentan and statins are also considered teratogenic and should be stopped before pregnancy. For women with mechanical valves taking warfarin, shared decision making will help guide the appropriate choice of anticoagulation in the first trimester. Beta blockers are generally considered safe in pregnancy. Women may frequently present during pregnancy with newly diagnosed or newly symptomatic valvular heart disease and collaborative care between MFM, cardiology, anesthesia, and other specialists is needed to reduce ongoing maternal, obstetric, and fetal risk.

RISK ASSESSMENT

The most common maternal complications of valvular heart disease during pregnancy are heart failure, arrhythmias, and thromboembolic complications. Postpartum hemorrhage can be a common complication for women on anticoagulation. Cardiac symptoms can be managed in many women with diuresis, medical therapy, and reducing level of physical activity. If symptoms are refractory to conservative management, valve intervention during pregnancy may be necessary. Percutaneous balloon valvuloplasty performed by experienced operators is preferred for stenotic lesions. Ideally these interventions should be performed after the fourth month in the second trimester to minimize radiation exposure during organogenesis.[6] Valve surgery with cardiopulmonary bypass performed during pregnancy is associated with rates of fetal death up to 30%, especially when surgery is emergent and/or performed at early gestational age.[11,12] If surgery is needed, however, the second trimester is the preferred time frame with use of high flow on cardiopulmonary bypass to provide adequate placental perfusion.[13]

Maternal cardiac risk can be estimated using the lesion specific modified World Health Organization (WHO) classification (**Table 1**).[6] Women with severe MS and severe symptomatic AS are considered to be at extremely high risk of maternal morbidity or mortality (WHO IV) and pregnancy is contraindicated. Most other types of valvular heart disease in pregnancy are considered to be moderate to high risk (WHO II-III). Those with regurgitant lesions such as aortic regurgitation and mitral regurgitation usually tolerate pregnancy well due to the decreased systemic afterload during pregnancy. Individualized risk can be further estimated using pregnancy-specific risk indices developed in large cohorts, including the CARPREG II and the ZAHARA models.[4,14,15] Contraception should be discussed with all women with valvular heart disease but highly effective contraception should be particularly recommended for women at high risk of pregnancy complications. Estrogen-containing contraception increases the risk of venous and arterial thrombosis and hypertension and should be avoided in women with cardiac disease, especially those at increased thrombotic risk. In such patients, long-acting progesterone-only methods

Table 1
Modified World Health Organization (WHO) classification of pregnancy risk

WHO Classification	Maternal Risk
WHO I Mild pulmonary stenosis Small patents ductus arteriosus (PDA) Mitral valve prolapse with mild mitral regurgitation Repaired simple lesions: ASD, VSD, PDA, anomalous pulmonary venous drainage Isolated atrial or ventricular ectopic beats	• Morbidity: little to no increased risk • Mortality: no increased risk
WHO II Uncorrected ASD or VSD Repaired Tetralogy of Fallot Most arrhythmias	• Morbidity: moderately increased risk • Mortality: mildly increased risk
WHO II-III Mild LV impairment (EF >45%) Hypertrophic cardiomyopathy Valvular heart disease not considered WHO I or IV Marfan syndrome, aorta <40 mm Bicuspid aortic valve, aorta <45 mm Repaired aortic coarctation	Risk varies based on individual patient • Morbidity: moderately to severely increased risk • Mortality: intermediate increased risk
WHO III Mechanical valve Moderate LV dysfunction (EF 30%–45%) PPCM with recovered LV function (EF ≥ 50%) Systemic right ventricle Fontan circulation Unrepaired Tetralogy of Fallot Marfan syndrome, aorta 40–45 mm Bicuspid aortic valve, aorta 45–50 mm Unrepaired cyanotic heart disease Other complex congenital heart disease	• Morbidity: severely increased risk • Mortality: significantly increased risk
WHO IV Severe mitral stenosis Severe symptomatic aortic stenosis Pulmonary arterial hypertension Severe LV dysfunction (EF <30% or NYHA class III-IV) PPCM with persistent LV dysfunction (EF <50%) Uncorrected severe aortic coarctation Marfan syndrome, aorta >45 mm Bicuspid aortic valve, aorta >50 mm	• Pregnancy is contraindicated due to extremely high risk of maternal mortality or severe maternal morbidity

Abbreviations: ASD, atrial septal defect; EF, ejection fraction; LV, left ventricle; NYHA, New York Heart Association; PPCM, peripartum cardiomyopathy; VSD, ventricular septal defect.
Adapted from Regitz-Zagrosek V, Roos-Hesselink JW, Bauersachs J, et al. 2018 ESC Guidelines for the management of cardiovascular diseases during pregnancy. Eur Heart J 2018;39(34):3165–3241; with permission.

are recommended, such as an intrauterine device or subdermal implants.[16]

DELIVERY CONSIDERATIONS

Unless indicated for obstetric indications, a vaginal delivery is preferred for most women with valvular heart disease.[1] Vaginal delivery is associated with less blood loss, more rapid recovery, and less thrombogenic and infectious risk. Patients at elevated risk of complications should discuss a delivery plan in consultation with a multidisciplinary team consisting of a MFM specialist, cardiologist, and obstetric anesthesiologist.

Women with stable cardiac disease can undergo full-term delivery at 39 weeks of gestation.[1] Good pain control with regional anesthesia during vaginal delivery can minimize the catecholamine release associated with sudden increases in heart rate and stroke volume. Epidural is preferred over spinal anesthesia due to lower rates of hypotension. Women with moderate to severe left-sided obstructive lesions may benefit from an assisted second stage of labor using forceps or vacuum, which shortens the time to delivery and minimizes the frequency and intensity of maternal effort with Valsalva maneuver, which transiently drops cardiac output. Cesarean delivery should be considered in women with severe heart failure (New York Heart Association [NYHA] class III-IV), high-risk aortic disease, and severe forms of pulmonary hypertension.[6] For women requiring delivery while fully anticoagulated on warfarin, Cesarean delivery should be considered to minimize the risk of fetal intracranial hemorrhage. Telemetry is recommended during labor and delivery and up to 24 hours after delivery in women at risk for developing arrhythmias. Women with severely stenotic or symptomatic valvular disease may require monitoring in a cardiac care or telemetry unit for at least 24 hours after delivery, with close monitoring of hemodynamics and volume status.

SPECIFIC VALVE LESIONS
Mitral Stenosis

MS is the most common valvular lesion managed during pregnancy and its prevalence is more common in areas of the world with a higher burden of rheumatic heart disease.[17] In some cases, MS may be congenital and due to a dysplastic valve or as a result of valve stenosis following an earlier intervention during childhood, as may be the case in patients with surgical repair of atrio-ventricular (AV) septal defects. During pregnancy, the physiologic increase in stroke volume and heart rate lead to higher gradients across the stenosed mitral valve and an increase in left atrial pressure. These changes can lead to worsening heart failure symptoms or the development of new symptoms in women who were previously asymptomatic. The hemodynamic changes of pregnancy can also lead to atrial arrhythmias, including atrial fibrillation, which can in turn precipitate pulmonary congestion.[18] In up to a quarter of women, pregnancy may be the first time a diagnosis of MS is made.[17,19]

Maternal outcomes
MS is associated with an increased risk of heart failure and atrial arrhythmias during pregnancy. Women with moderate or severe stenosis (mitral valve area (MVA) <1.5 cm^2), baseline maternal NYHA class III or IV, or a history of cardiac complications before pregnancy represent the groups at highest risk of maternal complications.[17,18,20] Most complications can be managed medically and rates of mitral valve intervention and maternal mortality are low, especially in North American and European cohorts.

Many women with MS will develop or experience progression of symptoms during pregnancy. Among 44 women with MS representing 46 pregnancies treated in California, 74% advanced $\geq$ 1 NYHA class during pregnancy.[19] Women with moderate or severe MS had high rates of developing heart failure or atrial arrhythmias, whereas women with mild MS had maternal outcomes similar to women without valvular disease (**Fig. 1**). In a Canadian cohort of 74 women representing 80 pregnancies, 31% developed pulmonary edema and 11% developed arrhythmias, with risk proportional to severity of stenosis.[18] Heart failure was managed medically in both cohorts and no maternal deaths were reported.

Similar rates of maternal complications were reported among the 273 women with MS participating in the International Registry of Pregnancy and Cardiac Disease (ROPAC).[17] In this cohort, 15 patients (5.9%) underwent mitral valve intervention including percutaneous balloon mitral commissurotomy (n = 14) and surgical valve replacement (n = 1). Most interventions occurred in women who were symptomatic before pregnancy. One woman with severe MS died during pregnancy and 2 died postpartum. Women with moderate and severe MS have high rates of preterm delivery and intrauterine growth restriction (IUGR).[19]

Management
The medical management of women who become symptomatic during pregnancy consists of beta blockers, diuretics, and activity restriction. Beta blockers slow the heart rate, lengthen diastolic filling time, and lower left atrial pressure.[21] Beta-1 selective agents, such as metoprolol, are preferred so as to avoid interfering with beta-2 mediated uterine relaxation. Furosemide should be used in patients with pulmonary edema or ongoing symptoms despite beta blockers. Women who develop atrial fibrillation should be anticoagulated, usually with low molecular weight heparin, unfractionated heparin, or warfarin depending on the trimester and clinical context. Anticoagulation should also be considered in women with severe MS and other risk factors for stroke, such as spontaneous echocardiographic contrast in the left

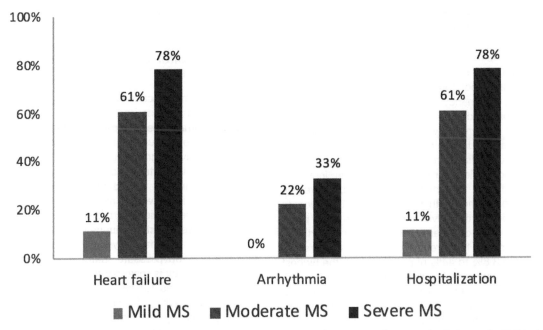

Fig. 1. Cardiac complication of MS according to severity. (*Adapted from* Hameed A, Karaalp IS, Tummala PP, Wani OR, Canetti M, Akhter MW, Goodwin M, Zapadinsky N, Elkayam U. The effect of valvular heart disease on maternal and fetal outcome of pregnancy. *J Am Coll Cardiol*. 2001;37:893–899; with permission.)

atrium, large left atrium (≥60 mL/m²), or congestive heart failure.[1] Rate control with beta blockers or digoxin should be used as an initial strategy, though many women will ultimately undergo electrical cardioversion (which is considered safe in pregnancy) due to ongoing symptoms, poor rate control, or hemodynamic instability.

Women who remain severely symptomatic despite adequate medical therapy and activity restriction may need to undergo mitral valve intervention during pregnancy. Percutaneous mitral balloon valvotomy (PMBV) can be safely performed during pregnancy and result in improved valve area and gradients.[11,22] Due to risk of ionizing radiation to the fetus, PMBV should be avoided during the first trimester, if possible, and performed by experienced operators. Surgical mitral valve replacement may be considered in women with refractory symptoms who are not candidates for PMBV but is associated with high rates of fetal mortality, estimated at 20% to 30%.[11,12]

Most women with MS can undergo a vaginal delivery with regional anesthesia, with preference for epidural placement.[23] An assisted second stage should be considered for women with moderate to severe stenosis. Cesarean delivery is reserved for obstetric indications and decompensated heart failure. Due to the hemodynamic shifts that occur postpartum, monitoring in a special care unit for at least 24 hours after delivery is recommended.

Careful preconception counseling of women with MS is critical in order to identify severity of stenosis, symptoms, and need for intervention before pregnancy. Similar to non-pregnant patients, the 2014 American Heart Association (AHA)/American College of Cardiology (ACC) Valvular Heart Disease Guidelines recommends PMBV, when feasible, in patients with severe symptomatic MS (Class I recommendation) before pregnancy. In order to avoid clinical decompensation and need for intervention during pregnancy. The AHA/ACC Guidelines also recommend PMBV in patients with severe MS who are asymptomatic (Class I recommendation). The decision to intervene in asymptomatic women before pregnancy should depend on valve area, exercise tolerance, and the presence of pulmonary hypertension, especially among women who are not candidates for PMBV.[6,23,24]

Aortic Stenosis

AS in pregnancy is most often caused by congenital bicuspid aortic valve and less commonly other congenital abnormalities or rheumatic heart disease.[24,25] Pregnancy is well tolerated in women with mild and moderate AS. Women with severe AS are at higher risk of developing cardiac complications, such as heart failure or atrial arrhythmias, however the risk of maternal mortality and need for aortic valve intervention during pregnancy is low. Women with congenital bicuspid valve or Marfan syndrome may have an associated aortopathy which further increases maternal risk and warrants additional monitoring before and during pregnancy. Pregnancy is contraindicated in women with bicuspid aortic valve when aortic dilation is >50 mm and in women with Marfan syndrome when aortic dilation is >45 mm.[6]

In a Canadian cohort of 39 women representing 49 pregnancies, cardiac complications, including heart failure or arrhythmias, were observed in 10% of women with severe AS. Only 1 woman required aortic valve intervention during pregnancy and no maternal deaths were reported.[25] Other series have reported that heart failure occurs in 3.8% to 44% of patients, with the highest rate observed in the smallest (n = 12) cohort.[19,26,27] Maternal complications are associated with severity of AS, especially when symptomatic, and maternal age >30 years.[26,27] Maternal mortality in contemporary cohorts and need for valvular intervention during pregnancy is low. Valve deterioration and need for aortic valve intervention may be higher in women with severe AS after pregnancy, although the causes for this are not well-understood.[25,26] Women with severe AS experience higher rates of preterm delivery, low birth weight, and fetal death.[19,26]

Management

Women who become symptomatic should be managed with activity restriction. Diuretics should be carefully used in women who develop pulmonary edema so as to avoid a sudden drop in preload. Women who remain symptomatic despite conservative management may need valvular intervention during pregnancy with a preference for percutaneous aortic balloon valvuloplasty if the valve anatomy is favorable and an experienced team is available. Percutaneous transcatheter aortic valve replacement for bicuspid severe AS has been successfully performed during pregnancy, and may be preferred over valvuloplasty if significant aortic regurgitation is present.[28] Women who develop severe symptoms early in pregnancy may consider pregnancy termination. Similar to patients with MS, vaginal delivery is the preferred mode of delivery with an assisted second stage for women with moderate to severe stenosis, though Cesarean delivery may be considered for patients with severe symptoms.[6,24] Regional anesthesia with an epidural is preferred for pain control but hemodynamics should be monitored closely to avoid a sudden drop in preload and systemic vascular resistance, which may poorly tolerated.

MITRAL REGURGITATION AND AORTIC REGURGITATION

The most common causes of mitral regurgitation (MR) during pregnancy are rheumatic heart disease and mitral valve prolapse. Patients with previously repaired (or unrepaired) AV septal defects may also have significant left-sided AV valve regurgitation. In contrast, aortic regurgitation (AR) is more commonly associated with congenital bicuspid aortic valve or aortopathy, and less commonly rheumatic heart disease. Both MR and AR are well tolerated during pregnancy, even if severe, due to the fall in systemic vascular resistance and blood pressure. Surgical intervention before pregnancy is reserved for women meeting routine indications for surgery, including severe symptomatic valve disease. Exercise testing before pregnancy can be considered to assess for exercise tolerance and symptoms.[29] Women who develop heart failure symptoms or left ventricular dysfunction can be treated with diuretics and vasodilators, such as hydralazine or nitrates, with care to avoid hypotension which can lead to placental hypoperfusion. Angiotensin-converting enzyme inhibitors and angiotensin receptor blockers are contraindicated during pregnancy.

PULMONIC STENOSIS

Pulmonic stenosis (PS) is most commonly a result of congenital valve disease but may also occur as a result of homograft calcification after a Ross procedure or prosthetic valve stenosis in patients with repaired tetralogy of Fallot. Mild and moderate PS are well tolerated during pregnancy. Severe PS is associated with high rates of hypertensive disorders, such as preeclampsia, preterm delivery, and thromboembolic complications.[30] Although severe PS may be well tolerated during pregnancy, some women may experience right ventricular heart failure or arrhythmias. As a result, women with severe PS, even if asymptomatic, should be considered for balloon valvuloplasty, surgical valvotomy, or percutaneous valve replacement before pregnancy.[31]

PULMONIC REGURGITATION

Pulmonic regurgitation (PR) may be secondary to prior tetralogy of Fallot repair, balloon valvuloplasty for isolated PS, or develop in patients with a prior right ventricle to pulmonary artery conduit. PR is generally well tolerated during pregnancy. Similar to the systemic vascular resistance, pulmonary vascular resistance also decreases during pregnancy. However, the increased plasma volume and CO associated with pregnancy can lead to right-sided heart failure symptoms in women with severe PR, especially in the presence of underlying right ventricular (RV) dysfunction, RV hypertrophy, or additional obstructive lesions such as branch pulmonary artery stenosis.[32,33] Right-sided heart failure can often be treated with diuretics and activity restriction. Valve intervention is rarely needed during pregnancy.[6] In women with severe PR before pregnancy who are symptomatic or have progressive RV dilatation or dysfunction, pulmonary valve replacement is recommended.[31]

TRICUSPID REGURGITATION

Isolated tricuspid regurgitation (TR) in young women is uncommon and, when present, occurs in the setting of Ebstein anomaly, rheumatic heart disease, or endocarditis. Patients with AV septal defects commonly have right-sided AV valve regurgitation. The hemodynamic changes of pregnancy are usually well tolerated in women with TR, even if severe. Ebstein anomaly is associated with atrial septal defect and Wolff-Parkinson-White syndrome. As a result, pregnancy may be associated with progressive cyanosis and/or arrhythmias in women at risk.[34] Ebstein anomaly is also associated with increased risk of preterm delivery.[35] Secondary TR can occur as a result of RV pressure or volume overload as a result of left-sided heart disease and pulmonary hypertension, cardiac conditions associated with significantly elevated maternal risk during pregnancy.

PROSTHETIC VALVES

Pregnancy is a prothrombotic state and is associated with an increased risk of valve thrombosis in women with prosthetic heart valves. Pregnant women with mechanical heart valves require careful anticoagulation management to prevent severe maternal morbidity while minimizing anticoagulation-related risk to the fetus. Although hypercoagulability risk increases throughout pregnancy and peaks in the immediate postpartum period, valve thrombosis frequently occurs in the first trimester and may be related to sub-therapeutic anticoagulation, underscoring the importance of preconception counseling.[36,37]

Anticoagulation

Warfarin is the standard of care for mechanical valves in non-pregnant patients to prevent thromboembolic complications. However,

warfarin crosses the placenta and is associated with an embryopathy, consisting of nasal hypoplasia, stippled epiphyses, and choanal atresia, when exposure occurs between 6 and 12 weeks of gestation.[37] Later exposure is associated with central nervous system abnormalities and intracranial hemorrhage. The most common fetal adverse even is miscarriage and fetal demise can occur at any gestational age.

Warfarin has a dose-dependent effect on fetal outcomes with the highest risk associated with daily warfarin doses >5 mg,[38] though lower risk with lower doses has not been demonstrated in all studies.[36] In a 2017 meta-analysis, the rate of livebirths among women taking ≤5 mg compared with >5 mg of warfarin daily was 83.6% versus 43.9%, respectively.[39] The rate of embryopathy/fetopathy was 2.3% with lower dose (≤5 mg) and 12.4% with higher dose (>5 mg) of warfarin. Women treated with low molecular weight heparin (LMWH) alone during pregnancy had the highest rate of livebirth at 92%.

LMWH does not cross the placenta and is therefore not associated with congenital malformations. Weight-based dosing is administered twice daily and cleared by the kidneys. Dose adjustment in response to peak anti-Xa levels is needed due to changes in renal clearance and volume of distribution over the course of pregnancy.[40] In contemporary studies, dose-adjusted LMWH is still associated with thromboembolic complication in 4% to 17% of pregnancies.[39,41,42]

Thromboembolic complications occur throughout pregnancy and may be related to sub-therapeutic anticoagulation during transition of anticoagulants, especially in the first trimester, or sub-therapeutic LMWH levels. Fixed dose LMWH is associated with significantly higher thromboembolic complications compared with dose-adjusted regimens.[43] The measurement of peak anti-Xa levels may not sufficiently assure adequate anticoagulation. Among pregnant women with peak anti-Xa levels within the recommended range of 0.8 to 1.2 U/mL, 57% had sub-therapeutic trough levels (<0.6 U/ml).[44] Low trough levels were still observed among women with peak anti-Xa levels at the upper range of 1.0 to 1.2 U/ml. Several small series have demonstrated favorable thromboembolic outcomes among women treated with close monitoring of both peak and trough anti-Xa levels, with peak levels targeted to 1 to 1.2 U/mL.[37]

Comparing Anticoagulation Strategies

Four anticoagulation strategies were compared in a meta-analysis of contemporary studies representing 800 pregnancies between 1974 and 2014.[42] Studies were excluded if fixed dose LMWH or unfractionated heparin (UFH) were used or if ball-in-cage valves were present in greater than 10% of reported pregnancies. Maternal risk was lowest in women using vitamin K antagonist (VKA) throughout pregnancy and 3-times-higher in women using alternative strategies, see **Table 2**. Maternal deaths were rare and adverse events were driven by systemic thromboembolism or valve thrombosis. Fetal risk was lowest in women using LMWH throughout pregnancy or LMWH plus VKA. Differences in fetal outcomes were driven by spontaneous abortions; congenital defects were uncommon. Women taking low-dose VKA throughout pregnancy had similar fetal outcomes compared with women taking LMWH or LMWH plus VKA. A similar meta-analysis (see **Table 2**) demonstrated that women treated with VKA throughout pregnancy had the lowest proportion of livebirths compared with women treated with LMWH (64.5% vs 92%) but had a lower risk of thromboembolic complications (2.7% vs 8.7).[39]

Management

Women with bioprosthetic and mechanical valves should be treated with a baby aspirin during the second and third trimesters. For women with mechanical valves, warfarin continued throughout pregnancy offers the lowest risk of maternal thromboembolic complications but carries a higher risk of miscarriage and embryopathy, as described previously. The 2014 ACC/AHA Valvular Heart Disease Guidelines and the 2018 ESC Pregnancy and Heart Disease Guidelines recommend continuing warfarin at doses ≤5 mg/d during the first trimester and transitioning to dose-adjusted LMWH or intravenous (IV) UFH when the daily dose is >5 mg/d, as summarized in **Table 3**.[6,45] Regardless of anticoagulant choice in the first trimester, treatment with warfarin is usually recommended in the 2nd and 3rd trimesters. Discontinuation of warfarin and starting IV UFH before planned vaginal delivery is recommended. Women who are therapeutically anticoagulated on warfarin and need to be delivered should undergo Cesarean delivery to minimize traumatic fetal hemorrhagic.

The AHA/ACC guidelines recommend targeting a peak anti-Xa level of 0.8 to 1.2 U/mL 4 to 6 hours after dosing for women treated with LMWH during pregnancy. Given the higher risk of thromboembolic complications in women with subtherapeutic anticoagulation, aiming for peak levels in the 1.0 to 1.2 U/mL range with trough levels greater than 0.6 U/mL may be reasonable, and is recommended in the 2018 ESC pregnancy and heart disease guidelines (see **Table 3**).[6] Because the safety profile of low-dose warfarin is based on a small number of studies and the risk of fetal loss is present throughout pregnancy, even at lower warfarin doses, some investigators advocate for using LMWH throughout pregnancy with

Table 2
Comparison of maternal and fetal risk with different anticoagulation strategies among women with mechanical valves

Anticoagulation Strategy	Steinberg et al[42]		D'Souza et al[39]	
	Maternal risk,[a] %	Fetal risk,[b] %	Maternal TE event,[c] %	Livebirths, %
VKA only	5	39	2.7	64.5
Low-dose VKA only	5	15		83.6
LMWH + VKA	16	16	8.3	89.5
UFH + VKA	16	34	6.1	72.4
LMWH only	15	14	8.7	92.0

Abbreviations: LMWH, low molecular weight heparin; TE, thromboembolic; UFH, unfractionated heparin; VKA, vitamin K antagonist.
[a] Maternal death, systemic TE, or valve failure resulting in heart failure, arrhythmia, or surgery.
[b] Spontaneous abortion, fetal death, or congenital defect.
[c] Valve thrombus or extravalvular TE event.
Data from D'Souza R, Ostro J, Shah PS, Silversides CK, Malinowski A, Murphy KE, Sermer M, Shehata N. Anticoagulation for pregnant women with mechanical heart valves: a systematic review and meta-analysis. *Eur Heart J.* 2017;38:1509–1516 and Steinberg ZL, Dominguez-Islas CP, Otto CM, Stout KK, Krieger EV. Maternal and Fetal Outcomes of Anticoagulation in Pregnant Women With Mechanical Heart Valves. *J Am Coll Cardiol.* 2017;69:2681–2691.

Table 3
Recommendations regarding anticoagulation strategy for mechanical valves during pregnancy

	1st Trimester	2nd and 3rd Trimesters	Peripartum
AHA/ACC guidelines[45]			
Warfarin dose ≤5 mg	Warfarin (IIa) or LMWH (IIb) or IV UFH (IIb)	Warfarin (I)	IV UFH (I)
Warfarin dose >5 mg	LMWH (IIa) or IV UFH (IIa)	Warfarin (I)	IV UFH (I)

- Aspirin is routinely recommended starting in 2nd trimester
- Target anti-Xa peak level: 0.8–1.2 U/ml 4–6 h post-dose (I)

	1st Trimester	2nd and 3rd Trimesters	Peripartum
ESC guidelines[6]			
Warfarin dose ≤5 mg	Warfarin (IIa) or LMWH (IIb) or IV UFH (IIb)	Warfarin (I)	IV UFH (I)
Warfarin dose >5 mg	Warfarin (IIb) or LMWH (IIa) or IV UFH (IIa)	Warfarin (IIa) or LMWH (IIb)	IV UFH (I)

- Aspirin is not routinely recommended
- Target anti-Xa peak level: 1.0–1.2 U/mL (mitral and right-sided valves) or 0.8–1.2 U/mL (aortic valves) 4–6 h post-dose (I). Target anti-Xa trough level: >0.6 U/mL (IIb)

Both LMWH and IV UFH refer to dose-adjusted rather than fixed dosing.
Abbreviations: AHA/ACC, American Heart Association/American College of Cardiology; IV UFH, intravenous unfractionated heparin; LMWH, low molecular weight heparin.
Data from Regitz-Zagrosek V, Roos-Hesselink JW, Bauersachs J, et al. 2018 ESC Guidelines for the management of cardiovascular diseases during pregnancy. *Eur Heart J.* 2018;39:3165–3241 and Nishimura RA, Otto CM, Bonow RO, et al. 2014 AHA/ACC Guideline for the Management of Patients With Valvular Heart Disease: A Report of the American College of Cardiology/American Heart Association Task Force on Practice Guidelines. J Am Coll Cardiol. 2014;63:e57–e185.

closely monitored anti-Xa levels.[46] Favorable clinical outcomes have been demonstrated in women treated with this strategy, but high levels of medication adherence and patient engagement are needed. This strategy may be desirable for women who are at otherwise low risk of thromboembolic complications (eg, mechanical valve in aortic position) or women who place higher value on avoiding potential fetal risk than maternal complications.

Valve thrombosis during pregnancy should be confirmed with transesophageal echocardiogram and treated first with heparin and, if needed, thrombolytic therapy for women with small thrombus and mild symptoms. Tissue-type plasminogen activator is associated with hemorrhagic complications but has been successfully used in pregnant women.[47]

Women presenting with large thrombus burden and more severe symptoms may require emergent surgery, which is associated with adverse maternal and fetal outcomes.

Choosing Prosthetic Valve Type Before Pregnancy

Mechanical heart valves offer superior hemodynamic profile and durability compared with bioprosthetic valves. Younger age at bioprosthetic valve implantation is associated with accelerated valve degeneration, which further shortens durability in women of reproductive age.[48] Preconception counseling regarding valve choice and implications for maternal and fetal risk in future pregnancies, especially for mechanical valves, is critically important and should be performed by a cardiologist familiar with treating pregnant patients with heart disease.

SUMMARY

Pregnancy in the setting of mild to moderate valvular heart disease is often well tolerated. Patients with severe mitral or severe symptomatic AS are at increased risk of severe maternal morbidity and mortality and pregnancy may be prohibitively high risk unless valve intervention is performed. Care by a multidisciplinary Pregnancy Heart Team consisting of MFM specialists and cardiologists can improve preconception counseling and coordinated pregnancy and postpartum care to minimize maternal and fetal complications.

CLINICS CARE POINTS

- Women with severe mitral stenosis and symptomatic severe aortic stenosis are at high risk of poor outcomes and should be evaluated for valvular intervention before conception.
- Mitral and aortic regurgitation are well tolerated during pregnancy.
- For women with mechanical valves, warfarin offers the lowest risk of maternal thromboembolic complications, whereas low molecular weight heparin offers the lowest fetal risk.
- Cardiac indications for Cesarean delivery include symptomatic heart failure and pulmonary hypertension.

ACKNOWLEDGMENTS

This study was supported by grants K12 HD085848 (Lewey) and R56 HL136730 (Levine) from the National Institutes of Health.

DISCLOSURE

The authors have nothing to disclose.

REFERENCES

1. ACOG practice bulletin No. 212: pregnancy and heart disease. Obstet Gynecol 2019;133:e320–56.
2. Petersen EE, Davis NL, Goodman D, et al. Vital Signs: pregnancy-related deaths, United States, 2011-2015, and strategies for prevention, 13 states, 2013-2017. MMWR Morb Mortal Wkly Rep 2019;68: 423–9.
3. Roos-Hesselink J, Baris L, Johnson M, et al. Pregnancy outcomes in women with cardiovascular disease: evolving trends over 10 years in the ESC Registry of Pregnancy and Cardiac disease (RO-PAC). Eur Heart J 2019;40:3848–55.
4. Siu SC, Sermer M, Colman JM, et al, Investigators on behalf of the CD in P (CARPREG). Prospective multicenter study of pregnancy outcomes in women with heart disease. Circulation 2001. Available at: https://www.ahajournals.org/doi/abs/10.1161/hc3001.093437.
5. Nanna M, Stergiopoulos K. Pregnancy complicated by valvular heart disease: an update. J Am Heart Assoc 2014;3:e000712.
6. Regitz-Zagrosek V, Roos-Hesselink JW, Bauersachs J, et al. 2018 ESC Guidelines for the management of cardiovascular diseases during pregnancy. Eur Heart J 2018;39:3165–241.
7. Sanghavi M, Rutherford JD. Cardiovascular physiology of pregnancy. Circulation 2014;130:1003–8.
8. Robson SC, Hunter S, Boys RJ, et al. Serial study of factors influencing changes in cardiac output during human pregnancy. Am J Physiol 1989;256:H1060–5.
9. Kamel H, Navi BB, Sriram N, et al. Risk of a thrombotic event after the 6-week postpartum period. N Engl J Med 2014;370:1307–15.
10. Mehta LS, Warnes CA, Bradley E, et al. American Heart Association Council on Clinical Cardiology; Council on Arteriosclerosis, Thrombosis and Vascular Biology; Council on Cardiovascular and Stroke Nursing; and Stroke Council. Cardiovascular Considerations in caring for pregnant patients: A Scientific Statement from the American Heart Association. Circulation 2020;141:e884–903.
11. de Souza JA, Martinez EE, Ambrose JA, et al. Percutaneous balloon mitral valvuloplasty in comparison with open mitral valve commissurotomy for mitral stenosis during pregnancy. J Am Coll Cardiol 2001;37:900–3.
12. John AS, Gurley F, Schaff HV, et al. Cardiopulmonary bypass during pregnancy. Ann Thorac Surg 2011; 91:1191–6.
13. Canobbio Mary M, Warnes Carole A, Aboulhosn J, et al. Management of pregnancy in patients with complex congenital heart disease: a scientific statement for healthcare professionals from the American Heart Association. Circulation 2017;135: e50–87.
14. Silversides CK, Grewal J, Mason J, et al. Pregnancy outcomes in women with heart disease: the CARPREG II study. J Am Coll Cardiol 2018; 71:2419–30.
15. Drenthen W, Boersma E, Balci A, et al. Predictors of pregnancy complications in women with congenital heart disease. Eur Heart J 2010;31: 2124–32.
16. Roos-Hesselink JW, Cornette J, Sliwa K, et al. Contraception and cardiovascular disease. Eur Heart J 2015;36:1728–34.
17. van Hagen IM, Thorne SA, Taha N, et al, ROPAC Investigators and EORP Team. Pregnancy outcomes in women with rheumatic mitral valve disease: results from the Registry of pregnancy and cardiac disease. Circulation 2018;137:806–16.
18. Silversides CK, Colman JM, Sermer M, et al. Cardiac risk in pregnant women with rheumatic mitral stenosis. Am J Cardiol 2003;91:1382–5.
19. Hameed A, Karaalp IS, Tummala PP, et al. The effect of valvular heart disease on maternal and fetal outcome of pregnancy. J Am Coll Cardiol 2001;37: 893–9.
20. Leśniak-Sobelga A, Tracz W, KostKiewicz M, et al. Clinical and echocardiographic assessment of pregnant women with valvular heart diseases– maternal and fetal outcome. Int J Cardiol 2004;94: 15–23.
21. al Kasab SM, Sabag T, al Zaibag M, et al. Beta-adrenergic receptor blockade in the management of pregnant women with mitral stenosis. Am J Obstet Gynecol 1990;163:37–40.

22. Joshi HS, Deshmukh JK, Prajapati JS, et al. Study of effectiveness and safety of percutaneous balloon mitral valvulotomy for treatment of pregnant patients with severe mitral stenosis. J Clin Diagn Res 2015;9: OC14–7.

23. Elkayam U, Goland S, Pieper PG, et al. High-risk cardiac disease in pregnancy. J Am Coll Cardiol 2016;68:396–410.

24. Elkayam U, Bitar F. Valvular heart disease and pregnancy: Part I: native valves. J Am Coll Cardiol 2005; 46:223–30.

25. Silversides CK, Colman JM, Sermer M, et al. Early and intermediate-term outcomes of pregnancy with congenital aortic stenosis. Am J Cardiol 2003;91: 1386–9.

26. Yap S-C, Drenthen W, Pieper PG, et al, ZAHARA Investigators. Risk of complications during pregnancy in women with congenital aortic stenosis. Int J Cardiol 2008;126:240–6.

27. Orwat S, Diller G-P, van Hagen IM, et al. Risk of pregnancy in moderate and severe aortic stenosis. J Am Coll Cardiol 2016;68:1727–37.

28. Hodson R, Kirker E, Swanson J, et al. Transcatheter aortic valve replacement during pregnancy. Circ Cardiovasc Interv 2016;9:e004006.

29. Nishimura RA, Otto CM, Bonow RO, et al. 2014 AHA/ACC Guideline for the Management of Patients With Valvular Heart Disease: A Report of the American College of Cardiology/American Heart Association Task Force on Practice Guidelines. J Am Coll Cardiol 2014;63:e57–e185.

30. Drenthen W, Pieper PG, Roos-Hesselink JW, et al, ZAHARA Investigators. Non-cardiac complications during pregnancy in women with isolated congenital pulmonary valvar stenosis. Heart 2006;92:1838–43.

31. Stout KK, Daniels CJ, Aboulhosn JA, et al. 2018 AHA/ACC guideline for the management of adults with congenital heart disease: a Report of the American College of Cardiology/American Heart Association Task Force on clinical Practice guidelines. Circulation 2019;139:e698–800.

32. Greutmann M, Von Klemperer K, Brooks R, et al. Pregnancy outcome in women with congenital heart disease and residual haemodynamic lesions of the right ventricular outflow tract. Eur Heart J 2010;31: 1764–70.

33. Khairy P, Ouyang DW, Fernandes SM, et al. Pregnancy outcomes in women with congenital heart disease. Circulation 2006;113:517–24.

34. Connolly HM, Warnes CA. Ebstein's anomaly: outcome of pregnancy. J Am Coll Cardiol 1994;23: 1194–8.

35. Lima F, Nie L, Yang J, et al. Postpartum cardiovascular outcomes among women with heart disease from A Nationwide study. Am J Cardiol 2019;123:2006–14.

36. van Hagen IM, Roos-Hesselink JW, Ruys TPE, et al, ROPAC Investigators and the EURObservational Research Programme (EORP) Team*. Pregnancy in women with a mechanical heart valve: data of the European Society of Cardiology Registry of Pregnancy and Cardiac Disease (ROPAC). Circulation 2015;132:132–42.

37. Alshawabkeh L, Economy KE, Valente AM. Anticoagulation during pregnancy. J Am Coll Cardiol 2016; 68:1804–13.

38. Vitale N, De Feo M, De Santo LS, et al. Dose-dependent fetal complications of warfarin in pregnant women with mechanical heart valves. J Am Coll Cardiol 1999;33:1637–41.

39. D'Souza R, Ostro J, Shah PS, et al. Anticoagulation for pregnant women with mechanical heart valves: a systematic review and meta-analysis. Eur Heart J 2017;38:1509–16.

40. Quinn J, Von Klemperer K, Brooks R, et al. Use of high intensity adjusted dose low molecular weight heparin in women with mechanical heart valves during pregnancy: a single-center experience. Haematologica 2009;94:1608–12.

41. Bhagra CJ, D'Souza R, Silversides CK. Valvular heart disease and pregnancy part II: management of prosthetic valves. Heart 2017;103: 244–52.

42. Steinberg ZL, Dominguez-Islas CP, Otto CM, et al. Maternal and fetal outcomes of anticoagulation in pregnant women with mechanical heart valves. J Am Coll Cardiol 2017;69:2681–91.

43. Oran B, Lee-Parritz A, Ansell J. Low molecular weight heparin for the prophylaxis of thromboembolism in women with prosthetic mechanical heart valves during pregnancy. Thromb Haemost 2004; 92:747–51.

44. Goland S, Schwartzenberg S, Fan J, et al. Monitoring of anti-Xa in pregnant patients with mechanical prosthetic valves receiving low-molecular-weight heparin: peak or trough levels? J Cardiovasc Pharmacol Ther 2014;19:451–6.

45. Nishimura RA, Otto CM, Bonow RO, et al. 2014 AHA/ACC guideline for the management of patients with valvular heart disease: a Report of the American College of Cardiology/American Heart Association Task Force on Practice guidelines. J Am Coll Cardiol 2014;63:e57–185.

46. Elkayam U. Anticoagulation therapy for pregnant women with mechanical prosthetic heart valves: how to improve safety? J Am Coll Cardiol 2017;69: 2692–5.

47. Özkan M, Çakal B, Karakoyun S, et al. Thrombolytic therapy for the treatment of prosthetic heart valve thrombosis in pregnancy with low-dose, slow infusion of tissue-type plasminogen activator. Circulation 2013;128:532–40.

48. Pibarot P, Dumesnil JG. Prosthetic heart valves: selection of the optimal prosthesis and long-term management. Circulation 2009;119:1034–48.

Delivering Coordinated Cardio-Obstetric Care from Preconception through Postpartum

Anna C. O'Kelly, MD, MPhil[a], Nandita Scott, MD[b], Doreen DeFaria Yeh, MD[b],*

KEYWORDS

- Cardio-obstetrics • Coordinated care • Maternal mortality • Congenital heart disease
- Cardiovascular disease

KEY POINTS

- Cardiovascular disease is a leading cause of maternal mortality globally and in the United States.
- A cardio-obstetrics team is a multidisciplinary, collaborative team that cares for women from the preconception through postpartum periods and is composed of cardiologists with training in cardio-obstetrics and adult congenital heart disease, maternal and fetal medicine specialists, anesthesiologists, and allied health care professionals.
- There are limited guidelines to standardize how cardio-obstetrics care is provided, and more work needs to be done.
- Cardio-obstetrics education needs to be better integrated in general cardiology training programs.

INTRODUCTION

Cardiovascular disease (CV) is a leading cause of maternal mortality globally.[1–4] It affects 1% to 4% of pregnancies in the United States[1–4] and is the most common cause of pregnancy-related mortality.[1–6] Although complications from congenital heart disease (CHD) account for some of this morbidity and mortality, acquired cardiovascular disease including cardiomyopathy and heart failure, ischemic heart disease, hypertensive disorders of pregnancy, arrhythmia, and stroke accounts for a much larger share.[1,3,4] Cardiovascular complications during pregnancy are associated with future CV disease.[7–10] Pregnancy is thus considered a vascular and hemodynamic "stress test" that allows for early identification of women who may be at increased future CV risk.

CV disease during pregnancy is an increasing cause of maternal mortality in the United States.[1–6] This growth is driven by many factors, including advances in the treatment of CHD, increasing comorbidities such as obesity and diabetes during pregnancy, advanced maternal age, and importantly inadequate access to health care.[1,11–14] The risk of CV complications during pregnancy disproportionately affects racial minorities,[2,5] and pregnancy-related mortality is 3 to 4 times higher in black than in white women.[5]

Developing a comprehensive cardio-obstetrics team is critical to optimizing preconception maternal health, manage CV complications as

a Department of Medicine, Massachusetts General Hospital and Harvard Medical School, Yawkey 5700, 55 Fruit Street, Boston, MA 02114, USA; b Division of Cardiology, Cardiovascular Disease and Pregnancy Program, Massachusetts General Hospital and Harvard Medical School, Yawkey 5700, 55 Fruit Street, Boston, MA 02114, USA
* Corresponding author. Cardiology Division, Massachusetts General Hospital, Yawkey 5700, 55 Fruit Street, Boston, MA 02114.
E-mail address: ddefariayeh@mgh.harvard.edu

Cardiol Clin 39 (2021) 163–173
https://doi.org/10.1016/j.ccl.2020.09.012

they arise during pregnancy, and ensure post-partum CV risk factors are addressed. The cardio-obstetrics team is a collaborative, multidisciplinary team composed of obstetricians-gynecologists and maternal and fetal medicine (MFM) specialists, cardiologists with subspecialty training and experience in cardio-obstetrics and adult congenital heart disease, anesthesiologists, primary care physicians, midlevel and allied health professionals, and may also include neonatologists and geneticists and is increasingly important in providing wraparound care for women at risk of CV complications peripartum.[1,11] This collaborative approach to maternal health is supported by both the American Heart Association and the American College of Obstetricians and Gynecologists (ACOG).[15]

This paper outlines the importance of coordinated preconception through postpartum care. It highlights the potential role of such care in mitigating CV risk factors and addressing disparities in CV disease distribution. It also addresses the role of cardiology fellowship programs in educating trainees about the field of cardio-obstetrics and how coordinated efforts between obstetrics and cardiology departments can create collaborative and multifaceted cardio-obstetrics programs.

PRECONCEPTION

The preconception period is an important window to optimize maternal health before pregnancy.[1,16–18] For women who plan their pregnancy and seek preconception care, preconception counseling can occur during an appointment with a primary care provider or obstetrician. For women with known congenital or acquired CV disease or who are at significant risk of CV complications during pregnancy, preconception counseling should be performed by the cardio-obstetrics team, especially a cardiologist with subspecialty expertise in CHD or cardio-obstetrics for careful evaluation and risk stratification.[18–20] Because almost half of pregnancies may be unplanned and unintended, preconception counseling should take place as part of routine evaluation of women of childbearing age in the primary care setting or cardiology office.[16,18] Unfortunately only half of reproductive age women receive counseling to address risks of future pregnancies and birth outcomes. The One Key Question initiative recommends providers caring for women of childbearing age ask "Would you like to become pregnant in the next year?" with the intention to identify women who may become pregnant and begin a conversation about their health and pregnancy risks.[21] For

many women, their initial pregnancy visit—either preconception or shortly after conception—may be the first time they have recently engaged with the health care system, and it can be a vital opportunity for welcoming them in a nonjudgmental and supportive way so as to encourage ongoing care. Regardless of whether pregnancies are planned or not, preconception care is a vital opportunity to discuss modifiable maternal risk factors including weight loss, blood pressure and diabetes management, screening for and treatment of any chronic conditions, and assessment of vaccination status.[3,16,18,20,22]

The preconception period is also an important opportunity to identify women who may be at higher risk of CV complications and refer them to appropriate subspecialty providers. Careful history-taking, specifically regarding any prior cardiac conditions or procedures and symptoms of exercise intolerance, is essential. A thorough physical examination should focus on assessing for cardiac abnormalities. Although soft systolic ejection murmurs are seen in greater than 90% of pregnant women,[23] any diastolic or loud murmurs (grade 3 or greater) are abnormal and should be further evaluated with echocardiography.[20,24] When in doubt, referral to a cardiologist with expertise in cardio-obstetrics is prudent.

For women at elevated CV risk, collaborative care between the members of the cardio-obstetrics team is essential. Cardiologists with training and expertise in cardio-obstetrics should play a primary role in risk stratification.[1,19,20,25,26] Numerous risk-stratification models exist and incorporate multiple factors including prior cardiac history and interventions, lesion-type if relevant, baseline functional status, and medication use.[20,27,28] Of these, the modified World Health Organization (WHO) model is endorsed by expert consensus.[20,29,30] Women with known cardiac lesions may require a baseline echocardiogram, electrocardiogram, and exercise stress test to assess functional status and appropriately risk stratify.[1,18,20,31]

In addition to these factors, there are certain maternal congenital and cardiac diseases in which pregnancy is contraindicated due to prohibitive risk. These include pulmonary artery hypertension, severe systemic ventricular dysfunction including from prior peripartum cardiomyopathy, severe left-sided obstructive disease, Eisenmenger syndrome, severe aortic dilatation particularly with Marfan syndrome, and poorly tolerated complex CHD.[19,20,32] For these especially high-risk lesions, early pregnancy termination is advised.[19,20,31]

Preconception counseling should also include discussion about medication safety both in pregnancy and post partum.[11,19,20,31] This includes the cessation of known teratogenic medications and transition to safer alternatives, as well as the initiation of beneficial medication such as prenatal vitamins and daily aspirin for women at risk of preeclampsia.[1,20,33]

For women with CHD, genetic testing and fetal risk of transmission should also be discussed.[18,19,31] The risk of transmission varies widely and by lesion-type, from 3% to 50%,[31,34] although it is considerably higher than the 0.3% to 1.2% risk of CHD in the general population.[34]

In emphasizing the importance of wraparound care, preconception counseling should also include anticipatory guidance about ongoing care throughout pregnancy and some of the postpartum changes women may experience.[35] This can include counseling on adjustments to early motherhood and challenges with self-care, as well as the importance of medication compliance and ongoing follow-up to mitigate CV risk. In particular, counseling on the importance of exercise and the prevention of excessive weight gain during and following pregnancy should begin in the prenatal period. Despite the known associations of excessive weight gain with both pregnancy complications and future CV disease,[36-40] only approximately 30% to 40% of women in the prenatal period receive counseling about weight management.[41-43] Furthermore, moderate physical activity during pregnancy reduces the risk of hypertensive disorders including preeclampsia[44-46] and gestational diabetes.[47-50]

PREGNANCY AND PERIPARTUM

Just as coordinated care is important in risk-stratifying and optimizing health before pregnancy, so too is coordinated care throughout pregnancy. Coordinated visits with cardiologists, MFM specialists, and allied health professionals allows for close monitoring and treatment of any CV complications that occur. Although there are no clear guidelines for follow-up frequency during pregnancy,[1] expert opinion is that women should meet at least once per trimester with their cardiologist and MFM.[31,51] A formalized delivery plan should be developed by the end of the second trimester or beginning of the third. Some models of cardio-obstetrics care include joint visits with both cardiologist and MFM specialist,[52] whereas others include monthly integrated meetings between MFM specialists and cardiologists to ensure ongoing communication and updated care.[51] At the authors' institution they hold monthly multidisciplinary cardio-obstetric meetings between MFM specialists, cardiologists with expertise in cardio-

obstetrics and CHD, anesthesiologists, and nurses to discuss all shared patients, detail plans for their upcoming deliveries, and provide documentation in the medical record for all providers to review when a women presents in labor (**Fig. 1**).

There are no guidelines for the frequency of imaging monitoring throughout pregnancy either, and often it is lesion and patient specific. Expert consensus recommends serial echocardiography be performed approximately every trimester for women with valvular disease and cardiomyopathy and more frequently in severe disease or if symptoms develop.[20,53-56] ACOG recommends ongoing surveillance every 4 to 6 weeks throughout pregnancy for women with congenital aortopathy including Marfan syndrome and bicuspid aortic valve.[1]

Delivery Planning

For women at high risk of CV events during delivery, decisions regarding timing, location, and mode of delivery should be reached early in pregnancy and with input from the patient's multidisciplinary cardio-obstetrics team. This should ideally occur no later than the end of the second or early in the third trimester of pregnancy.[57-59] Contingencies for possible obstetric and cardiac emergencies should be part of the preparation for labor and delivery.[59]

The patient's specific CV disease, whether congenital or acquired, her functional status, and risk of cardiac event should be primary factors in guiding discussions about delivery.[3,18,31] High-risk patients should be delivered at a tertiary care center.[19,20,31] Women who are especially high risk, such as those with pulmonary hypertension, may need to be hospitalized late in their second or early in their third trimester and closely monitored until delivery.[60] In general, planned vaginal delivery is preferred over cesarean delivery,[20,57,61,62] and cesarean delivery is generally only indicated by obstetric need.[20,57,60] In the absence of contraindications or spontaneous onset of labor, women with CV disease may be induced between 39 and 40 weeks gestation, although specific guidance should be directed by the cardio-obstetrics team.[1] Any medication changes indicated before delivery, including changes in anticoagulation, should also be discussed early in the pregnancy course.[1] Continuous pulse oximetry throughout delivery is generally advised, and invasive hemodynamic monitoring is very rarely indicated.[20,60] Continuous telemetry during delivery is generally not warranted given that most arrhythmias peripartum are both benign and rare,[63,64] though are more

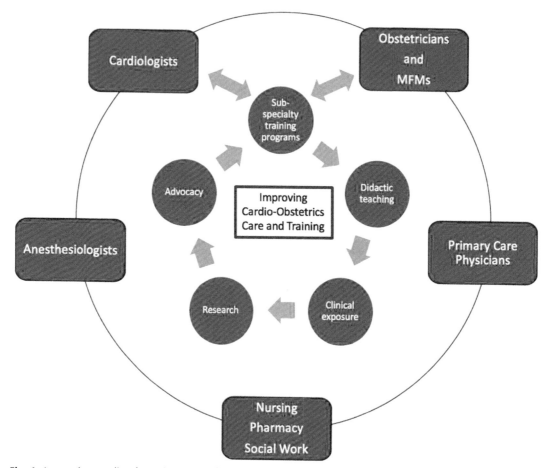

Fig. 1. Improving cardio-obstetrics care and training.

common in women with known arrhythmia before pregnancy.[65,66] In women with known arrhythmia or at risk of malignant arrhythmia including ventricular tachycardia, continuous telemetry during delivery may be considered and may require modifications to nursing staffing.[67–69]

With appropriate planning and specialist input, most women with CV disease have uncomplicated deliveries. It is estimated that only 1% to 3% of pregnancies in the United States require critical care management at the time of delivery.[58] Hemorrhage and hypertension are the most common reasons for intensive care unit admission peripartum, and 20% to 30% of patients have a nonobstetrical indication for admission.[58] When possible, it is best to decide on the need for intensive care before delivery.[58]

If pregnant women present hemodynamically unstable or in cardiogenic shock, urgent decision-making regarding management and delivery are essential.[20,70–72] This should be driven by the cardio-obstetrics team, with additional input from an advanced heart failure team,

interventional cardiology or cardiac surgery, intensivists, and neonatologists when needed.[20,70,72] Women may require urgent vasopressor support and rapid evaluation for advanced mechanical circulatory support,[20,70,71] and emergent delivery may be required regardless of gestational age.[20,69–71,73] If hospitals do not have on-call advanced heart failure or cardiac interventional/surgical resources, collaboration with tertiary centers is critical to ensure rapid transfer of care is facilitated in these time-sensitive situations.

POSTPARTUM

The postpartum period, which is generally considered to extend up to 1 year after delivery, allows not only for monitoring of postpartum complications but also for interventions to reduce future obstetric and CV risk.[74] For this reason, the postpartum period is often considered the "fourth trimester."[35] Importantly, women with known cardiac disease and CV complications of pregnancy require lifelong cardiac care.

The immediate postpartum period should be focused on ensuring hemodynamic safety before discharge from the hospital. With the significant hemodynamic shifts of delivery, women are at risk of heart failure and pulmonary edema, arrhythmia, stroke, acute coronary syndrome, aortic dissection, and death.[1,18,27,60,75–78] This is especially true for women with congenital or acquired CV disease.[4,11] Contraception for those desiring it should be discussed before discharge from the hospital.[1,11,35,79]

Although close postpartum monitoring after discharge is important, there are no guidelines to standardize the follow-up schedule. ACOG generally recommends initial follow-up with their obstetrician within approximately 3 weeks after delivery and a comprehensive postpartum visit within the first 12 weeks.[35] The WHO recommends follow-up at 3 days, 1 to 2 weeks, and 6 weeks post partum.[35,80]

Women with congenital or acquired CV disease should be followed more closely. ACOG recommends follow-up with a cardiologist or primary care provider within 7 to 14 days of delivery.[1] For women with hypertensive disorders of pregnancy, ACOG recommends a blood pressure check within 7 to 10 days after delivery and within 72 hours after delivery if severe hypertension.[35,81] Although in-person visits are ideal, new mothers may face challenges in coordinating numerous appointments both for themselves and their infants. At the authors' institution, they coordinate postpartum visits with pediatric visits when able. To reduce visit burden, these initial visits may be performed virtually in some circumstances or with visiting nurses. Follow-up visits are tracked and promptly rescheduled if missed or canceled, to support continued cardiac care. A subsequent 3-month follow-up visit to assess CV risk modification is advised.[1]

Cardiovascular risk factor modification in the postpartum period is especially important given the increase risk for future CV disease,[1,35,82,83] and any modifiable CV risk factors should be aggressively managed.[1,35,82,83] Both chronic hypertension and excessive weight gain during and following pregnancy mediate future CV disease.[39,40] Furthermore, women should be counseled that obstetric history is increasingly recognized as an integral part of their CV history[10,19,20,84] and that expert guidelines now include CV complications during pregnancy as disease-modifying factors that influence CV disease prevention strategies.[10,84] Collaboration between cardiologists and primary care physicians is essential.

Despite these recommendations, the postpartum period remains a high-risk period for women, and more than half of pregnancy-related deaths occur during this period.[1,3,35,85] Although the event rate of CV complications is fairly low (6%–12%),[86,87] their potential repercussions are devastating.[18,27,60,75–77] This is also a high-risk period for women to fall through the cracks of a fragmented health care system.[76] During the postpartum period, women are often transitioning from inpatient to outpatient care and out of the obstetrics space and into the primary care setting.[35,88] Furthermore, for numerous personal, logistical and systems-level reasons, women are frequently unable to seek care as recommended. Despite advised follow-up within the first 3 weeks, many women do not have first contact with their provider until 4 to 6 weeks post partum and are frequently without accessible guidance or support in the intervening weeks.[35] In addition, 40% of US women do not attend any postpartum follow-up appointments.[35] This is especially true of minority and socioeconomically disadvantaged women, which may contribute to disparities in CV risk factor management and disease burden.[35] Inconsistent health care insurance is one of the primary barriers to adequate continuity of care,[89,90] and many women in the United States lose their insurance after 42 days following delivery.[1] This is especially problematic for the disproportionate number of racial minorities who have CV complications during pregnancy and insecure health insurance.[3,5,91,92] Increasingly, virtual visits prove to be a helpful means of addressing challenges with facilitating both prenatal and postpartum care.[93–95] It is critical that women with known CV disease and CV complications of pregnancy are counseled early and often regarding the importance of lifelong cardiac care.

It is unclear how to best overcome these obstacles and provide appropriately focused, continuous postpartum care for women with CV disease.[96–98] Although specialty clinics can play an important role in the postpartum period,[96,97] relying on such clinics may be unrealistic for all women.[98] The postpartum period thus presents an especially important time for coordinated care between primary care physicians, cardiologists, and allied health professionals in ensuring that women's CV risk factors are appropriately addressed.

CARDIO-OBSTETRICS TEAM: WHAT HAS BEEN ACHIEVED AND WHAT REMAINS TO BE ACHIEVED

Delivering coordinated comprehensive multidisciplinary cardio-obstetric care from preconception through postpartum is critical in optimizing immediate and long-term maternal health. Despite the growing recognition of the relationship between peripartum CV complications and future CV risk, many physicians—including cardiologists—are insufficiently aware of this relationship and fail to include obstetric history in their assessment of CV risk or screen for future pregnancy.[12,99,100] Dedicated cardio-obstetrics teams can help to raise awareness about these issues and guide care in the dynamic period following pregnancy.

Creating a dedicated cardio-obstetrics team has many challenges. It requires longitudinal commitment from multiple specialists, and allied health care professionals, as well as commitment from institutional leadership. Often these teams develop organically, and there is no standard of care to guide how these teams should form, who should be included, when they should meet, and how they should best complement each other's roles. Many academic cardiology divisions,

however, now have focused heart centers for women (HCW) and/or adult CHD programs and these potentially offer a physical home for collaboration.[12]

As the cardio-obstetrics team plays an increasingly central role in caring for women with CV disease from preconception to postpartum and beyond, cardiologists need to be better trained in cardio-obstetrics. Most HCW have faculty who can support research in women's CV disease and cardio-obstetrics, but formal training and educational guidelines for CV trainees do not yet exist.[99,101,102] At the Massachusetts General Hospital a multipart didactic series has been implemented for general cardiology fellows that is offered throughout the academic year, in addition to required Women's Heart Health and adult CHD clinical rotations including peripartum management. In 2013 the authors' cardio-obstetrics program began a full-day Cardiovascular Disease and Pregnancy educational course for a

---

Box 1
Key questions that remain

Preconception

  How early should preconception counseling begin?

  How should those without health insurance best receive preconception counseling?

  What is the best preconception risk stratification test?

  How do we improve rates of preconception counseling and risk stratification, particularly among cardiologists?

Pregnancy and peripartum

  How often should a cardio-obstetrics team meet as a group, with patients? How can "visit burnout" best be prevented? When are virtual visits safe and appropriate?

  How frequently should echocardiography be performed throughout pregnancy?

Postpartum

  How to best predict who will require postpartum monitoring in the intensive care unit (ICU)?

  How can we facilitate keeping women in CV care long term?

  How should postpartum CV care best be provided for women with limited or no health insurance?

  What is the relative role of primary care physicians versus subspecialists in providing ongoing postpartum follow-up?

Cardio-Obstetrics teams: what we have achieved and what remains to be achieved

  How should cardio-obstetrics teams best collaborate? Is shared physical space important?

  How can we expand education content for trainees? How should exposure to and focused clinical training in cardio-obstetrics best be integrated in general cardiology fellowship programs?

  What role can cardiologists play in advocating for health policies to promote CV follow-up after pregnancy?

  How can cardiology and obstetrics professional societies best create joint cardio-obstetrics guidelines?

  How do cardiologists and obstetricians address the marked disparities that exist in maternal outcomes?

multidisciplinary audience including cardiology, obstetrics, and anesthesiology and included both trainees and practicing physicians and allied health providers. The University of Pennsylvania CV disease fellowship program has developed a focused woMen's CardiovAsCular HeAlth curriculum to facilitate formal training in identifying sex differences in the diagnosis and treatment of CV disease.[103] Standard educational requirements across all CV fellowship training programs is needed. By integrating more cardio-obstetrics experiences into general cardiology fellowship programs and offering dedicated subspecialty programs and training in the field, the next generation of general cardiologists can be better equipped with the knowledge to improve maternal mortality and address disparities in maternal and CV health.

There are additional systems-level changes that would further bolster these efforts. Government policies to support paid parental leave would potentially help women attend their postpartum medical appointments, and extending prenatal and postpartum health insurance would lessen the financial cost to do so.[35] Furthermore, additional data about CV disease during pregnancy would help develop guidelines and standards of care. One such solution is the Heart Outcomes in Pregnancy: Expectations for Mom and Baby Registry, which is a multicenter, multidisciplinary collaborative initiative to gather data about pregnant mothers with CV disease in the United States.[91] Such a coordinated initiative will catalyze the development of best practices and guidelines. Guidelines should be jointly developed and endorsed by expert groups in both obstetrics and cardiology.[15,99] Current guidelines are developed by either obstetric[1] or CV societies.[19,20,31] Joint efforts would both strengthen recommendations for caring for women during this critical time and further galvanize collaboration[99] (**Box 1**).

SUMMARY

Coordinated preconception through postpartum cardio-obstetrics care is necessary to optimize both maternal and fetal health. Maternal mortality in the United States is increasing, largely driven by increasing CV disease burden during pregnancy, and needs to be addressed emergently. Both for women with congenital and acquired heart disease, CV complications during pregnancy are associated with increased future risk of CV disease. Comprehensive cardio-obstetrics care is a powerful way of ensuring that women's CV risks before and during pregnancy are appropriately identified and treated and that they remain engaged in CV care long term to prevent future CV complications.

CLINICS CARE POINTS

- Preconception counseling is critical for all women with pre-existing structural or congenital heart disease, hypertension and ischemic heart disease.
- Patients with known or previously repaired congenital heart disease should be referred to adult congenital heart disease specialists for preconception and peripartum evaluation and management.
- Case review and multidisciplinary discussion of all pregnant women at high risk of cardiovascular complication should conducted regularly.

DISCLOSURE

None.

REFERENCES

1. Hollier L. ACOG practice bulletin No. 212: pregnancy and heart disease. Obstet Gynecol 2019; 133(5):e320–56.
2. Pregnancy mortality surveillance system | Maternal and infant health | CDC. 2020. Available at: https://www.cdc.gov/reproductivehealth/maternal-mortality/pregnancy-mortality-surveillance-system.htm. Accessed July 18, 2020.
3. Hameed AB, Lawton ES, McCain CL, et al. Pregnancy-related cardiovascular deaths in California: beyond peripartum cardiomyopathy. Am J Obstet Gynecol 2015;213(3):379.e1-10.
4. Briller J, Koch AR, Geller SE. Maternal cardiovascular mortality in Illinois, 2002-2011. Obstet Gynecol 2017;129(5):819-26.
5. Creanga AA, Syverson C, Seed K, et al. Pregnancy-related mortality in the United States, 2011–2013. Obstet Gynecol 2017;130(2):366–73.
6. MacDorman MF, Declercq E, Cabral H, et al. Is the United States maternal mortality rate increasing? Disentangling trends from measurement issues short title: U.S. Maternal mortality trends. Obstet Gynecol 2016;128(3):447–55.
7. Grandi SM, Filion KB, Yoon S, et al. Cardiovascular disease-related morbidity and mortality in women with a history of pregnancy complications: systematic review and meta-analysis. Circulation 2019; 139(8):1069–79.
8. Wu P, Gulati M, Kwok CS, et al. Preterm delivery and future risk of maternal cardiovascular disease: a systematic review and meta-analysis. J Am Heart Assoc 2018;7(2). https://doi.org/10.1161/JAHA.117.007809.

9. Gulati MM. Improving the cardiovascular health of women in the Nation: moving beyond the bikini boundaries. Circulation 2017;135(6):495–8.

10. Arnett Donna K, Blumenthal Roger S, Albert Michelle A, et al. 2019 ACC/AHA guideline on the primary prevention of cardiovascular disease: executive summary: a report of the American College of Cardiology/American Heart Association Task Force on clinical practice guidelines. Circulation 2019;140(11):e563–95.

11. Mehta Laxmi S, Warnes Carole A, Bradley Elisa, et al. Cardiovascular considerations in caring for pregnant patients: a scientific statement from the American Heart Association. Circulation 2020; 141(23):e884–903.

12. Lundberg Gina P, Mehta Laxmi S, Sanghani Rupa M, et al. Heart centers for women. Circulation 2018;138(11):1155–65.

13. Elkayam U, Goland S, Pieper PG, et al. High-risk cardiac disease in pregnancy: part I. J Am Coll Cardiol 2016;68(4):396–410.

14. Shapero KS, Desai NR, Elder RW, et al. Cardio-obstetrics: recognizing and managing cardiovascular complications of pregnancy. Cleve Clin J Med 2020;87(1):43–52.

15. Brown HL, Warner JJ, Gianos E, et al. Promoting risk identification and reduction of cardiovascular disease in women through collaboration with obstetricians and gynecologists: a presidential advisory from the American Heart Association and the American College of Obstetricians and Gynecologists. Circulation 2018;137(24). https://doi.org/10.1161/CIR.0000000000000582.

16. Farahi N, Zolotor A. Recommendations for preconception counseling and care. Am Fam Physician 2013;88(8):499–506.

17. Harville EW, Viikari JSA, Raitakari OT. Preconception cardiovascular risk factors and pregnancy outcome. Epidemiology 2011;22(5):724–30.

18. Clapp MA, Bernstein SN. Preconception counseling for women with cardiac disease. Curr Treat Options Cardiovasc Med 2017;19(9):67.

19. Stout KK, Daniels CJ, Aboulhosn JA, et al. 2018 AHA/ACC guideline for the management of adults with congenital heart disease: executive summary. J Am Coll Cardiol 2019;73(12):1494–563.

20. Regitz - Zagrosek V, Roos - Hesselink JW, Bauersachs J, et al. 2018 ESC Guidelines for the management of cardiovascular diseases during pregnancy. Eur Heart J 2018;39(34):3165–241.

21. Allen D, Hunter MS, Wood S, et al. One Key Question®: first things first in reproductive health. Matern Child Health J 2017;21(3):387–92.

22. Harrison CL, Brown WJ, Hayman M, et al. The role of physical activity in preconception, pregnancy and postpartum health. Semin Reprod Med 2016; 34(2):e28–37.

23. Cutforth R, MacDonald CB. Heart sounds and murmurs in pregnancy. Am Heart J 1966;71(6):741–7.

24. Stout KK, Otto CM. Pregnancy in women with valvular heart disease. Heart 2007;93(5):552–8.

25. Nanna M, Stergiopoulos K. Pregnancy complicated by valvular heart disease: an update. J Am Heart Assoc 2014;3(3). https://doi.org/10.1161/JAHA.113.000712.

26. Nishimura RA, Otto CM, Bonow RO, et al. 2014 AHA/ACC guideline for the management of patients with valvular heart disease: executive summary: a report of the American College of Cardiology/American Heart Association Task Force on practice guidelines. J Am Coll Cardiol 2014; 63(22):2438–88.

27. Siu SC, Sermer M, Colman JM, et al. Prospective multicenter study of pregnancy outcomes in women with heart disease. Circulation 2001; 104(5):515–21.

28. Drenthen W, Boersma E, Balci A, et al. Predictors of pregnancy complications in women with congenital heart disease. Eur Heart J 2010;31(17):2124–32.

29. Balci A, Sollie-Szarynska KM, van der Bijl AGL, et al. Prospective validation and assessment of cardiovascular and offspring risk models for pregnant women with congenital heart disease. Heart 2014;100(17):1373–81.

30. van Hagen IM, Boersma E, Johnson MR, et al. Global cardiac risk assessment in the Registry of Pregnancy and Cardiac disease: results of a registry from the European Society of Cardiology. Eur J Heart Fail 2016;18(5):523–33.

31. Canobbio MM, Warnes CA, Aboulhosn J, et al. Management of pregnancy in patients with complex congenital heart disease: a scientific statement for healthcare professionals from the American Heart Association. Circulation 2017; 135(8). https://doi.org/10.1161/CIR.0000000000000458.

32. Hemnes AR, Kiely DG, Cockrill BA, et al. Statement on pregnancy in pulmonary hypertension from the pulmonary vascular research institute. Pulm Circ 2015;5(3):435–65.

33. American College of Obstetricians and Gynecologists Committee Opinion. Low dose aspirin use during pregnancy. 2018;132(1):9.

34. Donofrio MT, Moon-Grady AJ, Hornberger LK, et al. Diagnosis and treatment of fetal cardiac disease: a scientific statement from the American Heart Association. Circulation 2014;129(21):2183–242.

35. American College of Obstetricians and Gynecologists Committee Opinion. Optimizing postpartum care. 2018;131(5):11.

36. Whitaker KM, Wilcox S, Liu J, et al. Patient and provider perceptions of weight gain, physical activity, and nutrition counseling during pregnancy: a qualitative study. Womens Health Issues 2016;26(1):116–22.

37. Hernandez DC. Gestational weight gain as a predictor of longitudinal body mass index transitions among socioeconomically disadvantaged women. J Womens Health 2012;21(10):1082–90.

38. Holland DJ, Kumbhani DJ, Ahmed SH, et al. Effects of treatment on exercise tolerance, cardiac function, and mortality in heart failure with preserved ejection fraction: a meta-analysis. J Am Coll Cardiol 2011;57(16):1676–86.

39. Honigberg MC, Zekavat SM, Aragam K, et al. Long-term cardiovascular risk in women with hypertension during pregnancy. J Am Coll Cardiol 2019;74(22):2743–54.

40. Timpka S, Stuart JJ, Tanz LJ, et al. Lifestyle in progression from hypertensive disorders of pregnancy to chronic hypertension in Nurses' Health Study II: observational cohort study. BMJ 2017;358.

41. Stotland N, Tsoh JY, Gerbert B. Prenatal weight gain: who is counseled? J Womens Health 2011; 21(6):695–701.

42. McDonald SD, Pullenayegum E, Taylor VH, et al. Despite 2009 guidelines, few women report being counseled correctly about weight gain during pregnancy. Am J Obstet Gynecol 2011;205(4): 333.e1-6.

43. McDonald SD, Park CK, Pullenayegum E, et al. Knowledge translation tool to improve pregnant women's awareness of gestational weight gain goals and risks of gaining outside recommendations: a non-randomized intervention study. BMC Pregnancy Childbirth 2015;15(1): 105.

44. Sorensen TK, Williams MA, Lee I-M, et al. Recreational physical activity during pregnancy and risk of preeclampsia. Hypertension 2003;41(6): 1273–80.

45. Barakat R, Pelaez M, Cordero Y, et al. Exercise during pregnancy protects against hypertension and macrosomia: randomized clinical trial. Am J Obstet Gynecol 2016;214(5):649.e1-8.

46. Farpour-Lambert NJ, Ells LJ, Martinez de Tejada B, et al. Obesity and weight gain in pregnancy and postpartum: an evidence review of lifestyle interventions to inform maternal and child health policies. Front Endocrinol 2018;9. https://doi.org/10.3389/fendo.2018.00546.

47. Tobias DK, Zhang C, Dam RM van, et al. Physical activity before and during pregnancy and risk of gestational diabetes mellitus: a meta-analysis. Diabetes Care 2011;34(1):223–9.

48. American College of Obstetricians and Gynecologists Committee Opinion. Physical activity and exercise during pregnancy and the postpartum period. 2020;135(4):11.

49. Aune D, Sen A, Henriksen T, et al. Physical activity and the risk of gestational diabetes mellitus: a systematic review and dose–response meta-analysis of epidemiological studies. Eur J Epidemiol 2016; 31(10):967–97.

50. Wang Z, Wang Z, Wang L, et al. Hypertensive disorders during pregnancy and risk of type 2 diabetes in later life: a systematic review and meta-analysis. Endocrine 2017;55(3):809–21.

51. Verma AK, Williams D, Nelson DM, et al. A cardio-obstetric approach to management of the complex pregnant cardiac patient. J Am Coll Cardiol Case Rep 2020;2(1):86–90.

52. Grodzinsky A, Florio K, Spertus JA, et al. Importance of the cardio-obstetrics team. Curr Treat Options Cardiovasc Med 2019;21(12):84.

53. O'Kelly AC, Sharma G, Vaught AJ, Zakaria S. The use of echocardiography and advanced cardiac ultrasonography during pregnancy. Curr Treat Options Cardiovasc Med 2019;21(11):71.

54. Castleman S, Ganapathy YH, Taki P, et al. Echocardiographic structure and function in hypertensive disorders of pregnancy: a systematic review. Circ Cardiovasc Imaging 2016;9(9):e004888.

55. Elkayam U. Risk of subsequent pregnancy in women with a history of peripartum cardiomyopathy. J Am Coll Cardiol 2014;64(15):1629–36.

56. Elkayam U, Bitar F. Valvular heart disease and pregnancy: Part I: Native valves. J Am Coll Cardiol 2005;46(2):223–30.

57. Goldszmidt E, Macarthur A, Silversides C, et al. Anesthetic management of a consecutive cohort of women with heart disease for labor and delivery. Int J Obstet Anesth 2010;19(3):266–72.

58. Practice bulletin No. 170: critical care in pregnancy. Obstet Gynecol 2016;128(4):e147–54.

59. Arendt KW, Lindley KJ. Obstetric anesthesia management of the patient with cardiac disease. Int J Obstet Anesth 2019;37:73–85.

60. Uebing A, Steer PJ, Yentis SM, et al. Pregnancy and congenital heart disease. BMJ 2006; 332(7538):401–6.

61. Liu S, Liston RM, Joseph KS, et al. Maternal mortality and severe morbidity associated with low-risk planned cesarean delivery versus planned vaginal delivery at term. CMAJ 2007;176(4):455–60.

62. Lau E, DeFaria Yeh D. Management of high risk cardiac conditions in pregnancy: anticoagulation, severe stenotic valvular disease and cardiomyopathy. Trends Cardiovasc Med 2019;29(3):155–61.

63. Li J-M, Nguyen C, Joglar JA, et al. Frequency and outcome of arrhythmias complicating admission during pregnancy: experience from a high-volume and ethnically-diverse obstetric service. Clin Cardiol 2008;31(11):538–41.

64. Vaidya VR, Arora S, Patel N, et al. Burden of arrhythmia in pregnancy. Circulation 2017;135(6): 619–21.

65. Silversides CK, Harris L, Haberer K, et al. Recurrence rates of arrhythmias during pregnancy in

women with previous tachyarrhythmia and impact on fetal and neonatal outcomes. Am J Cardiol 2006;97(8):1206–12.

66. Laksman Z, Harris L, Silversides CK. Cardiac arrhythmias during pregnancy: a clinical approach. Fetal Matern Med Rev 2011;22(2):123–43.

67. Roston TM, van der Werf C, Cheung CC, et al. Caring for the pregnant woman with an inherited arrhythmia syndrome. Heart Rhythm 2020;17(2):341–8.

68. Henry D, Gonzalez JM, Harris IS, et al. Maternal arrhythmia and perinatal outcomes. J Perinatology 2016;36(10):823–7.

69. Pieper PG. The pregnant woman with heart disease: management of pregnancy and delivery. Neth Heart J 2012;20(1):33–7.

70. Bauersachs J, König T, van der Meer P, et al. Pathophysiology, diagnosis and management of peripartum cardiomyopathy: a position statement from the Heart Failure Association of the European Society of Cardiology Study Group on peripartum cardiomyopathy. Eur J Heart Fail 2019;21(7): 827–43.

71. Mebazaa A, Yilmaz MB, Levy P, et al. Recommendations on pre-hospital & early hospital management of acute heart failure: a consensus paper from the Heart Failure Association of the European Society of Cardiology, the European Society of Emergency Medicine and the Society of Academic Emergency Medicine. Eur J Heart Fail 2015;17(6): 544–58.

72. Stergiopoulos K, Lima FV. Peripartum cardiomyopathy-diagnosis, management, and long term implications. Trends Cardiovasc Med 2019;29(3):164–73.

73. Grewal J, Silversides CK, Colman JM. Pregnancy in women with heart disease: risk assessment and management of heart failure. Heart Fail Clin 2014;10(1):117–29.

74. ICD-10: International Statistical Classification of diseases and related health problems. World Health Organization; 2011.

75. Hayward RM, Foster E, Tseng ZH. Maternal and fetal outcomes of admission for delivery in women with congenital heart disease. JAMA Cardiol 2017;2(6):664–71.

76. Karamlou T, Diggs BS, McCrindle BW, et al. A growing problem: maternal death and peripartum complications are higher in women with grown-up congenital heart disease. Ann Thorac Surg 2011;92(6):2193–9.

77. Thompson JL, Kuklina EV, Bateman BT, et al. Medical and obstetric outcomes among pregnant women with congenital heart disease. Obstet Gynecol 2015;126(2):346–54.

78. Connolly HM. Managing congenital heart disease in the obstetric patient. Semin Perinatol 2018; 42(1):39–48.

79. Committee opinion No. 654: reproductive life planning to reduce unintended pregnancy. Obstet Gynecol 2016;127(2):e66.

80. WHO | WHO recommendations on health promotion interventions for maternal and newborn health 2015. WHO. Available at: http://www.who.int/maternal_child_adolescent/documents/health-promotion-interventions/en/. Accessed July 21, 2020.

81. American College of Obstetricians and Gynecologists; Task Force on Hypertension in Pregnancy. Hypertension in pregnancy. Report of the American College of Obstetricians and Gynecologists' Task Force on Hypertension in Pregnancy. Obstet Gynecol 2013;122(5):1122–31.

82. Mosca LM, Barrett-Connor E, Kass Wenger N. Sex/gender differences in cardiovascular disease prevention: what a difference a decade makes. [Miscellaneous Article]. Circulation 2011;124(19): 2145–54.

83. Rich-Edwards JW, Fraser A, Lawlor DA, et al. Pregnancy characteristics and women's future cardiovascular health: an underused opportunity to improve women's health? Epidemiol Rev 2014; 36(1):57–70.

84. Grundy SM, Stone NJ, Bailey AL, et al. 2018 AHA/ACC/AACVPR/AAPA/ABC/ACPM/ADA/AGS/APhA/ASPC/NLA/PCNA guideline on the management of blood cholesterol. J Am Coll Cardiol 2019;73(24): e285–350.

85. Kassebaum NJ, Bertozzi-Villa A, Coggeshall MS, et al. Global, regional, and national levels and causes of maternal mortality during 1990–2013: a systematic analysis for the Global Burden of Disease Study 2013. Lancet 2014;384(9947): 980–1004.

86. Kampman MAM, Balci A, Groen H, et al. Cardiac function and cardiac events 1-year postpartum in women with congenital heart disease. Am Heart J 2015;169(2):298–304.

87. Balint OH, Siu SC, Mason J, et al. Cardiac outcomes after pregnancy in women with congenital heart disease. Heart 2010;96(20):1656–61.

88. Wise PH. Transforming preconceptional, prenatal, and interconceptional care into A comprehensive commitment to women's health. Womens Health Issues 2008;18(6):S13–8.

89. Gifford K, Walls J, Ranji U. Apr 27 IGP, 2017. Medicaid coverage of pregnancy and perinatal benefits: results from a state survey - introduction. The Henry J. Kaiser Family Foundation; 2017. Available at: https://www.kff.org/report-section/medicaid-coverage-of-pregnancy-and-perinatal-benefits-introduction/. Accessed May 5, 2020.

90. Prenatal and postpartum care (PPC). NCQA. Available at: https://www.ncqa.org/hedis/

measures/prenatal-and-postpartum-care-ppc/. Accessed May 5, 2020.

91. Grodzinsky A, Florio K, Spertus J, et al. Maternal mortality in the United States and the HOPE registry. Curr Treat Options Cardiovasc Med 2019;21(9): 42.

92. Moaddab A, Dildy GA, Brown HL, et al. Health care disparity and pregnancy-related mortality in the United States, 2005–2014. Obstet Gynecol 2018; 131(4):707–12.

93. Aziz A, Zork N, Aubey JJ, et al. Telehealth for high-risk pregnancies in the setting of the COVID-19 pandemic. Am J Perinatol 2020;37(8):800–8.

94. Harrison BJ, Hilton TN, Riviere RN, et al. Advanced maternal age: ethical and medical considerations for assisted reproductive technology. Int J Womens Health 2017. https://doi.org/10.2147/IJWH.S139578.

95. Zork NM, Aubey J, Yates H. Conversion and optimization of telehealth in obstetric care during the COVID-19 pandemic. Semin Perinatol 2020; 151300. https://doi.org/10.1016/j.semperi.2020.151300.

96. Smith GN, Pudwell J, Roddy M. The maternal health clinic: a new window of opportunity for early heart disease risk screening and intervention for women with pregnancy complications. J Obstet Gynaecol Can 2013;35(9):831–9.

97. Smith GN, Louis JM, Saade GR. Pregnancy and the postpartum period as an opportunity for cardiovascular risk identification and management. Obstet Gynecol 2019;134(4):851–62.

98. Park K, Wu P, Gulati M. Obstetrics and gynecological history: a missed opportunity for cardiovascular risk assessment. J Am Coll Cardiol Case Rep 2020;2(1):161–3.

99. Sharma G, Zakaria S, Michos ED, et al. Improving cardiovascular workforce competencies in cardio-obstetrics: current challenges and future directions. J Am Heart Assoc 2020;9(12):e015569.

100. Roberts JM, Catov JM. Pregnancy is a screening test for later life cardiovascular disease: now what? Research recommendations. Womens Health Issues 2012;22(2):e123–8.

101. Davis MB, Walsh MN. Cardio-obstetrics. Circ Cardiovasc Qual Outcomes 2019;12(2):e005417.

102. Halperin JL, Williams ES, Fuster V, et al. ACC 2015 core cardiovascular training statement (COCATS 4) (revision of COCATS 3). J Am Coll Cardiol 2015; 65(17):1721–3.

103. Reza N, Adusumalli S, Saybolt MD, et al. Implementing a women's cardiovascular health training program in a cardiovascular disease fellowship: the MUCHACHA curriculum. JACC Case Rep 2020;2(1):164–7.

Moving?

Make sure your subscription moves with you!

To notify us of your new address, find your **Clinics Account Number** (located on your mailing label above your name), and contact customer service at:

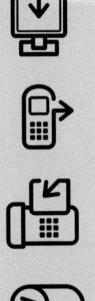

Email: journalscustomerservice-usa@elsevier.com

800-654-2452 (subscribers in the U.S. & Canada)
314-447-8871 (subscribers outside of the U.S. & Canada)

Fax number: 314-447-8029

Elsevier Health Sciences Division
Subscription Customer Service
3251 Riverport Lane
Maryland Heights, MO 63043

*To ensure uninterrupted delivery of your subscription, please notify us at least 4 weeks in advance of move.

Printed and bound by CPI Group (UK) Ltd, Croydon, CR0 4YY

03/10/2024

01040372-0019